Neurocinema—The Sequel

Neurocinema—The Sequel

A History of Neurology on Screen

Eelco F. M. Wijdicks, MD, PhD

Professor of Neurology
Professor of History of Medicine
Mayo College of Medicine

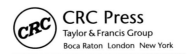

CRC Press
Taylor & Francis Group
Boca Raton London New York

CRC Press is an imprint of the
Taylor & Francis Group, an **informa** business

First edition published 2014
by CRC Press
6000 Broken Sound Parkway NW, Suite 300, Boca Raton, FL 33487-2742

2 Park Square, Milton Park, Abingdon, Oxon, OX14 4RN
CRC Press is an imprint of Taylor & Francis Group, LLC
© 2022 Taylor & Francis Group, LLC

Library of Congress Cataloging-in-Publication Data

Names: Wijdicks, Eelco F. M., 1954- author. | Wijdicks, Eelco F. M., 1954- Neurocinema. 2015.
Title: Neurocinema-the sequel : a history of neurology on screen / Eelco F.M. Wijdicks.
Description: First edition. | Boca Raton : CRC Press, 2022. | Sequel to Neurocinema : when film meets
    neurology / Eelco F.M. Wijdicks. 2015. | Includes bibliographical references and index
Identifiers: LCCN 2021045767 (print) | LCCN 2021045768 (ebook) | ISBN 9781032220055 (hardback) | ISBN
    9781032220024 (paperback) | ISBN 9781003270874 (ebook)
Subjects: MESH: Medicine in the Arts—history | Motion Pictures—history | Neurology—history | Nervous
    System Diseases | Neurologists | History, 20th Century | History, 21st Century
Classification: LCC RC346 (print) | LCC RC346 (ebook) | NLM WZ 331 | DDC 616.8—dc23
LC record available at https://lccn.loc.gov/2021045767
LC ebook record available at https://lccn.loc.gov/2021045768

ISBN: 978-1-032-22005-5 (hbk)
ISBN: 978-1-032-22002-4 (pbk)
ISBN: 978-1-003-27087-4 (ebk)

DOI: 10.1201/9781003270874

Typeset in Minion
by KnowledgeWorks Global Ltd.

Printed in the UK by Severn, Gloucester on responsibly sourced paper

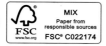

To Barbara

To our family and friends who go with us to our basement theater to experience and savor a film on the Big Screen

Contents

Preface to *Neurocinema— The Sequel*

Neurocinema grew out of a long fascination with cinema and, more specifically, neurology in cinema. The book's reception signified there is a field of study. The fictionalization of neurologic disease has been present since the early days of cinema but also has changed over the years, and there has been some increased prioritization. Currently, we see neurologically themed films regularly, and since the initial publication of *Neurocinema* in 2014, more films have appeared and almost yearly. Therefore, reworking and reimagining were needed; many chapters have been extensively revised, rewritten, and expanded. On all counts, *Neurocinema—The Sequel* is a different book. For one thing, it has become more academic with analytical perspectives and hundreds of footnotes. Knowing that the story of film and filmmaking is apocryphal and laden with folklore, I used a combination of primary sources, archives, available interviews, and memoirs to corroborate my interpretations. Few filmmakers in the past wanted to tell their story and explain the choices they made, and many felt that films have more impact when uncommitted. Another concern is that some of the accounts told by filmmakers were not truthful. To increase readability, I have carefully avoided obscure minutia and rhetorical flourishes. I added many great film quotes from creative, gifted screenwriters. Furthermore, I added innumerable nuggets that were not only interesting to me but provided more context. The book has a number of new, original observations sprinkled throughout the text. Three new chapters appear, including an introductory chapter comparing the real history of neurology with the "reel" history and explaining how selections were made and where parallels still exist. I have included recently available information on films in the silent era and a section highlighting the fascinating role of neurology in early educational film. These new chapters provide further context on the interaction of cinema and neurology and fill in important missing pieces of the bigger picture. One chapter discusses the overlap between psychiatry and neurology. This includes "functional neurology" (previously known as conversion disorder or, earlier, hysteria), in which symptoms are unexplained by neurologic disease and frankly unexplained by mental disease. Psychiatric manifestations of neurologic disease also entered screenplays and are discussed. Another new chapter reviews documentaries and fictional films on celebrities with neurologic diseases and how some families of the celebrity patients have used these films to maximal advantage to promote visibility and help foundations.

The account of *Neurocinema—The Sequel* is thematic. To attempt a methodical presentation of the subject, I have divided the book into three sections. After three introductory chapters on how medicine and neurology were covered in cinema over the years, chapters follow on neurologic diseases, the ethical quandaries posed by neurologic disease, and documentaries. The core of the book, including rating, in-depth discussion, and contextualization, is found in Chapters 4 through 8, followed by a chapter on follies and a final one where I indulge in speculation about how the brain responds when watching a film, particularly a neurofilm, but also how we can bring this collection to good use. A full filmography is included, and I will end by listing my personal favorites.

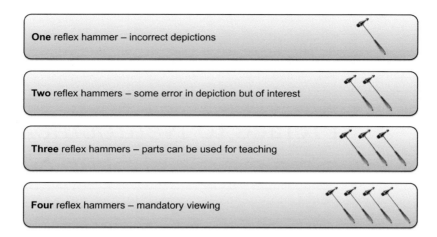

FIGURE   Rating of Neurocinema

One wonders how to judge (rate) these films. Rating films is subjective, idiosyncratic, and arcane. (For this edition, I re-reviewed portions of several films and changed my original rating in a few.) There are multitudes of rating systems, with fresh and rotten tomatoes and percentages for each critic used by Metacritic. Most known are Siskel and Ebert's "two-thumbs-up sign," which was a reliable indicator for many Americans. (Roger Ebert also used a 4-star rating system, and additionally for him, several qualified as a "great movie.") The benchmark film magazine *Cahiers du Cinéma* once famously had a rating system that included a black dot for "abominable." It remains a popular mug's game.

The neurologist's traditional tools are the reflex hammer (to test tendon and superficial reflexes) and a pin (to test sensation). In this book, the film's accuracy (rather than its very different cinematic significance) is appraised using a rating scale from one to four reflex hammers. The rating may apply to the entire work or may apply to the portrayal of the neurologist only. For a film to attain a rating of four reflex hammers, it must display an accurate representation of the disease (not necessarily from all angles but mostly). A film with three reflex hammers contains at least one teachable scene or some other interesting aspect. A film with two reflex hammers has many inaccuracies but remains richly interesting despite the inaccuracies (or because of them). One reflex hammer indicates a serious misrepresentation that should have little interest to any of us (Figure above). Films are rated if they tackle a neurologic subject but not if it surfaces only briefly and the topic does not return in significant manner.

And then there are irredeemably silly films; these require a separate rating system. The pinpricks indicate a representation that goes from bad to worse, but in some, the neurologist (and, I suppose, the viewer) must be genuinely impressed by the wild imagination. Thus, folly is qualified using a rating scale from one to three pinpricks because these movies are literally painful to watch (Figure below).

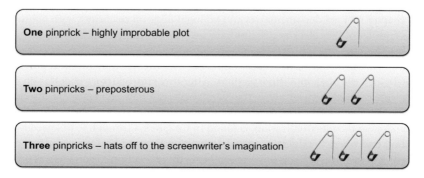

FIGURE (CONTINUED)   Rating of Neurocinema

I have rated over 180 films, and many of these are exemplary. A few made-for-TV films have been mentioned when they showed a major portrayal of neurologic disease or problematic professionalism. This brief crossover should be allowed because we can expect the boundaries between TV and cinema to blur over the next few years, certainly now that major film directors have taken an interest in directing TV series. (A comprehensive history of neurology in TV is another story and may be harder to tell because of a more frequent lack of serious depiction.)

The main premise of this book remains to select several films with each topic. My attitude is to be an internationalist, but I recognize there are films created and screened in large parts of the world that we will never see, and some may appear only briefly at far away international film festivals.

I tried to balance my praise and criticism. I summarize plots (avoiding unnecessary clutter by not going too deep into the narrative storylines) and analyze key scenes. Other films pertaining to the discussed topic will be briefly mentioned only if there are notably different observations. I hope the reader agrees that the history of neurology as seen through the lens of the filmmaker is fascinating and extraordinary. Their selections and history often contain an underlying meaning, which has guided my approach. I recognize that cinema as a medium can be analyzed in infinite ways and is open to academic study. In a way, it is a split-screen image—one cinema, the other the relationship of cinema with neurology. It is a review of the history of neurology as seen in film, starting in the early days of cinema, to what we now see in theaters and on streaming sites.

The major themes of this book continue to be how neurology was represented in the history of cinema and how neurologic topics emerged and then disappeared, with some staging a comeback in more recent films. These evolving topics have no connection with the contemporary history of neurology—hence, the subtitle *a* history of neurology and not *the* history of neurology. But my approach to medicine and cinema has remained accepting of what is offered—from miraculous improvements to lapses into sorrier states and cruel changes associated with degenerative neurologic disease. Rather than calling out outrageous representations of neurologic disease, my goal is to examine whether film—from a neurologic perspective—can provide insight and even debate. Films about neurology may acquaint the public with these disorders, and many are accurate representations of the consequences of specific neurologic disorders including the impact on social interactions and relationships. Films are best when they are very close to the real thing and "squirm-free." But even undeniably hokey films that are grotesquely successful may have some significance. Overall, cinematic representation of neurologic disease and its impact on caregivers is quite good, and many acclaimed filmmakers and stupendous actors participated in these productions. Some films teem with imaginary (and imaginative) images and are totally inaccurate, seemingly plausible for an unknowing audience, fantastical but cinematically beautiful, bracing, creative, innovative, and invigorating. The scene on the cover of this book, which shows a patient experiencing a "visual hallucination" due to a "seizure" while looking at his "frozen" neurologist, illustrates that premise well—the filmmaker as an esthete and neurologic-like symptoms used as allegorical framing. Of note, the actor David Niven was afflicted by serious neurologic disease—as an invented character (brain tumor) and later in his personal life (ALS).

Each of the films discussed in this book demands serious attention from those who see and manage neurologic patients and support their families. Many films come close to the subject matter, and there is little to luxuriate in. *Neurocinema—The Sequel* chronicles this archive of neurologic representation, drawing readers into a rich collection of cinematic wonders of permanent cultural and historical value.

Eelco F.M. Wijdicks

Preface to *Neurocinema*

Coma, stroke, seizures, and spinal cord injury are some of the conditions that appeal to screenwriters, and as we will find out, there are several feature films where neurologic disease unfurls as a plot element. Film directors know that neurologic disease impacts mind and motility. Equally important, these films say as much about the consequences as they say about the disorder.

It should be interesting to deconstruct the neurologic representation in film. There are obvious questions to ask: How are neurologic disorders shown, and how accurately are they depicted? How is the practice of the neurologist represented? How do documentaries handle these disorders? Do films have educational value for neurology residents, and can the topic bring about a deep discussion?

This book is organized by the main neurologic conditions after selecting over 100 films. I divided the material into chapters, which has discussions on neurologic disorders, moral and ethical quandaries in major neurologic illnesses, and neurology as a subject of a documentary, as well as silly neurology frequently used in science fiction. Neurologic disorders in film are not so easy to find, and even titles such as *Coma, Brain, Dementia 13*, and *Vertigo* are about different themes. The films were found after using a variety of library and internet resources, but the filmography mostly came from a personal file I kept over the years. The selection criteria I used were broad and inclusive, but naturally films must have well-defined scenes showing the acting out of a neurologic disorder and its consequences.

I decided to include documentary films, recognizing that documentary is not free of bias and sometimes they are what they are—overdramatizing and close to fiction. Films that only tangentially mentioned neurologic signs and symptoms (e.g., "honey, I have a headache" or some unclassifiable spell) were excluded. To do that was generally simple.

TV series such as *Grey's Anatomy, House MD,* and *ER* have inserted neurologic disorders in their stories, and the nature of films and series made for TV is changing. However, to maintain focus, films made for TV and TV series were also excluded, unless they involved crucial topics and I could not escape it. Finally, I have shied away from horror and slasher films because—I suppose—when it pertains to brains and gore, there is nothing we can learn here, and it is a dead end. I recognize this book inescapably remains a selection and cannot be exhaustive without the full availability of movies. (World cinema is thus underrepresented). All the described films should be available on DVD, YouTube, or media video streaming sites (e.g., Netflix, Hulu, and Amazon Prime Video).

The main premise of this book is to discuss a film (or two) that represents the salient aspects of a specific neurologic disorder and its impact. These films can be seen fully and not just for one clip. Plots are summarized, key scenes are analyzed, some shots are parsed, and hopefully, the book will illuminate what underlies the screenwriter's intention. I then compare it with other films that are worth watching, even if they contain a single pertinent scene. To provide further context, each chapter will have background information mostly aimed at physicians but with sufficient clarity to be accessible for the nonmedical reader. The purpose of these essays is to elaborate on what is shown, and it is up to the viewer to be fascinated, amused, or appalled by it. Each chapter has callouts with dialogue lines that were chosen to draw the reader into the film and to highlight the themes. It also accentuates the brilliant art of one-liner writing. (*Spoiler Alert*: because many of these reviews have details about the films, they probably should be read after the film is seen.)

What more can be done with this information? I decided to judge these films but avoided a fail/pass decision and rated them on an ordinal scale. The traditional tools used by the neurologist are the reflex hammer (to test tendon and superficial reflexes) and a pin (to test sensation). The film's accuracy is thus qualified using a rating scale from one to four reflex hammers. Folly and absurdity are qualified using a rating scale from one to three pinpricks because they are painful to watch. Rating a film four reflex hammers required an accurate representation and when there was simply no question about it. Rating a film with two or three reflex hammers required the presence of a teachable scene or some other interesting aspect. One reflex hammer indicated a serious misrepresentation. The pinpricks indicated—in a handful of unredeemable silly films—a representation that was bad to even worse.

Screenwriters and directors may deviate from reality to produce a certain effect. Thus, neurology may give way to the story and such an approach may all be permitted under the moniker "poetic license." At best it is just entertainment and there may even be situations—walking out of the theater—that the physician (or neurologist) may have to clarify what just happened. At worst a departure from the truth may result in misperceptions with the public. Some films are serious and comical at the same time, making it even more difficult to filter out deceit. I lack the credentials to judge the artistry of filmmaking, and I recognize the need for film directors to dramatize, the need to create a gripping and watchable film while skewing some of the reality, even after professional medical advice. I recognize that any art criticism is arbitrary and arguably pretentious. Some may say using such a scrutiny is not needed ("Hey, it's only a movie"), but gross misrepresentation of serious neurologic disease does no good to the lay public. The filmmakers that are the best not only entertain and amuse but also come face to face with the subject matter.

It may leave the reader wondering: where does the "Neurocinema critic" come in? Neurologists might anticipate being troubled by the portrayal, but there are a considerable number of films that are accurate representations of acute or chronic neurologic disease. Neurologic disease can be devastating, and many of us will be stirred by the images before them with some mordant dramas.

I think many of these films are mandatory viewing, not only for specialists in the neurosciences but for everyone else as well. Some documentaries are nearly impossible to watch, some fiction films are comical, but all have something to talk about. For me seeing a film is a fantastic experience, and I tell people. I am often asked, "Have you seen …?" or told, "You should see …!" and thus, it is only natural to combine my profession with an interest of mine and to write about neurologic representation in film. I have noticed early on that many films used acute neurology in their screenplays, and that clearly fits my subspecialty. I wanted to put together a series of important fiction films and documentaries which I think few of the readers have seen or even heard about. I hope the reader finds this collection of film critiques—summarized by the rubric NEUROCINEMA—informative and educational, serious, and amusing and that it will lead to watching or re-watching these celebrated films. It was a great pleasure to write about them.

Eelco F.M. Wijdicks

Acknowledgments

Seeing neurology through film requires close observation and recognition of proper representations. This can only be done through the help, criticism, and suggestions of colleagues with expertise other than mine. Many people have shared their knowledge with me; some send me emails to see a film I may have missed, and several filmmakers have been very helpful in providing material. Many of these suggestions took me to new discoveries.

A great number of libraries were consulted for historical material, and I am thankful to numerous librarians who kept digging for me. The following distributors have kindly provided stills for the films discussed: Ferndale Films/Hells Kitchen, Ltd; El Deseo, S.A.; Les Films du Losange; Music Box Films; eOne Publicity; PCH Films; and FameFlyNet. Permission has also been obtained from multiple other sources, and I received great assistance from Shari Chertok of Chertok Research, LLC (dba re:search), who secured permissions to use stills and other historical material. She has been a major resource and a delight to work with. The 35 added film stills will enhance understanding of the text.

Over the years I have published a good number of reviews of films with a neurologic topic for *The Lancet Neurology* and other medical journals, and these pieces are excerpted in his book. I have authored a trilogy of articles on the beginnings of neurology on screen in the history section of *Neurology,* and some material and ideas have, in some form, been re-used.

I sincerely thank Lea Dacy for providing all the secretarial and editorial assistance these projects need. She has been deeply involved and even suggested films I should investigate. Her creative impact on this work is undeniable.

The editorial team of CRC Press/Taylor & Francis ably assisted me in improving the prose. I thank Ashraf Reza, Project Manager of KnowledgeWorks Global Ltd and his team. I thank my editor, Miranda Bromage, with CRC Press/Taylor & Francis, for her encouragement, and Kyle Meyer for his guidance through the production process.

Neurocinema Collection

NEURODOCUMENTARIES

Alzheimer's Disease	You're Looking at Me Like I Live Here and I Don't, Genius of Marian, The Forgetting, Extreme Love
Amyotrophic Lateral Sclerosis	I Am Breathing, So Much So Fast, Living with Lew
Multiple Sclerosis	When I Walk
Poliomyelitis	A Paralyzing Fear, Martha in Lattimore
Huntington's Disease	Do You Really Want to Know?
Aphasia	Picturing Aphasia, Aphasia, After Words
Traumatic Brain Injury	The Crash Reel
Neurorehabilitation	Coma

NEUROPSYCHIATRY

Functional Neurology	War Neurosis, Let There Be Light, Shades of Gray, Safe, Persona, The Magician, Home of the Braves, Hollywood Ending
Autoimmune Encephalitis	Fire in Brain

NEUROCELEBRITIES

Multiple Sclerosis	Hilary and Jackie
Alzheimer's Disease	Iris, Glen Campbell, I'll be Me
Lewy Body Disease	Robin's Wish
Motor Neuron Disease	Pride of the Yankees, Brief History of Time
Brain Tumor	Rhapsody in Blue
Chronic Traumatic Encephalopathy	Muhammad Ali

NEUROFOLLIES

Mind the Mind	The Cell, Limitless, Lucy, Charly, The Dead Zone, Phenomenon, Donovan's Brain, Brain Waves, The Penalty
When Amnesia Actually Helps	50 First Dates, Clean Slate, Groundhog Day
The Violent Epileptic	The Terminal Man
Brain Transplantation	The Brain That Wouldn't Die, Crimson

Author Biography

Eelco Wijdicks is Professor of Neurology and Professor of History of Medicine at the Mayo Clinic College of Medicine. He established Neurocritical Care at Mayo Clinic and is a consultant neuro-intensivist in the Neurosciences Intensive Care Unit at Saint Marys Hospital (Mayo Clinic Campus Rochester). He has published commentary and criticism on medical and neurologic portrayal in film including *Neurocinema: When Film Meets Neurology* (CRC Press, 2014) and *Cinema, MD: A History of Medicine on Screen* (Oxford University Press, 2020).

1

Introducing the History of Medicine in Film

Cinema is a great way to explain the past.

Martin Scorsese (2012)[1]

In cinema, every thematic component and motif can be subject to scholarly criticism. At the heart of the matter is whether the history of social science in medicine could include an exploration of medicine in cinema. I think it should. I assume few would dispute that, viewed in the right way, the story of medical professionals treating diseases in and out of the hospital and over decades, the manifestations of acute and chronic medical and neurologic disease, and how they affect the patient, family, and public health, can be told in a cinematic language. Moving between fact and fiction, screenwriters and directors are common proselytizers for social change, and pointing out disgrace or scandal may easily extend to medical institutions and their workers. You might think, therefore, that cinema can recreate disease and, in neurocinema specifically, make us understand how damaged brains work—or rather do *not* work. We can look at a frame of reference and examine how films incorporating the practice of medicine create meaning.

The preservation of early film and the recently achieved, widespread availability to view film over various social media platforms have allowed us to look at a number of themes—the changing persona and status of the physician and the shifting patterns of disease. Medical bioethics entered the fray in the mid-1970s, but neurologic disease-related themes as a provocation for controversial decision-making were preferentially used in film as early as the 1940s; later, they surfaced occasionally as part of a biopic but always to advance the cause of self-determination. Trying to understand another human being with a medical death sentence was (and still is) a topic of morbid curiosity for serious filmmakers. Other common dramatic themes included the perceived "atrocities" perpetrated in psychiatric institutions, the consequences of major addictions, medical violations, medical monsters and "freaks of nature," and the all-too-common health disparities and lack of health equity. Historically, film may remind us that people can change (and societies with them).

No one enjoys going to the hospital, and we all fear bad news. In film, illness is often unexpected and accidental. Filmmakers often perceive medicine as health interrupted by illness followed by disability or death, and this topic is an endless source of ideas and fictional inventions. Screenwriters have inserted life-threatening disorders—for example, suddenly diagnosed terminal cancer—into the story to unnerve the audience and create tension in the narrative. Doctors in their white coats or surgical scrubs appear when the leading character in the film becomes ill. Over many years, their portrayal has evolved from the general family doctor to medical specialists, in parallel with the subspecialization of medicine itself. Currently, the medical specialties most preferred by screenwriters are surgeons, psychiatrists, and pediatricians.

---

[1] Queenan J. Interview: Good fellows: Martin Scorsese and Colonel Blimp. *The Guardian*. London: Guardian News & Media Limited; 2012.

DOI: 10.1201/9781003270874-1

Filmmakers also favor panic-causing epidemics and dystopian viral outbreaks. The social anguish and fury of these rapidly spreading diseases triggered filmmakers to tell a story. Before the onset of the COVID-19 with its devastating loss of life, these films were often belittled as scary mainstream movie entertainment with little or no scientific basis. We all believed that great epidemics belonged to the distant past.[2] Pandemics are serious, and initial disbelief and later persistent denial are always rampant with public health officials desperately trying to convey the real danger to the public and our leaders. This pandemic certainly caused us to feel like we were in a movie, and movies seem to mimic reality, although not quite.

Medicine can also serve as a topic of comedy, making fun of medical decisions and physicians. The silent era in cinema was particularly dominated by burlesques (using escaped "lunatics") outwitting dull (and incompetent) doctors. More recent films satirize the medical health system and the health insurance industry. Filmmakers are at pains to stress that a system and a process, rather than the individual, are to blame. In *Critical Condition* (1987), Richard Pryor impersonates a doctor; after being discovered, he decides that his only chance of avoiding prison is to plead insanity, which leads to a comical courtroom display of schizophrenia.

Medicine in film crosses all genres and is everywhere[3]. Yet, in the end, and in the bigger picture, medical diseases are rarely lauded. There are only 3 in Roger Ebert's 4-volume set of books on *The Great Movies*, comprising 300 reviews, and no entries in the magazine *Sight and Sound's* Top 50 poll of major international film critics. *Cahiers du Cinéma*, a film magazine posting the longest yearly best of listing, noted only three films. Not surprisingly, these focused on psychiatry.

For medical professionals, the representation of medicine—particularly in films of import—must be intriguing at the least. There are actors ready to take risks in roles that others would have avoided.[4] Here, we glimpse into the vast cinematic portrayal of diseases, doctors, and hospitals as a lead-in to the main topic of this book.

Portrayal of Hospitals: From Caring Nursing Sisters to Dilapidation and Disarray

For many decades, the hospital was for the impoverished and immobilized bedridden.[5] When the well-to-do fell ill, they typically were treated in their own homes and cared for by a trained physician. For those less privileged, a bed among strangers in a hospital ward was to be avoided and was a last resort. Hospitals were better known as charitable guest houses (almshouses) and evolved to organized institutions with some centers of excellence and scientific progress. The professionalization of nursing reshaped and refashioned hospital care. Some films depicted a caring environment with Catholic sisters serving the poor, as in *Umberto D*. In contrast, *The Hospital* is a place of mayhem where just about everything goes wrong (Figure 1.1).[6] Interior scenes are on soundstages, but the outside shots can feature known (albeit renamed) hospitals.

---

[2] Cases of AIDS peaked in the mid-1980s; indie films on AIDS came quickly with *Buddies* in 1985. However, it took Hollywood much longer to recognize the AIDS global epidemic (*Philadelphia*, 1993) than it took to seize on the storytelling potential of the COVID pandemic. *Corona* (Mostafa Keshvari, Level 33 entertainment 2020) was the first movie shown at film festivals. *Locked Down* (Liman D. Warner Bros. Pictures. January 14, 2021) focuses on how the lockdown altered people's daily lives including their livelihood and capacity for in-person socialization. A number of horror films have appeared and are planned (*Songbird; Covid-21*).

[3] See Wijdicks EFM. *Cinema, MD*. New York: Oxford University Press; 2020. The chapter titles reflect the most common themes screenwriters use when the practice of medicine becomes a large part of the narrative.

[4] Boris Karloff (the creature of Dr. Frankenstein) played a number of "mad doctors" in other horror films and most famously Dr. Savaard in *The Man They Could Not Hang* (1939) experimenting with bringing back the dead using an artificial heart and lung machine.

[5] See Risse GB. *Mending Bodies, Saving Souls: A History of Hospitals*. 1st ed. New York: Oxford University Press; 1999 and Rosenberg CE. *The Care of Strangers: The Rise of America's Hospitals*. Baltimore, MD: The Johns Hopkins University Press; 1987.

[6] De Sica V. *Umberto D*. Dear Film. January 20, 1952; Hiller A. *The Hospital*. United Artists. December 14, 1971.

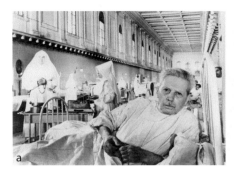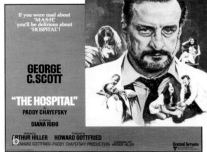

FIGURE 1.1 (a) The solemn hospital in *Umberto D* (Rizzoli Film, Alamy Stock Photo). (b) The pandemonium in a modern setting in *The Hospital* (Photofest).

In documentaries, the camera enters with the (presumed) permission of leadership and consent of patients and families. Between the late 1960s and early 1980s, Frederick Wiseman filmed hundreds of hours in an emergency department, an intensive care unit (ICU), and an asylum. These films have not lost any of their educational value.[7] Selected, anecdotal, but also baffling and "in your face," his films emphasize the lack of decent, universal healthcare and bias in patient care on the bases of gender, race, or socioeconomic status—issues applicable to today.

Film depictions of medicine often start in a racing ambulance.[8] The attendants wheel the patient's gurney into the emergency department, a scene of (sometimes bloody) chaos, with shouting physicians questioning who is in charge. Cardiopulmonary resuscitation has been shown in several films, and as expected, the intervention has spectacularly good outcomes, even after the physician has pronounced the patient dead.[9] Because medical cinema often involves trauma or a gunshot wound, the scene may change to the operating room or the intensive care area. For dramatic purposes and to create further tension, a blood-spattered surgeon may emerge from the operating room to tell distressing news to family members.[10]

ICUs or surgical trauma units usually show the actor after polytrauma—packed and in traction. Most remarkably, we hear the patient's heartbeat in the ICU just as it is in the operating room—becoming fast when the patient is in distress. Moreover, the ventilator shown in the ICU very much looks like the one used in the operating room (moving bellows included).

Medical institutions are not always depicted accurately. Veterans Affairs (VA) hospitals are commonly shown, usually in the war-film genre. VA hospitals are either appalling[11] or sites of frustrating bureaucracy.[12] The psychiatric hospital offers multiple opportunities to shock the audience. Sadly, many of these are undeservedly vicious attacks on mental health care and psychiatrists. *One Flew over the Cuckoo's Nest*[13] cemented a dramatic, negative depiction of psychiatric hospitals and staff. (Who does not remember Louise Fletcher as Nurse Ratched?) Most disturbing was the implication that electroconvulsive therapy and lobotomy were primarily employed to control patients' behavior.[14] *Shutter Island*,[15] a psychological horror film, shows the criminally insane in shackles. Patients are forcefully committed, and the patient population is either violent or non-violent but developmentally disabled. Set in the 1950s,

[7] Wijdicks EFM. Teaching Medicine through Film: Wiseman's Medical Trilogy Revisited. *BMC Med Educ.* 2019;19:387.

[8] Scorsese M. *Bringing Out the Dead.* Paramount Pictures. October 22, 1999.

[9] For example, Sturges J. *The Girl in White.* Metro-Goldwyn-Mayer. June 23, 1952.

[10] In *Fruitvale Station* (2013), a surgeon enters the waiting room and tells an anxiously waiting family, "He did not make it."

[11] For example, Ashby H. *Coming Home.* United Artists. February 15, 1978, or Stone O. *Born on the Fourth of July.* Universal Pictures. December 20, 1989.

[12] Deutch H. *Article 99.* Orion Pictures. March 13, 1992.

[13] Forman M. *One Flew over the Cuckoo's Nest.* United Artists. November 19, 1975.

[14] This was the first of Jack Nicholson's brilliant depictions of mental illness; the other one is in *The Shining* (Kubrick S. Warner Bros. May 23, 1980).

[15] Scorsese M. *Shutter Island.* Paramount Pictures. February 19, 2010.

the film capitalizes on the fear, paranoia, and secrecy of the Cold War era and emulates the film noir genre of the period.[16]

Many hospital-based dramas are notable for incompetent palliative care. A desperate mother (Oscar-awarded Shirley MacLaine) in *Terms of Endearment* (1983) demands that the nurses give her dying daughter morphine: "I don't see why she has to have this pain …. It's time for her shot, do you understand? Do something … My daughter is in pain!" Few are depicted as places of healing and comfort.

Portrayal of Physicians: From Adoration to Apprehension

In *The Good Doctor* (2011), Dr. Waylans (Rob Morrow) tells his colleague, "You know the secret of being a good doctor, don't you? … You act like one"—which leads to the question: can actors portray a good doctor? Films released in the 1930s and 1940s offered fine country doctors, simple and compassionate, who always put the patients first. Over time, portrayals dramatically changed, introducing major medical ethical issues such as mercy killing and abortion with physicians as instigators.

Historically, physicians in film have been male, attractive, and witty, although the sympathetic portrayal of the character varies depending on the needs of the script. When the white doctor enters the scene, he is usually meticulously dressed in a crisp white coat, but then his character shows.[17] The silver screen surgeons are portrayed as deus ex machina and certainly in the silent film era.

In the United States, the 1940s and 1950s are best remembered as the "Dr. Kildare era." Indeed, Kildare (both in his movie and TV iterations) and his celluloid colleagues were an idyllic depiction of hospitals and their physicians, nurses, and administrators. *Dr. Kildare's Wedding Day* (1941) offered this classic line: "Doctors doctor for 24 hours a day. The rest of the time he can't be a husband." Although the demands of their vocation may have excluded them from domestic bliss, film physicians worked tirelessly to ensure a Hollywood-style happy ending for their patients, ideally within a 90-minute run time. *The Country Doctor* shows a compassionate but scrappy physician (played by Jean Hersholt), who would later star as Dr. Christian on radio, TV, and six films. Older and grumpier than the smoothly handsome Kildare, Dr. Christian did not hesitate to tangle with officious bureaucrats or other nemeses to improve the well-being of his patients and neighbors (Figure 1.2).[18] It is rumored that the actor's demeanor as a kind and knowledgeable doctor resulted in mail sent to him by viewers asking for advice.

Japanese filmmaker Akiro Kurosawa featured physicians as the main characters in five of his films, and his physicians are notable for their dedication (despite lack of resources), rationality, and private lives that have been eclipsed by their professional lives. This is particularly true of *Red Beard*.[19] Elderly people in Japan still use the term "Red Beard" to describe a physician who is always available and unmotivated by financial incentives.

Other, less laudatory portrayals of the medical profession also suffer from distortion and inaccuracy. In *The Interns* (1962), which follows a group of young moving into practice, nurses are warned, "Never talk to the interns. They are all sex maniacs."

Film doctors gradually evolved from dedicated, solo general practitioners to arrogant, intimidating hot-shot surgeons. In *Doc Hollywood* (1991), Michael J. Fox proclaims, "Beverly Hills, plastic surgery, the most beautiful women in the world. What do these three things have in common? Answer: Me, in one week."

Gynecologists and obstetricians occasionally appear, even as the main actor in one movie—Richard Gere in Robert Altman's *Dr. T and the Women* (2000). Ingmar Bergman's *A Lesson in Love* (1954) is a comedy about the gynecologist Dr. Erneman, his extramarital affair, and reconciliation

---

[16] A likely inspiration was *Shock Corridor* (Fuller S. Allied Artists Pictures. September 11, 1963).

[17] Dans PE. *Doctors in the Movies: Boil the Water and Just Say Aah.* Bloomington, IL: Medi-Ed Press; 2000. Dans authored the first comprehensive, in-depth work on physicians in film, although his many novel observations of the medical profession on film were limited to Hollywood productions.

[18] Borst CG. "The Noblest Roman of Them All?" Professional versus Popular Views of America's Country Doctors. *J Hist Med Allied Sci.* 2021;76:78–100.

[19] Kurosawa A. *Red Beard*. Toho. April 3, 1965.

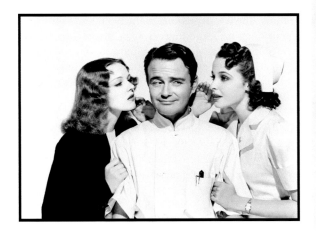
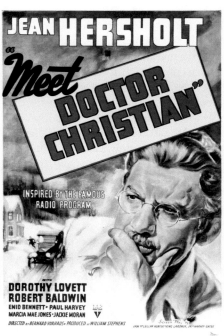

FIGURE 1.2   The first iconic doctors in film. The "perfect" one and heartthrob, heartthrob Dr. Kildare, played by Lew Ayres (left; TCD/Prod.DB/Alamy Stock Photo – Metro-Goldwyn Mayer) and the pensive one, Dr. Christian, played by Jean Hersholt (right; Poster Art, Jean Hersholt, 1939 Everett Collection, Inc. / Alamy Stock Photo).

with his wife. Repeatedly, women ask him if it is not "difficult" for a gynecologist to see attractive women. *Brink of Life* (1958) offers a more realistic and sympathetic portrayal of these specialists. Obstetricians, of course, get caught up in birthing traumas. *Rosemary's Baby* (1968) is the major representation of a scary pregnancy, rape fantasies, and other absurdities such as the gestation of a devil child. The horror film *Dead Ringers* (1988) portrays the speculum as an instrument of torture.

Given the many films on psychiatric disorders, the portrayal of psychiatrists has been well analyzed. They have been categorized as competent and caring (Dr. Bergen, played by Judd Hirsch in *Ordinary People* [1980]), neurotic and comical (Richard Dreyfuss as Dr. Marvin in *What about Bob?* [1991]), and serial killer (Dr. Hannibal Lecter, played by Anthony Hopkins in *Silence of the Lambs* [1991]). Hopkins again plays a psychiatrist (in this instance, an ethical one) in *Elyse* (2020), when he must treat a woman (Lisa Pepper) with a catatonic form of borderline personality disorder in a film directed by his spouse, Stella Hopkins.[20] Hitchcock cast Ingrid Bergman as a psychiatrist in *Spellbound* (1945).[21] Director John Huston's fascination with hypnosis and psychoanalysis gave us *Freud: The Secret Passion* (1962) and *Let There Be Light* (1946). Interestingly, Huston did not use any other physician in his work until the horror film *Phobia* (1980), where patients with phobias are killed by what they fear most.

The social and professional status of physicians is high. Quite a few surgeons drive sports cars and live in palatial country homes. Specialists' salaries enter the script, most notably in *Crisis* (1950), where the

---

[20] Hopkins delivered yet another stellar performance in *Elyse* (directed by his wife Stella Hopkins) the same year he won an Oscar for *The Father* (see Chapter 4). Of note, he elevates the tension when manipulated by his patient Elyse and fortunately recognizes counter-transference, but I suspect the audience is waiting for him to turn into Hannibal Lector at any time.

[21] In a memorable (albeit very non-PC) line, Dr. Peterson's mentor tells her, ".... women make the best psychoanalysts, till they fall in love. After that, they make the best patients."

neurosurgeon (Cary Grant) says, "My fee? I usually charge 10% of the patient's income." In *Drunken Angel* (1948), the physician says to his patient, "I warn you my fees are very high—I always overcharge people who eat and drink too much." But there are more peculiarities. Some films emphasize addictions by physicians or physicians practicing while intoxicated, such as the general surgeon (Alec Baldwin) in *Malice* (1993) and the heart surgeon (Kirk Harris) stealing drugs from the hospital to trade for cocaine in *Intoxicating* (2003).

Very few female doctors appear in early feature films. The few depictions in the 1930s and 1940s were demeaning (e.g., with patients refusing care by female doctors[22]), and these were principally secondary roles with unknown actresses and weak characterizations. Diversity in film was hard to find and closely reflected the attitude of medical societies and male practitioners. Few women were accepted into accredited training programs. Later films did show more female physicians, and several are neurologists (e.g., *Declaration of War*, *The Late Quartet*, and *The Father*, discussed in Chapter 4).[23]

Black or Asian physicians were nearly invisible in American, British, or European films. Supreme Pictures released *Am I Guilty?* (1940) and re-released it in 1945 as *Racket Doctor—Am I Guilty?* One of the so-called "race films" in the United States, specifically made for Blacks, it featured an all African American cast and a physician (Ralph Cooper) running a free clinic in Harlem. Better known are Sidney Poitier's physician portrayals in three films.[24] These served to highlight racial disparity or subconscious implicit racism. Until the 1950s, Black doctors were not admitted to the American Medical Association (AMA), and they still comprise only 3% of physicians. The documentary *Black Women in Medicine* (2016) highlights the unfinished work needed for equity.[25]

Screenwriters have toiled carefully over portrayals of specialists, and a brief summary of their (often amusing) specialty characterizations is shown in Table 1.1.

Nurses in film had subservient roles for many decades. Nurses were typically in awe of the doctors because "they always know best." Doctors were also seen as major marriage prospects and incited jealousy among the nurses. Often in the nurse–physician relationship, however, the nurse endured sexual harassment and verbal abuse. Gradually, relationships between physicians and nursing staff became confrontational on film. In *Critical Care* (1979), a nurse questions whether the care of a patient in a persistent vegetative state should continue. The physician answers, "It's important that we say that we did everything," to which the nurse replies, "That's doctor-speak for 'we put this patient through hell before he died.'"

Exploitive relationships are common in the movies, and physicians violating boundaries are sometimes used as a plot device. Virtually in every film involving doctors, there is a barrier between patient and doctor—only to be broken later—or the physician seeks a relationship with a family member (Diane Keaton in *Something's Gotta Give* [2003] and Keri Russell in *Waitress* [2007]). Also, in *Critical Care* (Chapter 4), the attending physician develops a sexual relationship with the daughter of a patient.

Although they are by no means common, some medical biographic films (biopics) have been made. Some have involved laboratory researchers (e.g., *The Story of Louis Pasteur* [1936], rabies and anthrax; *Dr. Ehrlich's Magic Bullet* [1940], syphilis). Heroic nurses have also appeared in films like *The White Angel* (1936), about Florence Nightingale; and *Sister Kenny* (1946, see Chapter 3). More recent biopics involve the psychiatry greats Freud and Jung (*A Dangerous Method*, 2011) and sexual researcher Alfred Kinsey (*Kinsey*, 2004).

---

[22] Bacon L. *Mary Stevens, M.D.* Warner Bros. Pictures. July 22, 1933.

[23] Dans PE, ed. Where Are All the Women Doctors? In: *Doctors in the Movies: Boil the Water and Just Say Aah.* Bloomington, IL: Medi-Ed Press; 2000:121–148.

[24] Mankiewicz JL. *No Way Out.* 20th Century Fox. August 16, 1950; Cornfield H. *Pressure Point.* United Artists. December 2, 1962; Kramer S. *Guess Who's Coming to Dinner.* Columbia Pictures. December 12, 1967. A new major work is Colorization : One Hundred Years of Black Films in a White World. Haygood W. New York: Knopf; 2021.

[25] Written and directed by filmmaker Crystal Emery, *Black Women in Medicine* is a documentary following the careers of four trail-blazing surgeons. Emery's motivation was to inspire more Blacks to enter the field of medicine with a goal of 7% by 2030. See Emery CR. *Black Women in Medicine.* American Public Television 2016 and Manning KD. Black Women in Medicine—A Documentary. *JAMA.* 2017;318:1306–1307.

TABLE 1.1   Characterization of Medical Specialties in Film in Quotables

Anesthesia	"Anesthesia is the easiest thing in the world until something goes wrong. It's 99 percent boredom and 1 percent scared-shitless panic." (*Coma* [1978])
Surgery	"A surgeon's job is to cut—get in, fix it, and get out." (*The Doctor* [1991])
	"You do not think much of surgeons. Not as much as they think of themselves." (*The Interns* [1962])
	"If this operation is a success, I have created a monster - a beautiful face and no heart." (*A Woman's Face* [1941])
Neurosurgery	"It is like Russian roulette. In one hand, you have a revolver called treatment and, the other side, a revolver called no treatment." (*The English Surgeon* [2007])
Intensive care	"Jesus brought Lazarus back from the dead, but he did it only once. People were amazed we did it every day." (*Critical Care* [1997])
Family medicine	"I am just a small-town doctor who pushes aspirin to the elderly." (*Eve's Bayou* [1997])
Dermatology	"The patient never gets better and never gets sick." (*Young Dr. Kildare* [1938])
Neurology	"What did the neurologist say? ... He does not know." (*Regarding Henry* [1991])
Psychiatry	"Evaluate, medicate, vacate." (*12 Monkeys* [1995])

Films have also focused on medical atrocities during the Holocaust, and some are unforgettable.[26] *The Boys from Brazil* (1978) is based on a science fiction novel in which a Nazi hunter, modeled after Simon Wiesenthal (Lawrence Olivier), tries to find Josef Mengele (Gregory Peck). We see Mengele injecting dark-skinned boys in Paraguay with a chemical that causes green eyes.

Portrayal of Diseases: From Unknowns to Knowns

Early cinematic descriptions of illness were vague. Detailed explanations of how disorders affect organs and functions came later. This lack of transparency was likely due to the Hays Code. There are many reasons why scriptwriters like disease. In films, unconventional diseases baffle doctors, frustrate families, and of course, threaten the life of the patient. Being forced helplessly to observe progressive deterioration is tragic. Moreover, the fears provoked by these diseases (e.g., isolation and dependency) are universal. Not understanding our environment when our mind betrays us—due to senility and dementia—is a recurrent topic. And finally, there is the loss of a loved one. Cinematic diseases run a similar course to reality, but the mortality rates are higher in film (*Love Story* [1970], *Terms of Endearment* [1983]).

Cinema has dealt with diseases in multifarious ways, but rarely have such films become classics. Kurosawa's *Ikiru* (1952), which deals with a man with inoperable gastric cancer, is a rare example of a film in which disease is the main theme. A full discussion of major medical diseases is outside the scope of this book, but Table 1.2 shows some of the more recognizable films. Doctors may also get sick (*The Doctor* [1991]), and directors often shape this into a life-changing event, which, of course, it often is.

Directors often find their topics for a screenplay when medicine interfaces with other disciplines, such as ethics and psychology. Bioethicists, psychologists, and sociologists have all written critiques of film with many themes suggested. For example, Dr. Isak Borg's character in Ingmar Bergman's *Wild Strawberries*.[27] Dr. Borg is an emeritus professor of bacteriology who reminisces about his life. The themes of pity and regret, guilt, family dysfunctionality, religious doubt, fear of failing exams, and fear of death have all been offered as explanations. Disease leads to death, and cinema found a way to personify death. In addition to a violent death from viruses, aliens, climate change, and nuclear Armageddon, studios made serious movies about disease and dying.

---

[26] In *Mr. Klein* (Losey J. Fox-Lira. October 27, 1976), for example, a doctor examines a woman to determine, in an official report, whether she is Jewish. He looks at examining her gums and jaw, measures her nostrils with a specially devised ruler, and inspects her naked body and gait.

[27] Bergman I. *Wild Strawberries*. AB Svensk Filmindustrie. December 26, 1957.

TABLE 1.2   Characterization of Medical Diseases in Film

Disorder	Film Examples
Cancer	*Ikiru* (1952) *Cries and Whispers* (1972) *The Barbarian Invasions* (2003) *Me and Earl and the Dying Girl* (2015)
HIV	*Philadelphia* (1993) *Absolutely Positive* (2012) *Dallas Buyers Club* (2013) *120 BPM* (2017)
Alcoholism	*Leaving Las Vegas* (1995) *Crazy Heart* (2009) *The Rum Diary* (2011)
Opioid addiction	*Ben is Back (2018)* *The Souvenir* (2019)
Viral epidemic	*Outbreak* (1995) *Contagion* (2011)
Myocardial infarction	*Something's Gotta Give* (2003)
Bipolar disorder, schizophrenia	*Mr. Jones* (1993) *A Beautiful Mind* (2001) *Take Shelter* (2011)
Multiple personalities	*The Three Faces of Eve* (1957) *Zelig* (1983) *Split* (2015)

Early European filmmakers wondered if we could ask Death a favor. Directors Victor Sjöström and Ingmar Bergman both asked if the Grim Reaper would entertain debate. Postponement through negotiation was a major theme. *The Phantom Carriage* and *The Seventh Seal* personify death to great effect, invariably as a cloaked and hooded elderly male.[28] In Fritz Lang's film *Destiny*, a woman in love can only get her dying lover back if she saves a life or finds another soul to replace her lover in death, even going so far as to offer her child. Cinema has dealt with grief, and lack of resolution is common in recent films (*Don't Look Now*, *Three Colors, Blue*, *Manchester by the Sea*, and *Antichrist*). Death in the movies is often agonizing, and many explore common themes of despair, the randomness of fate, and everything associated with trying to come to grips with it. In cinema, death from illness is unavoidable and non-negotiable. Our current reality is not much better. We are not often confronted with a "good death," sudden and painless, as in *The Godfather*, where Vito Corleone gracefully collapses from a cardiac arrest in the tall tomato plants while playing with little Anthony. The boy laughs as he is unaware of mortality.

End Credits

I began with a claim that Medicine in film can be approached and studied from many angles.[29] We can break it up into depictions of disorders, specialists, medical institutions, and medical biographies. Many films are provocative (often involving psychiatric depictions), doctors are not always good supporters of

---

[28] Sjöström V. *The Phantom Carriage*. AB Svensk Filmindustri. January 1, 1921; Bergman I. *The Seventh Seal*. AB Svensk Filmindustri. February 16, 1957.

[29] A number of edited collections have been published. In addition to Dans 2000 (previously cited), see Colt H, Quadrelli S, Friedman L, eds. *The Picture of Health: Medical Ethics and the Movies*. 1st ed. New York: Oxford University Press; 2011; Gabbard GO, Gabbard K. *Psychiatry and the Cinema*. Washington, DC: American Psychiatric Press, Inc.; 1999; Glasser B. *Medicinema: Doctors in Films*. Paperback ed. London: Radcliffe Publishing Ltd; 2010; Harper G, Moor A, Calman KF, eds. *Signs of Life: Cinema and Medicine*. London: Wallflower Press; 2005; Robinson DJ. *Reel Psychiatry: Movie Portrayals of Psychiatric Conditions*. Port Huron, MI: Rapid Psychler Press; 2003; and Shapshay S, ed. *Bioethics at the Movies*. Baltimore, MD: Johns Hopkins University Press; 2009.

patients, and surgeons indulge in a bit of hubris. Celluloid physicians emerged early in cinema.[30] As medicine became more sophisticated, cinema took notice and changed in parallel. The family physician became a hospital specialist, primarily saving lives, but then physicians' vulnerability (and misjudgments) entered screenplays. Film doctors can be caricatures who do very little actual doctoring. Many specialties are absent in film, probably because they are less understood or provide no inspiration for a plot line, but psychiatrists, gynecologists, and surgeons appear frequently, perhaps because their specialties are more provocative. Physicians unwilling to consider alternative explanations are a common theme. Their bedside manners are often patronizing, but there are examples of kindness and compassion, too. The audience may cynically say that these characterizations imitate life as we know it, and physicians definitely do not lead an altogether ascetic lifestyle. Some say that Dr. Hill (Alec Baldwin in *Malice*, 1993) is a caricature; don't bank on it.[31] When asked in a deposition if he has a God complex, Dr. Hill tells a prosecuting lawyer, "I have an MD from Harvard, and I am board certified in cardiothoracic medicine and trauma surgery. I have been awarded citations from seven different medical boards in New England, and I am never sick at sea." Then he concludes, "you ask me if I have a God complex. Let me tell you something: I am God" (Figure 1.3).

Films do show the evolution of specialization—from the family doctor (Dr. Christian) and general internist (Dr. Kildare) to battle surgeons (Hawkeye Pierce), neurosurgeons, gynecologists, and the many psychiatrists played by many renowned actors. Some filmmakers habitually feature physicians. Bergman's filmography features 16 physicians in 13 films.[32] Bergman's comparably prolific peers—in a similar, active three-decade lifespan—made infrequent use of physicians. *Patch Adams* (based on the clownish physician who comforted gravely sick children), with a protagonist meant to be lovable but who indulged in a nearly intolerable amount of vulgarity, was another aberration of modern cinema.[33]

I think that the medicine of cinema follows a set of principles, but filmmakers are more interested in communicating a cinematic mood than presenting a realistic construction of the science of medicine. With these provisos in mind, the early, perfect movie doctors may have raised public expectations. But more modern filmmakers also uphold some of the more recognizable caricatures. Representations of physicians mingle arrogance, bewilderment, and self-destructiveness with many outright archaic behaviors in their profession or private lives. None of them pass muster, and there is little to be said about the authenticity of the doctor. Nursing staff also cannot escape coarse stereotypes, and sexualization is very common. Film nurses must be attractive and vulnerable to misogynists and shallow fantasies. Many nurses are offended, while others laugh it off.

Generally, the premise must be deeply affecting and shocking to drive the storyline. Medicine is also awash with plot devices to kill off characters (e.g., coma or terminal illness) or cause them pain and suffering (e.g., aggressive cancer, extreme mental illness, or a massive pandemic). Impairment as isolation and alienation has been a classic theme for playwrights and has found its way into film. Disability is often championed and even given new meaning. Finally, some filmmakers seek to highlight systemic bias in the care of patients on the bases of gender, race, sexual orientation, and socioeconomic strata.

Filmmakers and cinephiles understand that cinema became a niche medium when TV sets appeared in living rooms. Movies and TV series have always been very different in scope and quality, and this is also

---

[30] Cashman CR. Golden Ages and Silver Screens: The Construction of the Physician Hero in 1930–1940 American Cinema. *J Med Humanit*. 2019;40:553–568.

[31] The actual prevalence of his type of behavior is unknown and hopefully diminishing. Work is being done to change it. See Myers CG, Lu-Myers Y, Ghaferi AA. Excising the "Surgeon Ego" to Accelerate Progress in the Culture of Surgery. *BMJ*. 2018;363:k4537.

[32] Wijdicks EF. The bedside Manners of Ingmar Bergman's Celluloid Physicians. *Hektoen International*. 2020. Bergman created physicians who were revered in their profession but detached in their human relationships; only a few were likable. Generally, Bergman's portrayal of physicians leaves a bad impression.

[33] Patch Adams was a physician (and clown) who founded the Gesundheit Institute, a free community hospital in Hillsboro, West Virginia, which specializes in holistic medicine. According to its website, it is "1) no charge; 2) no health insurance reimbursement; 3) no malpractice insurance; 4) 3- to 4-hour initial interview with the patient; 5) home as hospital; 6) integration of all the healing arts; 7) integration of medicine with performance arts, arts and crafts, nature, agriculture, education, recreation, and social service; and 8) the health of the staff is as important as the health of the patient."

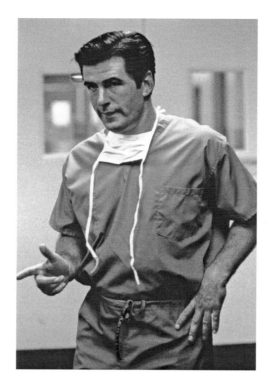

FIGURE 1.3   The movie surgeon with a disdainful hauteur (Dr. Hill played by Alec Baldwin; Photofest).

reflected in their representations of medicine. Later medical dramas such as *Marcus Welby MD*, *ER*, *Grey's Anatomy*, and *House MD* progressively tackled complex topics and introduced polarizing plot lines.[34] Exaggeration seems far more prevalent with TV series than film.[35] The lines between cinema and TV are blurring with directors crossing over because streaming giants provide the funds for high-budget drama. The previous confrontation has given way to reciprocal cooperation. Television is increasingly becoming a writer's medium and attracts major actors. Television allows a lot more time to expand on a topic and provide a more detailed back story. A case in point is the recent Netflix series *Nurse Ratched* with many kooky twists and, of course, her cruel authority. Whether these series will change the representation of psychiatry is an appropriate question to ask.

Film is often remembered by key moments but more often by catchphrases that stick in mind forever. (British actors have allegedly complained that taxi drivers shout these lines at them.) In medical movies, little of the dialogue approaches authenticity, and medical professionals seldom recognize the choice of words, nuance, exposition, and relation dynamics. We cannot expect screenwriters to ask healthcare workers for tutorials in medical lingo. Screenwriters may do extensive research on the subject matter but

---

[34] Brinkley J. Physicians Have an Image Problem—It's Too Good. *New York Times*. February 10, 1985; Week in Review. "Jim Snyder, an officer with the St. Paul Fire and Marine Insurance Company, which writes more medical malpractice policies than any other company, says his industry calls this the 'Marcus Welby syndrome,' after the television-series doctor who never seemed to lose a patient. It's apparent to us that with all the advances in medicine, he said, an awful lot of people now have this belief."

[35] Some of these series spawned explanatory books, including several by Andrew Holz, the former CNN medical correspondent. See Holtz A. *The Medical Science of House, M.D.: The Facts Behind the Addictive Medical Drama.* Paperback ed. New York: The Berkley Publishing Group; 2006; Holtz A. *The Real Grey's Anatomy: A Behind-the-Scenes Look at the Real Lives of Surgical Residents.* New York: The Berkley Publishing Co.; 2010; and Holtz A. *House M.D. vs. Reality: Fact and Fiction in the Hit Television Series.* New York: The Berkley Publishing Company; 2011.

seldom interview medical professionals. So, while none of us actually talk like Hawkeye Pierce, House, or behave as anyone in the cast of *Grey's Anatomy* (and, it is hoped, few of us emulate them), it stings if actors portraying medical professionals demean us. We wonder why the resulting image is so deficient and mortifying.

It is impossible to catalog the entire body of work of medicine in cinema,[36] but the allure of neurosciences is noteworthy, and thus films with the neurologic and psychiatric disease have positioned themselves quite visibly in this collection of medically themed films. In the next chapters, we will see how the specialty of neurology, in all its grandeur, is portrayed and used.

---

[36] Some attempt in Wijdicks EFM. *Cinema, MD*. New York: Oxford University Press; 2020.

2

Introducing the History of
Neurology in Film

Your memory's all shot to pieces—you can't concentrate. Look at your bridge scores! And you're irritable because your nerves are all on edge. You won't admit it, but you can't deny it, can you?

Dr. Steele in "Dark Victory" (1939)

Portraying a human being (Bette Davis) ignoring her symptoms but facing the ultimate reality and meeting it squarely is what made *Dark Victory (1939)* ⚔, successful and memorable. Some would interpret this story line as the quintessence of sacrifice. Bette Davis proclaimed: "it's a victory because we're not afraid." There was a risk with its production—Jack Warner famously asked, "Who wants to watch some dame go blind?"—but it filled the coffers for Warner Bros Pictures. *Dark Victory* should be considered one of the very first films in which a progressive neurologic disease plays a major role in the narrative and plot. The film not only depicts a progressive, rapidly fatal brain tumor but also advocates withholding information from the patient and even suggests the possibility of a close, amorous physician–patient relationship. Although it might have been a common perception, it was very rare at the time for physicians to withhold information, and most physicians were, as they should be, forthcoming. (Having a romantic entanglement with a patient was also not regarded favorably in the 1950s and is still considered unethical and a reason for sanctions or termination.) The film offers a highly unusual presentation of a brain tumor, which usually presents with a behavioral change or a seizure. *Dark Victory* was mythical and, early in the history of cinema, confronted the audience with the mystery of neurologic disease. It would be the start of neurologic disease emerging in screenplays.

If we decide that an actual history of medicine in film exists—even one marred by the uneven selection of topics by filmmakers—the next objective is to provide a synthesis of Neurology in Cinema throughout the years and to look at it with some magnification. Contrary to what the history of neurology on film suggests, a true account of the historical development of neurology is complex; the new specialty was interrelated with other disciplines (i.e., neurosurgery and psychiatry). Clinical (defining best care) and scientific (neuroimaging) advancements provided a major impetus that further delineated and matured the specialty. (It is misguided to portray the history of neurology, as some medical historians have done, as a synopsis of neurologic personalities and whether they deserved an eponym.[1]) Once independent from the other two disciplines, neurology advanced rather quickly and was recognized in many European countries followed by the United Kingdom and the United States. Each country has a story to tell, and because few of them overlap, all contributed to what eventually became the outline and fabric of our specialty. In film, we can recognize a timeline of single themes, with some emerging briefly while others stay as a recurrent theme. A few disappeared early only to return after a long interval away from the screen.

Several other observations can be made at the onset. Because cinema was only introduced in the early 20th century, one can expect a proclivity for showing neurology in the "modern" age. But the turn

---

[1] Tyler K, York GK, Steinberg DA, et al. Part 2: History of 20th Century Neurology: Decade by Decade. *Ann Neurol.* 2003;53(Suppl 4):S27–S45. doi: 10.1002/ana.1346

DOI: 10.1201/9781003270874-2   13

of the century was also an important era for neurology. The history of the neurosciences—a word that only emerged in the mid-1960s in manuscript titles—can be compartmentalized as several centuries of anatomic discoveries. The anatomical clinical approach of Charcot in the late 1800s was associated with therapeutic nihilism—disorders were intractable or self-limiting. But then, in the 20th century, physiologic (mechanistic) discoveries were plentiful, and in fact, the Nobel Prize in Medicine started to include work in physiology. All this escaped cinema as well as the screenwriters who developed ideas for movies. Exceptions are biopics on some scientists steadily laboring in their laboratories with their microscopes, whose contributions were immeasurably important (see Chapter 1).

Cinema has steered away from depicting the maturation of neurology as a cumulation of inventive physicians. Reputable neurologists, deserving a place in our specialty's pantheon, are conspicuously absent (see Chapter 3). Neurologic disorders, however, have percolated through educational films and fictional feature films. More recently, neurologic disorders became the main topic of documentaries discussing complicated ethical issues (e.g., progressive neurologic disease prompting the patient to decide when to become chronically dependent on machines and the dilemma of whether to pursue DNA testing).

This book discusses distinguished films that premiered during the heyday of cinema, but neurocinema has continued to this day with more cinematic offerings every year. The unforeseen changes and ups and downs of neurologic disease must have attracted screenwriters. Meanwhile, actors and directors had to figure out how to portray the manifestations of these diseases. Neurology (and psychiatry) affects mind or motion in various ways and with various degrees of severity, which may account for the interest it generates in the film industry.

Neurology on the Move—The Very Early Years

In the beginning, movies were simply science projects, and educational films grew out of advances of photography. It all started in 1872, when the photographer Eadweard Muybridge was commissioned to prove an expensive bet for retired governor and horse breeder Leland Stanford. Stanford claimed that horses have all four hooves off the ground when in full gallop rather than moving through a rocking movement. Muybridge was able to prove the hypothesis and later published his photographs in two popular books, *Animals in Motion* (1899) and *The Human Figure in Motion* (1901).[2] In one of the greatest developments of nineteenth-century photography, stills shown at speeds of up to 1/2000th of a second resembled a movie because the process is basically identical. Prepared in collaboration with the physician–neurologist Francis Dercum, Muybridge's *The Human Figure in Motion* contained photographs of a number of neurologic movements diagnosed as locomotor ataxia but also included choreoballistic movement, a spastic, high-stepping gait caused by multiple sclerosis, poliomyelitis, and tabes dorsalis (Figure 2.1). Dercum used some of these plates in his neurology textbook.[3,4,5] After projection of film became more robust, several physicians started to film neurologic patients. Between July 1898 and 1901, Romanian professor Gheorghe Marinescu made several science films in his neurology clinic. Remarkably, his very first films compared stroke-associated hemiplegia with functional weakness

---

[2] There is a bizarre claim that Muybridge's traumatic head injury "unveiled his artistic and inventive genius," i.e., unleashed a compulsive behavior that led to his admittedly unusual pursuits. Manjila S, Gagandeep Singh G, Alkhachroum AM, Ramos-Estebanez C. Understanding Edward Muybridge: Historical Review of Behavioral Alterations after a 19th-Century Head Injury and Their Multifactorial Influence on Human Life and Culture. *Neurosurg Focus.* 2015;39:E4.

[3] Lanska DJ. The Dercum-Muybridge Collaboration for Sequential Photography of Neurologic Disorders. *Neurology.* 2013;81:1550–1554.

[4] Lanska DJ. The Dercum-Muybridge Collaboration and the Study of Pathologic Gaits Using Sequential Photography. *J Hist Neurosci.* 2016;25:23–38.

[5] Some clinical histories of the photographed patients were discovered in 2017 and provided subtext to the pictures; see Noble G. Clinical Histories Animate Muybridge and Dercum's Original Photographic Study of Neurologic Gait. *Neurology.* 2021;97:1026–1030.

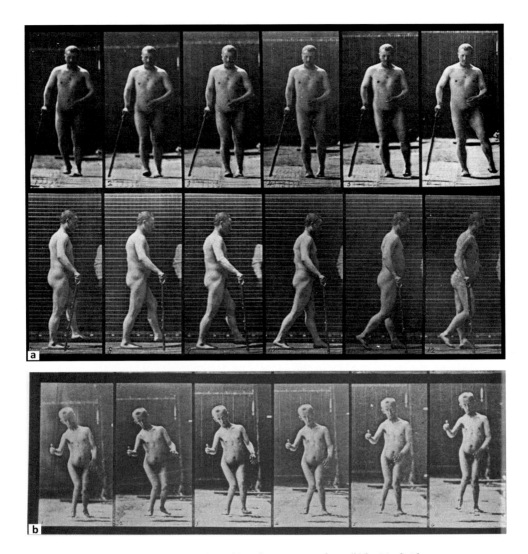

FIGURE 2.1 Photographed gaits of hemiplegia (a) and spastic paraplegia (b) by Muybridge.

(no circular movement and elevation of the hip but dragging of the leg with all muscles paralyzed and the remarkable success of hypnosis—a clip can be found on YouTube). The films are *Walking Troubles of Organic Hemiplegia* (1898), *The Walking Troubles of Organic Paraplegies* (1899), *A Case of Hysteric Hemiplegia Healed Through Hypnosis* (1899), *The Walking Troubles of Progressive Locomotion Ataxy* (1900), and *Illnesses of the Muscles* (1901).

Auguste Lumiere, one of the founders of cinema, saw Marinescu's science films and admired his fortitude but also lamented that few physicians were filming their patients.[6,7,8] However, a decade later,

[6] Podoll K. History of Scientific and Popular Educational Films in Neurology and Psychiatry in Germany 1985–1929. *Fortschr Neurol Psychiatr.* 2000;68:523–529.

[7] Podoll K, Luning J. History of Scientific Research Films in Neurology in Germany 1895–1929. *Fortschr Neurol Psychiatr.* 1998;66:122–132.

[8] Barboi AC, Goetz CG, Musetoiu R. The Origins of Scientific Cinematography and Early Medical Applications. *Neurology.* 2004;62:2082–2086.

several neurologists were filming in the United States (Walter Greenough Chase, Theodore Weisenburg), Germany (Paul Schuster), France (Albert Londe), Belgium (Arthur Van Gehuchten), and Italy (Camillo Negro).[9] These "film libraries" were actually a mix of psychiatry and neurology and in keeping with the scope of the specialty in Europe. Deciding how to use them was even more difficult because there was little if any interpretative text. Functional behavior and neurology from brain lesions were hard to distinguish unless a detailed comparison was made such as with Gheorghe Marinescu. Most shockingly, around 1908, Chase's films on epilepsy and status epilepticus were offered to the public at "one-cent" vaudeville parlors and as carnival sideshow attractions.[10,11]

At least one surgeon was very interested in filming. Eugène-Louis Doyen was a "renaissance man" who practiced neurosurgery. On July 1898, he presented the very first film on a craniotomy at the British Medical Association in Edinburgh. One year later, he launched his own private journal, the *Revue critique de méde-cine et de chirurgie* (Figure 2.2). On the first pages of the inaugural issue, he promoted the future potential of cinematography in teaching. For Doyen, it was not only to show off his surgical skills for his colleagues but also to show surgery in real time for students taught only on cadavers: "When I watched one of my surgeries on screen for the first time I realized to what extent I was unaware of myself (...) I've corrected, I've perfected, and I've simplified what needed to be; in such a way that the cinematograph helped me to perfect my surgical technique considerably." But also according to Doyen, one could not understand a new surgical procedure by reading about it, or even by watching it being performed by any other surgeon; one had to see the master and he advocated speed and simplification of surgery. His films showed the surgeon's demeanor ("undis-tracted," "concentration" and "self-confidence"). All his films were considered lost, but then ten were recently found in the Cinemateca Portuguesa-Museu do Cinema. Four film segments show temporal craniotomies. Doyen demonstrates his newly invented, motorized electric drill, and the clips show improved surgical techniques of lifting the bone flap and stripping of the dura. Doyen pierces or prods the dura to check for subdural blood. The reason for one of the craniotomies was epidural bleeding over the temporal dura. These films clearly were made to demonstrate new technology and his own advancements in surgical skills with creating burr holes and using a side-cutting saw to ensure safely stripping away of the dura. Historically, perhaps the most interesting person to watch is the assistant, who repeatedly gives the patient what is presumably chloroform on a handkerchief; this was a commonly used pain control method before Morton's ether inhalation (Figure 2.2). At the time, filming in an operating room was nearly impossible due to the light-insensitive (slow) films of short duration as well as the difficulties in creating adequate lighting in the window-less operating rooms. A good documentation of Doyen's films and the comments of his peers is available.[12] Doyen has a strong claim on being the first in filming a craniotomy. However, subsequent evidence revealed that the Polish cinematographer Boleslaw Matuszewski filmed surgeries in Saint Peterburg and Warsaw in the late 1890s; these allegedly included neurosurgical procedures. Baltic German surgeon Ernst von Bergmann also filmed some of his surgeries (amputations), but no records exist of a neurosurgical procedure.

A major document in the neurology of education cinema is the film *War Neurosis*.[13] From 1917 to 1918, Major Arthur Hurst filmed shell-shocked patients home from war. He recorded soldiers who suffered from intractable movement disorders. It was the first time that a comment on therapy was included. The film had intertitles that recommended "persuasion and re-education" but also used hypnotism and electric shock treatment in more severe cases.[14]

---

[9] Tosi V. *Cinema Before Cinema: The Origins of Scientific Cinematography.* Paperback ed. New York: Wallflower Press; 2006.

[10] Viva la dance. Epileptic Seizures, No. 1-8. Penn State University Libraries Catalog; 1905.

[11] Cartwright L. *Screening the Body: Tracing Medicine's Visual Culture.* Minneapolis: University of Minnesota Press; 1995.

[12] See Baptista T. Il faut voire le Maître: A Recent Restoration of Surgical Films by E.-L. Doyen (1859–1916). *J Film Preserv.* 2005;70:42–50; Doyen E-L. Le cinématographe et l'enseignement de la chirurgie. *Revue critique de médecine et de chirur-gie.* 1899;1:1–6. I had the opportunity to see these film clips in their entirety.

[13] Hurst A, Symns JLM. War Neuroses: Netley Hospital, 1917 [1 film reel: Silent, black and white, 16 mm]. Wellcome Trust; 1918.

[14] The most comprehensive treatise on this film is by Jones E. War Neuroses and Arthur Hurst: A Pioneering Medical Film about the Treatment of Psychiatric Battle Casualties. *J Hist Med Allied Sci.* 2012;67:345–373.

Dᴿ DOYEN

Le Cinématographe et l'Enseignement de la Chirurgie

Les projections animées ont été tout d'abord considérées comme une simple récréation.

On n'enregistrait que des scènes de courte durée : un rouleau pelliculaire de 18 mètres au pas Lumière ou Edison et à la vitesse de seize images par seconde durait exactement une minute.

La trépidation de l'image, très fatigante pour les spectateurs, lorsqu'il s'agissait de scènes quelconques, devenait intolérable si l'on voulait représenter un sujet compliqué.

Les conditions d'éclairage, difficiles à réaliser dans des locaux fermés, ne permettaient d'obtenir des négatifs vigoureux qu'en plein air ou dans un atelier spécialement aménagé.

Lorsqu'il y a quelques années j'ai voulu appliquer la cinématographie à l'enseignement de la chirurgie, ces obstacles étaient irréductibles.

Les pellicules ne possédaient pas une sensibilité suffisante pour les objectifs les plus rapides dont on disposait alors et les appareils en usage ne permettaient pas d'enregistrer pratiquement des scènes d'une certaine durée.

Il eût été facile de photographier en plein air des opé-

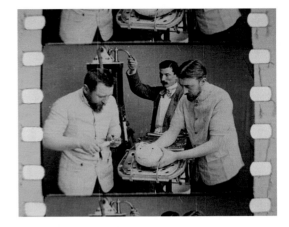

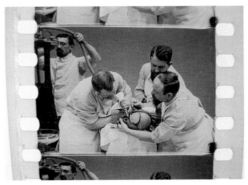

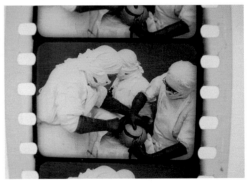

FIGURE 2.2 Doyen's paper on surgical cinematography and celluloid frames of craniotomy from Doyen's films. (Les Opérations sur la cavité crânienne SP 330 and SP 323. Kindly provided by Tiago Baptista and courtesy of Cinemateca Portuguesa-Museu do Cinema.)

For others who filmed neurology, the main goal was documentation rather than clinical monitoring over time or reviewing the effects of therapeutic interventions. They are monotonously similar. How many were done remains unknown (many may still be found) because countless film clips were lost due to fires or degradation of celluloid. For modern neurologists, these early films are curiosities with little or no teaching value. Nevertheless, they comprise an important cultural heritage despite their uncertain medical significance. Some were incorrectly interpreted. For example, recent analyses of certain gait patterns (the quadrupedal gait or walking on all fours) refuted Dercum's interpretation that humans walked like baboons.[15]

---

[15] Lanska DJ. A Human Quadrupedal Gait Following Poliomyelitis: From the Dercum-Muybridge Collaboration (1885). *Neurology.* 2016;86:872–876. This is an elegant study of the stop-motion photos of a child photographed by Muybridge with poliomyelitis walking on all fours (also known at the time as "hand walkers").

During nearly a century of teaching, neurology through film has been done sporadically by enthusiasts and collectors. Some films became curiosities when they showed neurologic manifestation from long-eradicated disorders (e.g., movement disorders and respiratory hiccups with encephalitis lethargica and tabetic gait). For example, Philip Goodhart, who was chief of the Neurological Service at Montefiore Hospital in New York City, produced an annotated collection of teaching films together with Drs. T.J. Putnam and B.H. Balser, *Neurological Cinematographic Atlas*, which other medical institutions could use for teaching purposes. Films, recording (dubious) animal studies, were studied to discover how removal of certain parts of the brain affected gait.[16] There must be an overabundance of teaching films in major academic institutions throughout the world, but this is not the focal point of this book. Obviously, filming neurologic diseases has become far more prevalent since the availability of video capabilities on smartphones. This all-too-easy technology has now made any physician a potential archivist of film clips of neurologic manifestations. Appropriate consent and protection of images remain the most important issue and, when published, the filmmaker must document consent from the patient or family.

Neurology before the Talkies

Cinema started with silent film. Before "talkies," symbols and gestures, and particularly the close-ups, carried the plot supplemented by title cards. Silent films relied on tropes and clichés to portray the practice of medicine, and today this largely forgotten, nearly lost art form (only 20% of original silent film production survives) reveals how medicine was perceived at the beginning of the 20th century. The major themes of fear of physicians, infections, and surgery quickly evolved from comedic pretexts to more serious considerations of medical ethics. Heroic surgical portrayals represented the progress of medicine, but movie surgeons could be unpredictable and overly eager to try experimental, unproven procedures. During the silent film era, heroic surgical portrayals falsely represented the progress of medicine. Surgeons healed paraplegics (*Stella Maris*, 1918) and restored sight to the blind (*Journey into the Night*, 1921).

Inability to walk is one of the first clear medical-neurologic themes in film, and it would return in many films over the years. Notably, Mary Pickford plays a paraplegic in both in *Stella Maris* and *Pollyanna* (Figure 2.3). The opening intertitle of *Stella Maris* (1918) 🎞 states, "Stella Maris, paralyzed from childhood, has been tenderly shielded from all the sordidness and misery of life." Stella Maris only knows the world as a paradise. A brilliant surgeon operates so she can walk again. Now she sees the world as full of poverty and pain and is determined to do something about it. Mary Pickford would reprise this role in *Pollyanna* (1920) 🎞, based upon Eleanor H. Porter's beloved children's book. Mary Pickford plays Pollyanna Whittier, the ever-so optimistic girl who always looks at the bright side ("the glad game" "there is something about everything that you can be glad about"). She becomes paralyzed after being hit by a car while saving a little child. Again, a surgeon enters the room, and on the intertitle, we read, "I am going to make you well because you have faith in me." She walks again after a few attempts with crutches. The movie was highly praised and considered an ideal family film.

Amnesia was another major neurologic theme in silent films, often after a traumatic head injury. Amnesia refers to the loss of memories, such as facts, information, and experiences. Forgetting one's identity is a common plot device. In one of the earliest lost films, *Garden of Lies* (1915), predictable complications ensue when a doctor hires a new husband to jog the memory of an amnesic bride. In also lost *The Right of Way* (1915), a nearly drowned, drunken lawyer loses his memory but is cured by an operation, which leads to complications when he remembers his prior life. On the IMDB database, we can

---

[16] The neurologist Derek Denny-Brown left behind films on approximately 450 monkeys with lesions made in nearly every part of the brain. He also left behind films of patients with movement disorders from Huntington's disease, Wilson's disease, and encephalitis lethargica. See Vilensky JA, Gilman S. The Denny-Brown Collection. *Neurology*. 1990;40:1636; Vilensky JA, Gilman S, Dec EM. The Denny-Brown Collection: A Research and Teaching Resource. *Ann Neurol*. 1994;36:247–251.

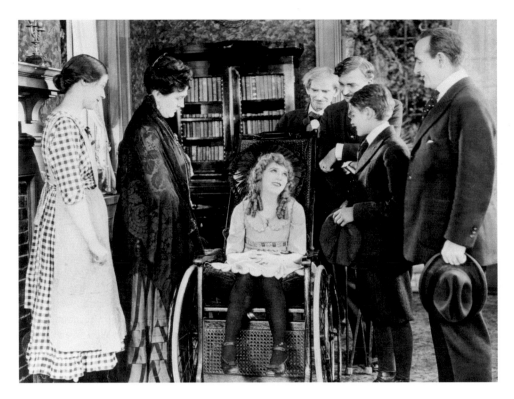

FIGURE 2.3   Mary Pickford as paraplegic in *Stella Maris* (Everett Collection, Inc.).

find over 60 amnesia-driven releases in the 1910s, 50 in the 1920s, and at least 40 in the 1930s. However, there is little verification of the actual manifestations of amnesia because not many films are available for scrutiny. Amnesia is rare in real life but remains relatively common in movies, typically, after trauma to the brain. Baxendale's original observation was that "one of the most neurologically bizarre features of cinematic amnesia is the universal embrace of the 'two is better than one' approach when it comes to traumatic head injury"[17]—that is, the amnesic deficit disappears after a second blow to the head. Exceptional among these films on amnesia was Léonce Perret's *The Mystery of the Kador Cliffs* (1912). In this film, the medium cures a young woman in an akinetic-amnestic state by staging a "reality re-enactment" that allows the patient to relive and confront trauma with immediate good results. Trauma may result in a personality change for the worse, such as in *The Back Trail* (1924) and *De Luxe Annie* (1918). We will revisit this topic in Chapter 4.

The Beginnings of Neurocinema

More than a decade after the first "talkies" were shown in theaters, films entirely devoted to a specific neurologic illness finally began to appear (*Dark Victory* [1939] and *Ich Klage An* [1941]). It is tempting to look at the entire collection of neurologic representation on film and to discover a theme. There are three central questions: Which topics came first and why? Which topics became a staple of fiction film cinema? Which topics most interested documentary makers? To be sure, screenwriters discovered that neurologic disease makes good monsters, causes paralysis, causes strange behavior, and when it strikes, it changes a plot in a very dramatic way. In its early representation, *Neurocinema* emerged as

[17] Baxendale S. Memories Aren't Made of This: Amnesia at the Movies. *BMJ*. 2004;329(7480):1480–1483. doi: 10.1136/bmj.329.7480.1480

(1) a diseased criminal brain, (2) a show of neurologic grotesques, and (3) a relentless disease that dehumanizes its sufferer and raises the question, "Who wants to live that way?"[18]

Ironically, one of the first introductions of neurology into the "talkies" was James Whale's *Frankenstein* (1931), with a new (and lasting) narrative as well as a new Universal Studios monster. Curiously, Whale made the monster mute. In the film, the brain taken from a criminal was inserted in a cadaveric body that became the monster *of* (better *by*) Frankenstein. During a brain-cutting scene in the film, macroscopically obvious anatomical differences from normal were pointed out, and the abnormalities in the frontal lobe gyri suggested a lack of inhibition and impulsivity. James Whale's classic depiction of Frankenstein established the idea that structural brain abnormalities were linked to monstrous, murderous behavior. According to film lore, Whale consulted a "brain specialist," who may have suggested the frontal-lobe connection, but no further details have surfaced.

A second film the following year introduced a developmental neurologic disorder; ironically, it was the hard-to-understand microcephaly[19] ("pinhead") in *Freaks* (1932) ◄◄ . Schlitzie (Simon Metz) was male but was dressed as a female and, in circuses, was known as "The Monkey Girl." Schlitzie worked for several circuses including Barnum & Bailey and Ringling Bros. Schlitzie's ancestors are unknown, and there is a high likelihood he was (illegally) sold to a circus. He could speak a few words and simple phrases but, more often, would simply parrot what he heard other people say. MGM created one of the most notorious displays of microcephaly (Figure 2.4). Nonetheless, the initial intent was to present Schlitzie as a sympathetic character because many in the audience would perceive him as deficient, which could easily cause revulsion. Perhaps that was the theme Hollywood was after, but we will not know. (He also appeared in 1932's *The Island of Lost Souls*, an early adaptation of H.G. Wells' *The Island of Dr. Moreau*, as one of the "manimals").

Neurologic diseases causing facial and hand deformities were occasionally introduced. An actor who used his "shocking face" (due to acromegaly from a pituitary tumor) was Rondo Hatton. He devoted himself to playing "the creeper," a serial killer. At least two other actors with a related disorder, gigantism,[20] played monsters— Eddie Carmel (The Jewish Giant) and André René Roussimoff (André the Giant). They portrayed brute strength but reduced intelligence. Several other actors have put their disorder to "good use," including Richard Kiel, who also had gigantism; he played the villain Jaws in *The Spy Who Loved Me* (1977).

Just as important in the development of cinema was the alleged contempt for disability, and this was perhaps partly fed by the early debate on eugenics, both in Germany and in the United States. The first film that introduced a progressive neurologic disease that could "justify" active euthanasia was *Ich Klage An* (1941) ◄◄◄ . The protagonists are Professor Thomas Heyt and his wife Hanna. Hanna asks for assistance in dying when she eventually learns of her exaggeratedly inaccurate prognosis,[21] ideally before she becomes "deaf, blind, and idiotic" from multiple sclerosis. Scenes in which she suffers excruciating pain and dramatic attacks of dyspnea suggest that she is beyond help. At this point, her husband ends it after providing her a "soothing drink." (See Chapter 5 for more discussion on the major ethical discussion in the final trial scene with point-and-counterpoint discussions on mercy killing.)

In the United States, just after the Second World War, the film *An Act of Murder* (1948) ◄◄◄ introduces Cathy, wife of a judge, who develops violent headaches and misses a glass when picking it up. She consults a family friend ("a distinguished neurologist and brain surgeon"), who examines her, performs an X-ray and even an encephalogram, and subsequently tells her it is "nothing organic." However, after she leaves and he closes the door of the office, a close-up shows him suddenly

---

[18] It was then a small step to explore neuroethics and introduce "passive" (stand down and no interventions) and "active" euthanasia (swallowing or injecting a lethal drug).

[19] Microcephaly (among other cases of static encephalopathy) was a major circus attraction. See Mateen FJ, Boes CJ. "Pinheads": The Exhibition of Neurologic Disorders at "The Greatest Show on Earth." *Neurology.* 2010;75:2028–2032.

[20] Also caused by a pituitary tumor that overproduces growth hormone and starts in early adulthood.

[21] The choice of multiple sclerosis (MS) as an example of rationalizing euthanasia was understandable at the time, but we now know depression goes hand in hand with the disease, and sometimes MS is benign for many years.

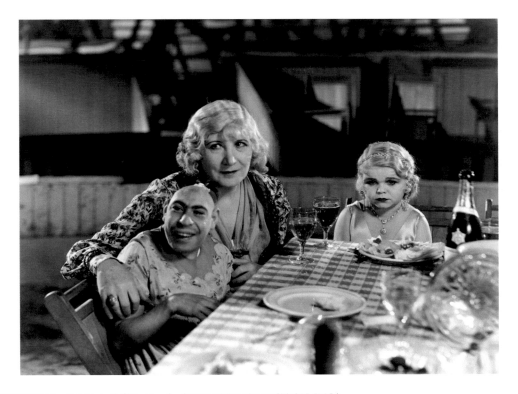

FIGURE 2.4 Schlitzie (left) in *Freaks*. (EVERETT COLLECTION, INC.)

terribly worried; he orders copies of the record to be sent to colleagues scattered over the United States ("leaders in the field"). Subsequently, the physician calls her husband, who is informed that "this is a neoplastic condition" and "[The] intracranial pressure undoubtedly will get worse. It is inoperable and will lead to painful spasms." In the final scene, Cathy develops hemiparesis. As they drive to get medication from the pharmacy to treat her excruciating pain, the husband impulsively yet deliberately crashes the car. She dies instantly, but he survives and decides to turn himself in: "I committed an act of murder and must be tried for it." The trial judge dismisses the murder charge but tells him he is "legally innocent but morally guilty." The topic of self-determination or physician-assisted suicide was not used again in film for more than 40 years until the 1980s, with *Whose Life Is It Anyway?* (1981), and again, much later, *Mar Adentro* (2004) and *You Do Not Know Jack* (2010). Each of these films raises key questions about this ethical quandary. I will revisit these films in Chapter 5.

Neurocinema Coming of Age

Classification needs have permeated all art forms including film. It aids interpretation and scholarship, and generally, we all understand what is meant by drama, romance, crime, horror, science fiction, adventure, and fantasy. Neurologic themes and developing disorders can be found in all of them but rarely generically. Neurology apparently adjusted to genres rather than becoming its own.

In the United States, neurologic disorders first appeared in cinema during the classic period of "film noir"—generally between 1935 and 1950. Brain tumors during this early period of neurocinema were commonly used. It has been speculated that brain tumors are not mutilating, which may have resulted in Hollywood filmmakers between 1930 and 1950 preferring it to other types of cancer.[22] Very few films

---

[22] Lederer SE. Dark Victory: Cancer and Popular Hollywood Film. *Bull Hist Med.* 2007;81:94–115.

used cancer as a major theme. In two earlier films, *Symphony of Six Million* (1932) and *Klondike* (1932), brain tumors were mentioned in the plot but did not play a central part in the film. We already came across *Dark Victory* (1939), but there was also *Rhapsody in Blue* (1945; see Chapter 7) and, as just mentioned, *An Act of Murder* (1948). In *Crisis* (1950), Cary Grant plays a neurosurgeon who operates on a brain tumor in a Latin American dictator. The most controversial film was *No Way Out* (1950) ◄◄◄, directed by Joseph L. Mankiewicz and the film debut of Sidney Poitier, where a spinal tap is performed to confirm a patient's brain tumor. Ray Biddle (Richard Widmark), a racist crook, accuses an African American doctor, Luther Brooks (Sydney Poitier), of intentionally killing his brother Johnny. Brooks claims that Johnny's death was the inadvertent result of a spinal tap he had performed to treat what he believed was an undiagnosed brain tumor. When Luther requests an autopsy to prove his case (he is later exonerated), Ray refuses to allow his brother to be "cut up like a log." The film not only reintroduced a brain tumor but also major racism. Poitier's debut as a Black physician in a major confrontational film was quite explicit and not shown in the South.

Later films would use several neurologic disorders (as this book will show), but some presentations offered an exceptional fascination. When it comes to dementia-related memory loss, comical situations mix with sadness and closely approximate the real thing. The fascination with coma (do they hear? do they dream? do they fight as in a nightmare?) poses valid questions for family members, and thus, expectedly, screenwriters ask themselves the same questions while writing the narrative. However, most films show actors playing comatose patients as "sleeping beauties" ready to awaken and resume their pre-coma lives. For some reason, neurology was rarely used in material in malpractice and egregious violations of patients' integrity and autonomy. The social revolution of the 1960s quickly ended any filmmaking tendency to glorify medicine, and perceptions quickly evolved from awe to suspicion to disdain. We can now look at a large body of film and analyze what these films mean to a viewer (without getting hung up on accuracy), what they do to the perception of neurologic disease (without getting bogged down by its most egregious presentations), and how they could open up a forum for discussion.

Parallels between Neurology and Cinema History

Several scholars agree that film in the first half of the 20th century was one of the most productive forms of media in the United States and elsewhere.[23,24] Cinema history is closely linked to changes in social culture, and filmmakers were influenced by changes in social structure. They did not turn their eyes to medicine except sporadically. Which aspects of neurology interested them? Neurologic disorders were well known (albeit not well understood), and their trajectory (misery and more misery) was tragically misunderstood. In film, poliomyelitis became curable or very manageable (it was not), and seizures were misinterpreted as supernatural possession in abject creatures who were once pretty girls (*The Exorcism of Emily Rose* [2005]).[25,26] Hollywood was not ready for hopeless, incurable illness on screen for some time. The few presentations that appeared were wrapped in a love story with no visible deterioration in functional status (*Love Story* [1970]). Later, filmmakers speculated about what could be happening to the perception of persons with certain disorders. Van Sant decided to use dreamy landscapes to show narcolepsy in *My Own Private Idaho* (1991) and created, for the first time, a pseudoseizure in a drug store to divert attention from the druggie stealing pills out of the storage room (*Drugstore Cowboy* [1989]). As the specialty of neurology developed treatment options, cinematic treatment of neurologic disorders was either implausibly spectacular (*Awakenings* [1990]) or riddled with scary side effects (homicidal sleepwalking in *Side Effects* [2013]).

[23] Sklar R. *Movie-Made America: A Cultural History of American Movies.* Revised and updated ed. New York: Vintage Books; 1994.

[24] Cousins M. *The Story of Film.* Revised ed. London: Pavilion; 2020.

[25] Baxendale S. Epilepsy at the Movies: Possession to Presidential Assassination. *Lancet Neurol.* 2003;2:764–770.

[26] Baxendale S. Epilepsy on the Silver Screen in the 21st Century. *Epilepsy Behav.* 2016;57:270–274.

Even more intellectual filmmakers such as Haneke did not shy away from showing coercion into questionable surgery after a questionable event with eventually poor results because it is just a wonderfully frightening theme. He must have pondered the consequences of certain medical care choices. *Amour* (2012) shows a complication of surgery of the carotid artery after a "warning stroke" and more strokes without any mention of therapeutic options. *The Diving Bell and the Butterfly* (2007) explored stroke as a constant threat of crumbling away until there is no vitality left but also used the major cinematic opportunity to speculate what the protagonist was trying to remember (i.e., bacchanals and orgies). Even epidemics causing massive killing did interest several filmmakers. Fear of the unknown, as well as the uncertainty of a threat we do not understand, remains a fantastic resource, even in the 2011 film *Contagion* by Steven Soderbergh. The film uses a made-up virus loosely modeled after a Nipah virus outbreak. Encephalitis lethargica was also pandemic through 1918, both in Europe and the United States, and resulted in *Awakenings,* based on the book by Oliver Sacks. Movies have also offered serious depictions of the poliomyelitis epidemics.

Neurology subspecialization was intrinsic to many universities, and divided neurology simply into investigational specialties such as neuropathology, neurophysiology, and neuroradiology. The movies took notice, and in many films, we see CT scanners, EEGs, and brains at autopsy. These investigations are visually attractive but also disturbing; going through a CT scanner in blue-tinted rooms with red laser lines lining up heads and bodies made the experience even more claustrophobic. Scans were then shown in offices with physicians pointing out the troubles. All of this coincided well with the times, but its use underscored the assumption that these studies were intimidating and, hopefully, avoidable. Specialization also changed practice, and neurology abounds with experts in epilepsy, movement disorders, peripheral nerve disorders, stroke and, much later, intensive care or acute neurology in some countries. None of this was of particular interest to filmmakers, who were already happy to show a bloody, sloppy brain on a wooden plank during autopsy. (Brains are cut after fixation and are stiff and brown in appearance.)

End Credits

Cinema had a wonky start and, of course, grew out of photography by studying movements the eye could not see. Muybridge's kinetic photographs were analytic searching for the nature of movement.[27] There is no single person who started cinema, and frankly, there is no single "father of neurology" either. Cinema certainly did not start as a major source of entertainment. It was a competitive, undisciplined, scientific race with many familiar names (e.g., Edison, Lumiere, Eastman, Marey, Muybridge) and others more obscure (e.g., Le Prince, Friese Greene, Doublier). It led to new industries ("the kinescopes and vitascopes") and the birth of movie theaters, each with more successively elaborate construction and ornamentation, in the 1920s. All this reinvention was very American. This segued into a more familiar innovative Hollywood production complex. The majors were the big five (Fox, MGM, Paramount, RKO, and Warner Brothers) and the little three (Columbia, United Artists, and Universal Pictures). As we will see, most eventually produced a film with neurology as a major theme.

We can attempt to construct some timeline (Figure 2.5). Medical themes did appear sporadically, and many had to do with dysfunction of the mind or brain. But only after cinema became more progressive after the Second World War, allowing realism into film and dismantling romantic cinema, did we start to see the consequences of neurologic disease, predominantly, the devastating effects of a brain tumor and paralysis associated with traumatic spine injury and poliomyelitis. Scholars agree that Cinema

---

[27] Muybridge's work inspired an opera (*The Photographer*, 1982) by Philip Glass, which choreographed the movements with music. Muybridge also inspired many other artists such as Degas. Strikingly, his methods returned to the screen in 1999 in *The Matrix*, in which motion is broken down and one moment in time is depicted from different angles.

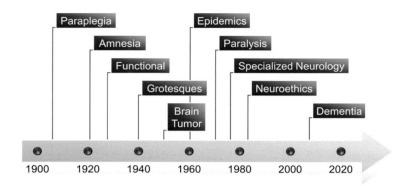

FIGURE 2.5   Timeline of Neurology in film.

became self-conscious in the 1950s and 1970s[28] and essentially became imaginative, creative work that agitates and thrills without educating. No preference for neurologic topics was seen in the decades that followed, but ageism and a lost sense of purpose, as well as the fear of dementia and disabling stroke, have appeared more frequently in the last decade. The older generation became a life drama to deal with. Actors playing characters with a disability often received Oscar nominations (over 5% of all nominations) and won statuettes approximately half of the time, but Oscars for portraying a neurologic disease were uncommon with the very notable recent exception of Alzheimer's disease in a short period of time (Julianne Moore for best actress in *Still Alice* in 2015, and Anthony Hopkins for best actor in *The Father* in 2021).

Admittedly Neurocinema is a portmanteau term whose artistic value can be questioned by healthcare workers. We are seeing dramatic improvements in portrayal, but these resulted from cinema adopting a more realistic style. A more disquieting issue is that we recognize so little of our specialty; indeed, some would want to look away. Filmmakers do not often know what to make of neurology, and films will not always deepen our understanding.

---

[28] See Biskind P. *Easy Riders, Raging Bulls: How the Sex-Drugs-and Rock 'N' Roll Generation Saved Hollywood.* 1st ed. London: Bloomsbury Pub Ltd.; 1998.

3

The Neurologist in Film

Those damned neurologists; they think they can run the world.

EDtv, 1999

Medicine is specialized, and expertise is divided over multiple areas. Physicians have a good idea of what these fields of medicine entail. For everyone else, the question is: what is a neurologist? The American Academy of Neurology (AAN) defines a neurologist as "a medical doctor with specialized training in diagnosing, treating, and managing disorders of the brain and nervous system." According to the AAN website, the disorders that neurologists treat are Alzheimer's disease and other dementias, brain injury and concussion, stroke, brain tumors, epilepsy, migraine and other headaches, multiple sclerosis, myasthenia gravis, peripheral neuropathy, chronic and acute such as Guillain-Barré syndrome, amyotrophic lateral sclerosis, Parkinson's disease and other movement disorders, sleep disorders, and spinal cord injury. Many neurologists have been trained in a subspecialty, and acute neurologic disorders are often seen by neurointensivists, neurohospitalists, vascular neurologists, and epileptologists.

We do not know how much information screenwriters have available when neurologic disorders are considered (or which sources they consult). Similarly, moviegoers—when they see neurologists and neurologic disease on the screen—may be largely incognizant of this part of medicine. I often hear the question "so what is neurology exactly?"

How do neurologists come across in cinema? Not surprisingly, neurologists were previously shown in a subsidiary role, not as protagonists. Typical examples are actors playing Alzheimer's disease patients visiting the (presumed) neurology office. These non-distinct physicians behind a desk ask questions about orientation and the day of the week and then conclude there is a problem (or give their card and instruct patients to call when it gets worse). Perhaps the evaluation of a neurologic symptom does not move a narrative forward. Little may be known of neurologists, partly because this specialty is relatively new. The same may apply to neurosurgeons, an even newer specialty. It could be the result of "neurophobia"—neurology is just too mysterious (an attitude shared by some medical students).[1] Or it could simply be that screenwriters prefer to portray surgeons, psychiatrists, and family doctors, or they may just prefer to keep the doctor's specialty unknown.

Clinical neurology knows many founders. In the United Kingdom, Thomas Willis (1621–1675) coined the term *neurology* in his book *Cerebri Anatome*, followed by John Hughlings Jackson (1835–1911), who added many ideas to what would become a neurologic approach. In the United States, development of the field came later and was modeled after French and British neurology, with the first role models being William Hammond (1828–1900), who wrote the first American textbook of neurology, *A Treatise on*

---

[1] Neurophobia (frustration with neurologic diagnosis starting with medical students and with other specialists, who may send patients to neurologists with nondescript observations) is a global phenomenon. See Jozefowicz RF. Neurophobia: The Fear of Neurology among Medical Students. *Arch Neurol.* Apr 1994;51(4):328–329. McGovern E, Louapre C, Cassereau J, et al. NeuroQ: A Neurophobia Screening Tool Assesses How Roleplay Challenges Neurophobia. *J Neurol Sci.* Feb 15 2021;421:117320.

DOI: 10.1201/9781003270874-3

Diseases of the Nervous System, and Silas Weir Mitchell (1829–1914). Many American neurologists also briefly trained in London at the National Hospital for the Paralysed and Epileptic in Queen Square.

History records a long line of "famous neurologists," with some made venerable by eponyms that celebrated their discovery (e.g., Parkinson, Brown-Séquard, Guillain-Barré, Miller-Fisher)[2] or by advancing knowledge of a specific neurologic disease but without any other distinction other than their highly significant body of work (e.g., Kinnier Wilson, Raymond Adams, Fred Plum). Moreover, many early "neurologists" were general internists with an interest in neurology. Such was the case at the Mayo Clinic, where I currently practice. Dr. Walter Sheldon, hired in 1913, is considered the first Mayo neurologist, but both Mayo brothers dabbled in it and published neurologic papers (William, on infantile spinal paralysis or poliomyelitis; Charles, on cerebral aneurysms). "Neurologists" were often neuroscientists. Dr. Alois Alzheimer, whose name is inextricably linked to neurology, was a pathologist. Some have made a compelling argument that the world's best-known neurologist is James Parkinson.[3] In the end, for many others, achieving fame as a neurologist can be pretty much due to anything including accidental or unintentional factors.

Oddly enough, when the canon of films involving medical issues is examined, there are quite a few cinematic depictions of neurologists, but the portrayal is seldom flattering. When neurologists appear on the screen, they usually run the full spectrum of caricatures and clichés. So, before we immerse ourselves in the discussion of cinematic depictions of a wide variety of neurologic disorders, let us look at the cinematic traits of the neurologist. As we will see, neurologists are generally not depicted as go-getters; rather, they seem to move quite slowly and deliberately. Cinema has not yet found a way to present clinical and academic neurologists to the audience, and we are currently stuck with one film on one of the founders and one documentary film about an eccentric clinical neurologist with phenomenal observational skills and inimitable writings on case histories but with paltry academic output.[4]

The Legendary Charcot

Neurologists often had a psychiatry practice, and, given the link of neurology with psychiatry and particularly with hysteria, this caught the attention of at least one filmmaker. A feature film, *Augustine* (2012), ◄◄◄◄ directed by Alice Winocour, is devoted fully to Dr. Jean-Martin Charcot (1825–1893), chair of Clinique des Maladies du Système Nerveux at La Salpêtrière (Figure 3.1), arguably the most influential neurologist of all. He was widely consulted, and his ideas were universally accepted and never questioned—at least not in France at the time.

Although Charcot's contributions to neurology are legendary (two eponyms as well as seminal descriptions of amyotrophic lateral sclerosis and multiple sclerosis), his studies of female hysteria cemented his international fame. For Charcot, the neurologist, *hystérie* was a *névrose functionelle* and not psychiatry, and for a long time, he was convinced there was a structural basis for the symptoms. (The hypothesis that the unconscious drives behavior would have to wait for Freud.) Charcot was widely known for his well-attended clinical demonstrations showing the effects of touching—usually by his assistants—of certain skin areas that could induce a hysterical attack. Charcot's treatment of young afflicted women (and, less often, men) included hypnosis and, most memorably, the *compresseur ovarien* (an abdominal vice with a knob applying pressure to the ovary), and both hypnosis and ovarian pressure

---

[2] There always will be someone who described the clinical phenomenon before the person who was eventually attached to a disorder. (The French were quick to grab credit but, in many instances, were also highly deserving.) Sometimes, there is a lasting gripe by the descendants about who should be named first (e.g., Eaton-Lambert or Lambert-Eaton syndrome).

[3] Stern G. Epagogic Eponyms. *Pract Neurol*. 2014;14(4):280–282.

[4] Oliver Sacks, known for many books and voluminous notes on his patients, rarely published in academic peer-reviewed journals. Most of his early observations appear as letters concerning encephalitis lethargica (see Chapter 4) or philosophical thoughts on the mind and behavior. Since 1972 his writings were books, magazine articles, and newspaper essays.

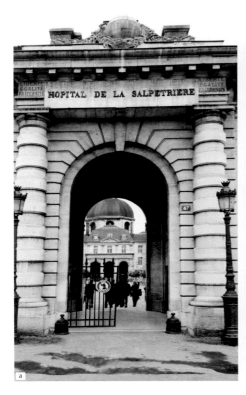
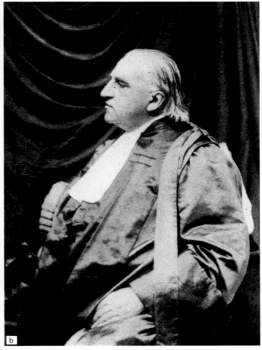

FIGURE 3.1 (a) Entrance of l'hôpital de la Salpêtrière in Paris. (b) Jean-Martin Charcot.

appeared to stop the spells. For Charcot, the gynecological organs acted up. Charcot, his school, and the hysterical attacks have been described in numerous books, but most writers have taken a significant artistic license. Neurologist Lees summarized it well.

> With his close friend and colleague, Alfred Vulpian, he set about analyzing the illnesses of all 2635 female residents under their care and would spend the 31 years up until his death observing the unfolding of nervous diseases.[5]

Charcot was particularly good at diagnosis on the spot and would tell his eager listeners that he could diagnose Parkinson's disease on the streets of Paris, Rome, and Amsterdam and did not need a medical history.

In *Augustine*, Charcot, played by the great actor Vincent Lindon, is surrounded by admiring neurologists, further increasing his standing. The neurologist Bourneville (who discovered the disorder tuberous sclerosis) is present but has no significant dialogue. Charcot and his patient Augustine are the focus of the film. The manifestations of *la Grande hystérie* are played by Soko (French actress Stéphanie Sokolinski), and we get quite a show. There is loud applause by all the attending neurologists after each hysterical attack. The movie shows hypnosis with a tuning fork and the patient following a small mirror that results in a spell (Figure 3.2). The hysterical attacks are well done and very real, with a typical *arc-de-cercle* (arching body backward).

Augustine also shows important aspects of the neurologic examination in a patient with so-called functional (unexplained by disease) symptoms and is of interest because examination of these patients is quite common for neurologists (see Chapter 8). It shows the exact symmetric loss of sensation (dramatically indicated in this film with a big red pencil by Charcot), patches of hypo- and hypersensitivity,

---

[5] For a wonderful description of Charcot's methods, see Lees AJ. In Search of Charcot's Second Sight. *Lancet Neurol.* 2021;20(6):424–425.

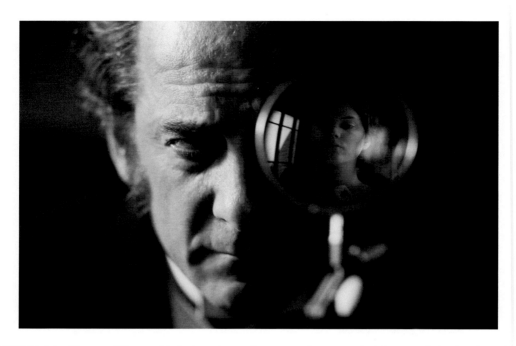

FIGURE 3.2 Charcot (Vincent Lindon) trying to hypnotize Augustine (Stéphanie Sokolinski aka Soko). (Photos provided courtesy of Music Box Films: Charcot © Dharamsala Photo. J.C. Lother Charcot and Augustine: © Dharamsala Photo.)

loss of smell in one nostril only, different types of color blindness in each eye, and a forcefully closed eye due to unilateral blepharospasm, called here "the hysterical wink." Augustine also displays a hysterical contracture.

The movie suggests that Charcot was sexually attracted to Augustine and that this attraction at some point would overwhelm him. *Augustine* is based on a real patient of Charcot, but that is where the comparison ends, and as the sexual undertones are developed, the film becomes nothing but a psycho-erotic thriller. The film may be a distorted, overblown view of a chauvinist doctor's behavior with sexual domination, and this might have been director Winocour's intended main topic. (Ten years earlier, the playwright Anna Furse wrote the play *Augustine [Big hysteria]* with similar feministic themes.) La Salpêtrière was a public women's hospital, and the physicians were all male, but even if Charcot's behavior was authoritarian, one cannot conclude misogyny. (A similar suggestion of erotic transference was made in John Huston's film *Freud* [1962], where Sigmund Freud massages the back of the completely undressed patient Dora—one of his other famous case histories.)

Obviously, *Augustine* is a must-see for neurologists. After all, how often do we get to see one of the pioneers of neurology on-screen? But I have a hunch that in future period films, the neurologist's link to psychiatry could potentially typecast these early giants in the field.

Neurologists On Screen

A few spring to mind. Portrayals have included the aloof neuroscientist studying a never-before-seen neurologic disease (Bill Murray in *The Royal Tenenbaums* [2001]), the uncompassionate curmudgeon (Patrick Chesnais in *The Diving Bell and the Butterfly* [2007]), the glib, unethical researcher (Gene Hackman in *Extreme Measures* [1996]), and other displays of unprofessional behavior. In some films, it is unclear whether the physician is a neurologist, general surgeon, or neurosurgeon, and their practices are not clearly shown. As we will see, one of the first neurologic examinations performed in a Hollywood

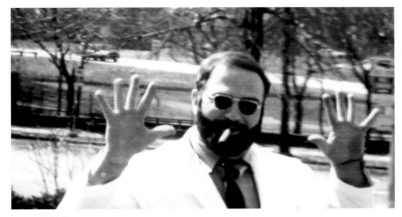

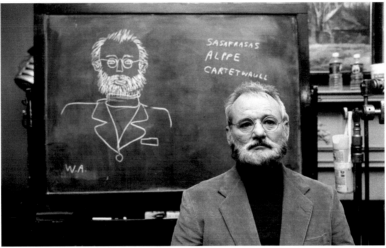

FIGURE 3.3   Oliver Sacks (top) and Bill Murray (below) as a neurologist modeled after Oliver Sacks in *The Royal Tenenbaums.* (Everett Collection, Inc.)

film was, strangely enough, performed by a neurosurgeon. Let's have a look at the fictional portrayal of celluloid neurologists and one neurologist with a peculiar kind of fame recently celebrated with a documentary.[6]

The "Most Famous Neurologist"

A new documentary by Eric Burns on the late Oliver Sacks (*Oliver Sacks: My Own Life,* 2019, 〰〰) provides great insight into the life and work of the "most famous neurologist."[7] Oliver Sacks was a Professor of Neurology at New York University's School of Medicine after receiving his medical degree from Queen's College at Oxford University and completing his residency at University of California,Los Angeles (UCLA) (Figure 3.3).

---

[6] Wijdicks EFM. The Neurologist in Film: From Sacks to Charcot. *Lancet Neurol.* 2014;13(1):33. doi:10.1016/S14744422(13)70243-6

[7] The neurologist Lewis Rowland recalls that when he proposed to ask Oliver Sacks to speak at the Decade of the Brain he met with pushback: "We need a prominent neurologist not a story teller," to which Rowland replied, "but this storyteller happens to be the most famous neurologist" (Rowland LP. In Memoriam: Oliver Sacks, MD (July 9, 1933 to August 30, 2015). *JAMA Neurol.* 2016;73(2):246–247.

In the documentary, Sacks tells his audience that his mission has always been to ask, "who are you?" Sacks called himself a clinical neurologist and added that (emulating the philosopher Thomas Nagel) "much of my life is trying to imagine what it's like to be another sentient being, what it is like to be a bat, what it is like to be an octopus, what it's like to be anyone else; for that matter, what it is like to be another human being." When asked why he became a neurologist, Sacks said that "neurology is the only branch of medicine that could sustain a thinking man." His personal life may not have been exemplary, and he used drugs liberally during his UCLA neurology residency and was "constantly disruptive." According to science writer and surgeon Atul Gawande, Sacks was "deeply an outsider floating in and out of the periphery," and "a supreme F***up multiple times along the way." Later, Gawande is far more laudatory and declares Sacks was the most important person in his [Gawande's] life because of his remarkable humanity. Another criticism mentioned in the film is that he exploited his patients, which is correctly rebuked as "a low blow," and this criticism has been fierce. (His book on face blindness or prosopagnosia, *The Man Who Mistook His Wife for a Hat*, was sarcastically changed to "the man who mistook his patients for a literary career" by the geneticist Tom Shakespeare.) His editor emphasized that his case histories were his major contribution to medicine, but appreciation was not readily forthcoming. She added (with a tone of disdain and by rolling her eyes): "the medical word needed science and statistics."

Oliver Sacks certainly had a repertoire of bizarre stories to share. For example, his mother, a gynecologist, once brought home an anencephalic corpse for ten-year-old Oliver to dissect. (Several other accounts, even more outlandish, cannot be repeated in this book.)

The documentary has great footage of patients with the rare disease of encephalitis lethargica that gave him some acclaim (see Chapter 4). Patient motility is shown both before and after L dopa, with major side effects ("hell dopa"), and the documentary allows us a glimpse of his meticulous notes on patients. When seen in his younger years, he bears a striking resemblance to actor Robin Williams (see Chapter 4). The documentary also mentions that 80% of neurology residency applicants at Columbia choose to specialize in neurology because of Oliver Sacks's books.[8] In the end, he is celebrated as a great neurologist who was able to write about neurologic disease as nobody else could or perhaps would. Sacks was a cheerleader for the specialty, and his assessment of very unusual neurologic manifestations—many of which are not seen by many neurologists—can be downright intoxicating. Oliver Sacks said once, "I could have written a book on each patient, and they'd each be worthy of it."[9]

Some book reviews of other authors writing on similar topics or medical mysteries might include a blurb hailing "the new Oliver Sacks" or "joining the ranks of Oliver Sacks" or "a true descendent of Oliver Sacks," but in reality, Sacks was a very unique, sensitive, indeed humanistic, charismatic individual with great observational talents. His patients were also unique despite his colorful presentations, and several of his seemingly improbably dramatic stories became feature films duly discussed in this book (see Chapter 4). Sack was unrivaled and *sui generis* or in his own words cited in this documentary: "there will be nobody like us when we are gone, but then there is nobody like anyone ever. When people die, they cannot be replaced. They leave holes that cannot be filled. It is the genetic and neural fate of every human being to be a unique individual, to find his own path, to live his own life, [and] to die his own death."

The neurologist Oliver Sacks also served as a model in two major feature films. In *Awakenings* (1990), Oliver Sacks is Dr. Sayer, played by Robin Williams. His character is the bearded, spectacled,

---

[8] This claim is very much overblown. A recent study on resident's applicant statements from Columbia University noted that stroke, epilepsy, and dementia were most mentioned and, far less prominently, persons such as Sherlock Holmes and Oliver Sacks (Grzebinski S, Cheung H, Sanky C, Ouyang J, Krieger S. Educational Research: Why Medical Students Choose Neurology: A Computational Linguistics Analysis of Personal Statements. *Neurology* 2021;97:e103-e108. Nonetheless, Sacks is mentioned regularly, although less frequently in recent years after his death (Chris Boes, personal communication).

[9] Cited from Weschler L. *And How Are You, Dr. Sacks? A Biographical Memoir of Oliver Sacks.* New York: Farrar, Strauss and Giroux; 2019:108.

coy neurologist discovering a cure for encephalitis lethargica. (According to Oliver Sacks, after Robin Williams spent some time with him, the actor started to look like his identical twin brother with the same mannerisms.) In *The Royal Tenenbaums (2001)* ⫷⫷ , the much nerdier and marvelously eccentric Raleigh St. Clair (played by Bill Murray, Figure 3.3) is undoubtedly modeled after Oliver Sacks, and the film also features a riff on his work, which usually contains highly unusual neurologic cases. In *The Royal Tenenbaums*, Dr. St. Clair writes a book entitled *The Peculiar Neurodegenerative Inhabitants of the Kazawa Atoll* and is seen studying a rare disorder of amnesia, dyslexia, and color blindness combined with a highly acute sense of hearing—a hilariously preposterous combination of clinical signs. It bears some resemblance to studies in the Chamorro people in Guam who died of amyotrophic lateral sclerosis/Parkinsonism dementia complex that was attributed to a yet unidentified neurotoxin.[10]

The Other Neurologists (and, from time to time, a Neurosurgeon)

Apart from these Sacks-inspired satires, in most other films, the neurologist is like any physician, but sympathetic depictions are few and far between. After reviewing many films, I found information to discuss the portrayal of communication skills, diagnostic competence, and even the neurologic examination. Here are some tidbits to illustrate that. (It should be noted that films with a compelling portrayal of neurologic disease may have not-so-compelling neurologists.)

First, how does the neurologist relay information? In *Declaration of War* (2011) ⫷⫷⫷⫷ , the parents of a child afflicted with a brainstem tumor are approached by a pediatric neurologist who, to say the least, is not overflowing with compassion and who treats them with opprobrium. She barges into the room with her entourage, looks at the child, tells the parents the child needs a CT scan, leaves, and has an assistant explain the details. Later, her inexplicable medical jargon and pompous attitude totally confuse the distraught parents.

The neurologist in *Goodbye, Lenin!* (2003) ⫷ explains coma after resuscitation and leaves the family with the uncertainty of the patient ever awakening again. When the patient awakens after being comatose for eight months, they are again told that outcome still may be problematic.

After Iris (*Iris*, 2001, ⫷⫷⫷⫷) completes a word-naming test, the neurologist tells her that her dementia is *implacable*. After Iris asks what he means, he says it's *inexorable*. She tells him that it won't win, and he counters, "It will win."

The neurologist in *A Song for Martin* (2001) ⫷⫷⫷⫷ suggests to the patient with Alzheimer's and his spouse that it is best not to use medication. Instead, they should try mental gymnastics and love.

In the film *Go Now* (1995) ⫷⫷⫷⫷ , the neurologist of a patient with suspected multiple sclerosis shuffles papers while eating a sandwich and cannot find test results. He says, "No results here … bit of a cock up." He then suggests that the patient return to the office in a month, stating, "I am on holiday."

In *Garden State* (2004) ⫷ , neurologist Dr. Cohen sees the protagonist for brief, intense, split-second headaches. (The setting is a room filled with diplomas and achievements and hilariously extending deep to the ceiling.) "Mr. Andrew Largeman, there is absolutely nothing wrong with you…just kidding… How would I know that? What can I do for you today?"

From these depictions of communication with families, we can only conclude that the neurologist is authoritarian, aloof, unrealistic, without compassion, and unprofessional. However, some good ones stand out. In *The Dreamlife of Angels* (1998) ⫷⫷⫷⫷ , the neurologist played by Jean-Michel Lemayeux explains coma quite well to a visiting friend. "She is unconscious, she can't communicate. She can't talk or move. She won't answer you. We are watching for any sign of her waking or of an improvement." He asks the friend to watch for changes in her condition, and he provides compassionate support. In a more

---

[10] Cox PA, Sacks OW. Cycad Neurotoxins, Consumption of Flying Foxes, and ALS-PDC Disease in Guam. *Neurology.* 2002;58:956–959; Murch SJ, Cox PA, Banack SA, Steele JC, Sacks OW. Occurrence of b-methylamino-l-alanine (BMAA) in ALS/PDC Patients from Guam. *Acta Neurol Scand.* 2004;110:267–269.

recent portrayal on coma (*The Descendants*, 2011) , a neurologist explains catastrophic brain injury well. "She will never be the way she was, Matt. We know that now. She may last several days to weeks."

Second, how is the diagnostic competence of the neurologist portrayed? The neurologist's competency is questioned by the patient or the family in some films (*Go Now* [1995] and *Memories of Tomorrow* [2006]), most notably in the film *A Late Quartet* (2012) , where the neurologist suggests a diagnosis of Parkinson's disease on the basis of a few simple clinical tests. In *Memories of Tomorrow* (2006) , the neurologist is young and seemingly inexperienced. When the neurologist tells the patient (Ken Watanabe) he has early Alzheimer's disease, the patient asks him how many years he has been practicing and laughs out loud at the neurologist when he hears it is only ten years. The neurologist in this film is all business, prim and proper, and in a neat, uncluttered office. After the second visit, the patient is told the positron emission tomography (PET) scan is diagnostic for Alzheimer's disease. The patient runs out of the office to a ledge on the roof of the hospital to commit suicide. The neurologist convinces him not to jump and to "have hope."

In *The Savages* (2007) , Mr. Savage (Philip Bosco), disoriented and agitated, is restrained in the hospital, while his children, Jon and Wendy (played by Laura Linney and the late Philip Seymour Hoffman) decide how to put him in a nursing home. The neurologist believes that his disinhibition, aggression, masked facies, and blank stare are more likely Parkinson's disease. When the children ask him what to expect, he tells them he will likely die from cardiac complications. Soon they are seen reading books on the basics of dementia and Parkinson's disease, but the real diagnosis is never revealed to the flustered children.

These examples illustrate that cinematic depictions of the neurologist's diagnostic skills and competence are based in a constant uncertainty about the diagnosis and a lack of transparency for family members. Neurologists sound rather vague and discombobulated.

Third, how is the neurologic examination portrayed in film? The neurologic examination shown is fragmented, out of order, and bizarre. This is to be expected. As moviegoers know, a physical examination in film often consists of a doctor arriving with a large bag, listening to the patient, and stating with great certainty what is wrong or, equally often, that there is no cause for concern. However, in contrast, the neurologic examination has always been elusive for non-neurologists and, thus, screenwriters. Not so much the tendon reflexes—reflex hammers are ubiquitously used by doctors in film, but filmmakers tend to focus on the abnormal mental examination, and most of what we see in film is strange. Directors use some elements of the mental status examination without an understanding of what these elements test and what they mean. Physicians and neurologists will be amused. A few examples follow.

In *Dark Victory* (1939) , the neurologic exam by neurosurgeon Dr. Steele (George Brent) is shown. "Please squeeze my hand." He tests reflexes (normal) and sensory testing (alternating the use of a piece of silk and a rough cloth). The neurologic examination is one of the first in Hollywood but, ironically, performed by a neurosurgeon (Figure 3.4). The next depiction is in *Crisis* (1950) , in which Cary Grant plays Dr. Ferguson, a neurosurgeon. He asks his patient to stretch out his arms, and his left arm (holding a cigarette) starts to drift downward followed by a loud cry, cramp, head turn, and unconsciousness for several seconds. He then performs a funduscopic examination ("There is great pressure") and finds a visual-field defect.

In *Reversal of Fortune* (1990) , Sunny von Bülow (played by Glenn Close) is found in a diabetic coma. She is examined by a nervous neurologist in the emergency department, who calls for an EEG (and not a CT scan) after performing a funduscopy.

The most interesting depiction of a full neurologic examination (and the neurologist's behavior in an acute setting) is in *The Death of Mr. Lazarescu* (2005) . The examination, however, is a bit all over the place. The film is about Mr. Lazarescu (Chapter 5), who has been complaining of headache and abdominal pain the entire day but does not receive treatment. After being dismissed from a crowded emergency room, he arrives at another hospital, and one of the staff notes an asymmetry in his response. She calls the neurologist—Dr. Dragos Popescu (played by Adrian Titieni). When he enters

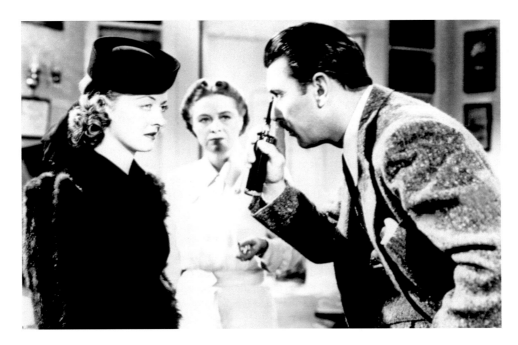

FIGURE 3.4   One of the first neurologic examinations in Hollywood (and ironically by a neurosurgeon). Bette Davis and George Brent as Dr. Frederick Steele in *Dark Victory*. (Note: Neurologists will recognize the wrong position of the ophthalmoscope, i.e., looking with left eye for left eye and looking with right eye for right eye.) (Everett Collection, Inc.)

the emergency room, he does not introduce himself and asks for the patient's name. He sits down at the bedside and immediately has him repeat an impossibly complex phrase ("Thirty-three storks on the roof of Mr. Kogalniceaunu"). He then follows by testing forehead sensation, eye tracking, pupil reflexes to light, finger-to-nose testing (the patient misses on the right), finger-strength testing by asking him to squeeze, testing for drift (mild drift on the right), testing leg strength by having him bend his knees (he has a subtle weakness), and asking him to walk. Although the medic advises that Lazarescu can neither walk nor stand, the neurologist ignores her warning, and the patient nearly falls to the ground. Then he goes back to testing speech and shows him his wristwatch and asks him what it is. With a wrong answer, he then surprisingly concludes there is a subdural hematoma and tells the nurse, with whom he flirts by rubbing her shoulders and calling her *mi amor*, that it is urgent. He tells the patient he might have a blood clot on the brain but also not to worry because the operation is simple and can be compared with surgery for appendicitis. Surely, for neurologists, this depiction of a neurologic examination goes way beyond taking a few liberties; indeed, it is all over the place, farcical, and a serious misrepresentation of how we obtain information that can lead to localization in a certain part of the brain.

We do not know how actors playing neurologists are instructed. If a reflex hammer is used, it is handled as a hammer and not with a loose swing moving the hammer and wrist through a 45- to 60-degree arc. There is tapping with a reflex hammer on muscles rather than tendons in *The Death of Mr. Lazarescu*. George Brent, as Dr. Frederick Steele in *Dark Victory*, has a clumsy use of the ophthalmoscope (Figure 3.4).

But parts of the neurologic examination are surprisingly well done in other films. In *The Men* (1950), an accurate sensory examination is shown. Marlon Brando, as Bud, is a paraplegic tested by Dr. Brock, a presumed neurologist. A safety pin is touched to the skin with the dull and sharp sides, and the doctor even simulates a touch without touching the skin to determine if the patient is guessing. Most remarkable is the testing of visual fields and the use of a car key to obtain a Babinski sign by neurologist Dr. Reeves in *A Matter of Life and Death* (1948). This performance (the sharp car key in particular) strongly suggests that the directors sought some neurologic advice.

Moreover, there is a very real depiction of pinpoint pupils in *The Man with the Golden Arm*.[11] At the outset of the movie, Frankie Machine (Frank Sinatra) is a fully rehabilitated heroin addict. When his spouse comes close to light his cigarette, she sees his pinpoint pupils from opioid use and knows he is using again. Although one of the most neurodiagnostic films in cinema, it does not even include a physician in its cast of characters. Of course, there is more; I will mention other notable observations in the films discussed in the next chapters.

It is seldom known whether neurologists have been consulted by filmmakers for advice or what advice they have been given. This information may appear in the closing credits, but often only a hospital or department is mentioned without naming specific consultants. Some films are based on patient stories remembered by a neurologist—notably, the case histories of Oliver Sacks—but the inspiration for other screenplays remains largely unexplored.

The entertainment industry, science, and medicine have organized cooperation between two organizations: Hollywood, Health & Society, and The Science & Entertainment Exchange. These organizations provide scientists and physicians the opportunity to explain biology to the screenwriter. The storyline remains mostly untouched, and advisers do not rewrite or edit scripts. Directors may still decide how to present their story, despite having received better, updated information. Whether these organizations are needed or will be helpful in future neurology projects is unknown.

End Credits

Reviewing these films is a stark reminder of stereotypical neurologist, who appears as an intellectual, aloof neuroscientist, and head-scratcher far from deferential and not much different from his counterpart, the psychiatrist. This is understandable because both specialties have similar roots. *Augustine,* the cinematic portrayal of one of the founders of neurology, Jean-Martin Charcot, is very much worth watching as a period piece and for parts of the neurologic examination of the patient with imagined neurologic illness.

Neurologists' offices and studies are typically spacious, with large, cluttered desks and ceiling-high bookcases packed with medical textbooks. This is not unlike any major intellectual in the last century with large collections of books. Filmmakers would pack these offices to show how learned physicians were. An illustrative example is Dr. Reeves's office in *A Matter of Life and Death* (1946), which is packed with books and other neurologic paraphernalia on his desk, stacks of opened books on side tables, and drawings of the brain as wall decorations (Figure 3.5).

One film deserves special mention because it shows a kind and helpful neurologist finally showing up after many misfires. In *Lorenzo's Oil* (1991) ✦ , the young boy Lorenzo is first seen by a pediatric neurologist, who finds nothing wrong. "The EEG is normal, skull x-ray is normal, CT is normal. I do not know what to tell you. This boy is neurologically intact." When the parents suggest some parasitic infection, the neurologist looks surprised and skeptical. Another pediatric neurologist suggests that "it could be any one of a dozen things," and admits him for tests. (The scene shows a hearing test with tuning fork, pupil reflex, electroencephalography [EEG], and CT scan, all with an intense operatic soundtrack.) But a second opinion is a relief. The diagnosis (adrenoleukodystrophy) is revealed by Professor Nikolais—replete with bowtie—sitting behind a grand desk in a grand office. The pediatric neurologist, Professor Nikolais (Peter Ustinov impersonating Hugo Moser), in *Lorenzo's Oil* (Figure 3.6), is a compassionate neurologist taking the time to listen to the parents, answering questions, and explaining complex genetics (see Chapter 4). But he is the exception.

Cinema has chosen Oliver Sacks as the archetypal neurologist, and we can expect most neurologists to be unhappy with that representation. The overriding theme in so many films involving his patient stories—which are undeniably cinematic—is that the neurologist is able to find something no other

---

[11] Preminger O. *The Man with the Golden Arm.* United Artists. December 15, 1955.

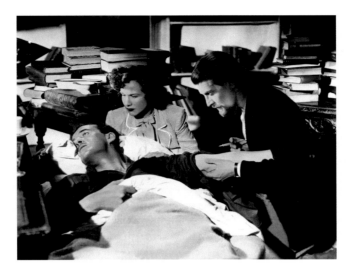

FIGURE 3.5 Dr. Reeves in his study with a very large number of opened and stacked books in *A Matter of Life and Death*. Peter (David Niven) was asked to stay with him so he could observe a spell. In this scene, he treats Peter's spell. (See cover for Peter in the middle of a spell with hallucinations.) (Everett Collection, Inc.)

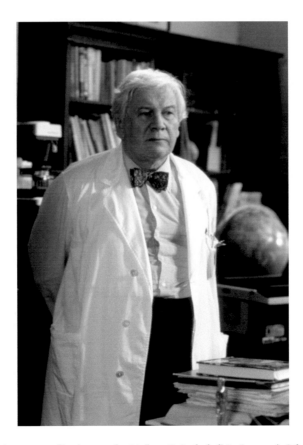

FIGURE 3.6 Peter Ustinov as a pediatric neurologist (bowtie included) in *Lorenzo's Oil*. (Everett Collection, Inc.)

physician has considered and is able to bring out clinical manifestations that are no less than astounding.[12] We know we are much different, and our practices are much different. Neurology is one of the most fascinating specialties—but not that fascinating. Oliver Sacks was not a wackadoodle but a serious writer and compassionate neurologist spending inordinate time with his patients; indeed, someone to whom we can aspire.

In films depicting the modern neurologist, the scenes—when seen together—may even illustrate another theme. In several films, the neurologist is condescending. Diagnostic skills are way off, and often there is uncertainty about what is going on. The skill of neurologic examination predictably often does not make sense.

Do these films help us to understand the neurologist any better? Sadly, of course, they do not, and there is a worrisome verisimilitude. In film, it is hard to feel a kinship toward neurologists, and almost never does a fiction film provide a useful insight into our current practice. In most films on neurologic practitioners, there is little focus on diversity and equity, and we are mostly seeing elderly white specialists and professors dressed to a tee. Dr. Nadir, played by the Indian-born Madhur Jaffrey in *A Late Quartet* (2012), is an exception. Nonmedical viewers will continue to ask what a neurologist really "does." We, as neurologists, will have to wait for a better depiction of our field with its many subspecialties and its many disorders that require timely recognition and complex management, even if there is no curative treatment. These disorders and their portrayal in cinema—right or wrong—are the focus of the next few chapters.

---

[12] In *Awakenings*, Sacks throws a ball to catatonic patients, which is unexpectedly caught most of the time by the patient's outstretched arm. This is an unrealistic representation of extreme Parkinsonian symptoms in encephalitis lethargica; most patients are more likely to flinch when a ball is thrown at them. See also Chapter 8 suggesting that the drawing of a clock test and finding spatial neglect is a pivotal test in autoimmune encephalitis.

4

The Neurologic Disorders in Film

Mrs. Turner, your husband is incredibly lucky. The bullet wound to the head caused minimal damage. See, it hit the right frontal lobe. That's the only part of the brain that has redundant systems. I mean, if you're going to get shot in the head, that's the way to do it.

Regarding Henry (1991)

He has no idea what he is saying. Basically, imagine if you took all of his thoughts, put them in a blender and then just pour them out.

Every 21 Seconds (2017)

Main Themes

When specifically asked, neurologists will anticipate that the film portrayal of neurologic disorders is inaccurate, perhaps even absurd. Theatrical portrayal by its very nature is always somewhat contrived, and embellishment of a new neurologic handicap might be expected in the art form we are discussing here. Indeed, there is exaggeration, but this chapter will show that the portrayal of the major syndromes and clinical signs can approach reality quite closely, and it often is deeply affecting. Many films (i.e., directors and screenwriters) have earned their renown for a good reason.

The main themes in *Neurocinema—The Sequel* are sudden confrontation with a major neurologic illness, disability from chronic neurologic disease, and inability to resume a normal life. What is the impact of neurologic disease on relationships, work, skill, and even creativity? How does the drama before us articulate the seriousness and the vicissitudes of certain neurologic disorders? Acute neurologic conditions produce sudden plot twists and are thus frequently used in screenplays.

Neurologic disease is portrayed in several scenarios. The first and most visible one is a film based on or inspired by a true story. These films come naturally because the story is often well researched and has originated from a personal memoir. Examples are *Reversal of Fortune, The Sea Inside, Lorenzo's Oil, My Left Foot, Iris*, and more recently, *The Intouchables*. All these films have distinct qualities; the neurologic disorder is a vital thread, but doing it right requires a great actor. Beyond those examples are several more underappreciated, less frequently seen films chiefly concerned with a specific topic that drives the plot, for example, *A Late Quartet, Side Effects*, and *The Tic Code*.

Finally, there is a category where neurology is fleetingly mentioned in one or two scenes, maybe briefly as part of the story, but not as part of the main plot. Some have memorable moments, and examples of films in this category include *Steel Magnolias, The Dreamlife of Angels, The Lookout, Barbara*, and *Drugstore Cowboy*. I will look at each of these categories. Neurology can be either portrayed by signs and symptoms or by revealing the entire disorder.

DOI: 10.1201/9781003270874-4

Neurologic Signs and Symptoms

In many feature films, neurologic signs and symptoms are highlighted without too much explanation in the plot about the cause. Headaches are headaches, amnesia is amnesia, seizures are seizures. Filmmakers have made use of signs and symptoms suggesting a neurologic problem without going into much detail. Coma is mostly violent trauma to the brain, including gunshot wounds, and we can easily imagine where it leads.

Notably, some films use musicians with deteriorating skills. We see them playing the cello (*Hilary and Jackie, A Late Quartet*), piano (*Ich Klage An, You Are Not You*), or directing an orchestra (*A Song for Martin*). Neurologic signs and symptoms lead to a clinical diagnosis, and often there are no specific laboratory tests. In *Late Quartet*, the meeting with the neurologist is a notable scene because Peter is surprised that it is a clinical assessment and not a laboratory test with a positive or negative result. When he questions whether the diagnosis really can be made without tests, she answers: "I am afraid I can." Peter's response ("wow!") accurately reflects the common surprise of patients when they are so quickly and confidently diagnosed with a neurologic illness. (The surprise may also be the sudden realization of a life-changing illness).

So how do actors render neurologic disease? Artistic credibility and authenticity are much debated. Actors often have difficulty portraying the major clinical features of a neurologic disease or symptom. Very few actors have been able to imitate aphasia, and most act out speech abnormalities as a combination of grunting, clenched teeth, or drunken speech. As we will see, Haneke decided not only to have the protagonist in *Amour* stop speaking but also to have her stare, which is more suggestive of a seizure than a stroke. Walking with a spastic, paralyzed leg is easier, but some actors use the cane incorrectly, even on the same side as the paralysis (e.g., *A Simple Life*). Portraying a seizure is difficult for most actors (but not for Gwyneth Paltrow in *Contagion*) and often involves exaggerated eye quiver, sudden upward eye deviation, and "fish out of the water" flailing movements with quick resolution. As we will see, presenting a prolonged comatose state is problematic, with many actors looking well-groomed and stunningly fit.

Of course, it matters which actor is suitable for a role. The character portrayed remains a synthesis of the actor playing the part and the character itself. The audience knows they are seeing an actor, not a patient. Anthony Hopkins thought his age of 83 made it easier for him to play the challenges of memory loss and dementia, and thus, he could better relate to its manifestations.[1]

Props such as a mouthpiece have been used to mimic bulbar spastic speech (*You're Not You*) and Alka Seltzer or toothpaste to mimic frothing at the mouth with a seizure (*Drugstore Cowboy*). Filmmakers use a variety of cinematic techniques to show confusion (having the camera turning 360 degrees around a person), seizures (loud, shrieking sounds), and visual disturbances (zooming in and out and blurring of the camera lens), but none approaches the personal experience of being struck by a neurologic disorder. Many are obvious mood-conditioning techniques and computer-generated imagery.[2]

Actors may spend time with patients who have had an acute brain injury, such as stroke patients in rehabilitation centers and, through close observation, may acquire knowledge about their limitations.[3] Such visits may provide insight, but it is impossible to bring actors into a hospital ward (or a neurologic intensive care unit with seriously ill patients). Screenwriters may contact patient support groups, and I suspect these sources supply most of their information. Let's review the major presenting neurologic signs and symptoms in movies.[4]

---

[1] Buchanan K. Anthony Hopkins Makes It Look Simple. (And Maybe It Should Be.) *The New York Times.* November 22, 2020. In other interviews, he said he just played his father who was fearful of dying.

[2] See *Electricity* (2014), where director Bryn Higgins makes seizures coming from the "occipital temporal region" look like a nightmarish dream with bold flashing lights.

[3] De Niro worked with a patient in his mid-forties with Parkinson's disease when researching his character Leonard with encephalitis lethargica (*Awakenings*, 1990). His highs and lows, different stages, and the effects on his body helped de Niro to play the frozen state of severe hypokinesis. He also visited patients in Highland Hospital in London.

[4] Patients (and certainly screenwriters) do not know whether certain symptoms are neurological. Indeed, some symptoms that seem non-neurological could be neurological. Clinicians must sort this out with pointed questioning. This lack of understanding might explain why earlier films used abnormal vision and dizziness for all sorts of neurologic diseases.

Coma

Films featuring actors who are unresponsive, unconscious, and in prolonged coma have been plentiful since the early days of moviemaking. Let us ignore the numerous plots where someone is beaten unconscious and concentrate on patients cared for in hospitals. These films are about coma, simply defined as a state in which the patient is unaware of his surroundings, does not awaken in response to a strong stimulus or pinch, and does not speak or open eyes. When the arms move, the responses are withdrawal or reflexive. Movements, when they do occur, are never purposeful, and some patients do not move at all. Coma is thus most simply summarized as an unreceptive and unresponsive state. Comatose patients do not awaken, speak, or open their eyes to a loud voice or pinch. Sleeping patients awaken quickly. None of the patients in the more affected states demonstrate any content (i.e., an awareness of what is happening in one's surroundings). The level of consciousness these patients experience remains difficult for us to know. However, when we ask later if they remember that episode, most of them do not.[5] In the movies, it seems that prolonged sleeping is not easily differentiated from prolonged coma or even death. Perhaps one of the earliest depictions of coma is Disney's *Snow White and the Seven Dwarfs* (1937), in which the dwarfs assume she has died and place her in a glass coffin. It is unclear if the Prince revitalizes her or kisses her out of her permanent slumber or "sleeping death." In *Sleeping Beauty*, the entire kingdom goes into suspended animation for 100 years. For less fanciful portrayals of coma, let us look at films from the 1970s onward,[6] beginning with the most notable.

Reversal of Fortune (1990) ◄◄◄◄ , directed by Barbet Schroeder, stars Jeremy Irons, who received Golden Globe for Best Actor, and Glenn Close. *Reversal of Fortune* is the true story of Sunny and Claus von Bülow, her "comas," and how her condition and Claus' murder charge played out in the courts. Sunny von Bülow (Glenn Close) has several bouts of diabetic coma and does not awaken from the third one. She is found lying in the bathroom with her husband (Jeremy Irons) reacting indifferently because he expects her to wake up (as she did twice before). "Please call an ambulance," is spoken matter-of-factly, without any sense of urgency. Sunny ends up in the emergency room; she is examined by a neurologist, who calls out for an electroencephalogram (EEG) while doing a fundoscopy. However, we do not hear any results,[7] and she remains in a vegetative state. She is shown lying immobile with eyes closed, a tracheostomy, and accurate positioning of her arms and wrists to mimic contractures. For dramatic effect, the mise-en-scène is a single hospital bed set in dazzling blue, adding to the loneliness and devastation. In real life, Sunny von Bülow died nearly 28 years later, remaining all the while in a persistent vegetative state (PVS) while attended by private nurses on New York's Upper East Side.

DIALOGUE

Reversal of Fortune

Sunny von Bülow

I never woke from this coma, and I never will—I am in what doctors call a persistent vegetative state—a vegetable. According to medical experts, I could stay like this for a very long time—brain dead—body better than ever.

---

[5] See Wijdicks EF. The Bare Essentials: Coma. *Pract Neurol.* 2010;10:51–60; and Wijdicks EF *Guide to the Comatose Patient. Expert Advice for Families and Caregivers.* Rochester, MN: Mayo Clinic Press; 2022.

[6] See also Wijdicks EF, Wijdicks CA. The Portrayal of Coma in Contemporary Motion Pictures. *Neurology.* 2006; 66:1300–1303.

[7] An amusing scene. I do not know what the neurologist saw in the fundus to suggest the need for an EEG in a diabetic coma. It seems to illustrate diagnostic chaos. The flustered neurologist certainly has an unexpected approach to coma in an emergency room.

The film shows each of these hypoglycemic comas well. (In a voiceover, Glenn Close as Sunny narrates and recounts each of these comas—"first coma," "second coma.") There is mention of bradycardia and hypothermia, so common in these types of comas. Claus von Bülow instructs the maid to "get something warm, a blanket or anything you can find." However, in the film, she does not awaken despite (unknown) medical care ("all this activity was pointless"). The sensational trial of Claus von Bülow (Jeremy Irons)—guilty twice, acquitted eventually—is the major part of the movie. The film implies that Sunny von Bülow's earlier episodes of diabetic hypoglycemic coma involved the use of needles (possibly prepared by Claus or at his directions) containing barbiturates and Valium as well as insulin. This film presents a very accurate portrayal of diabetic coma. This is an uncomfortable reality when there is long-lasting hypoglycemia and the patient does not awaken from irreversible brain injury.

Talk to Her (2002) ✖✖ , written and directed by Pedro Almodóvar and starring Javier Cámara, Darío Grandinetti, Leonor Watling, Geraldine Chaplin, and Rosario Flores, received an Academy Award for Best Original Screenplay, Golden Globe Award for Best Foreign Language Film, and BAFTA Award for Best Film Not in English Language and for Best Original Screenplay. *Talk to Her* involves two male–female relationships, with both female characters in PVS. The management of and recovery from PVS is pivotal in this film. The title of the film refers to talking to (or "with"[8]) a patient in PVS. Major topics are discussed in this film, and all are incorrectly depicted. Cinematically, many critics consider the film as a career highlight for Almodóvar, known for high, operatic melodrama and vivid colorations; even allowing for poetic license and accepting the caveat that we cannot always take neurologic content too literally, I must call out these neurologic inaccuracies in many scenes. Early in the movie, we are introduced to one of the patients (four years in PVS) showing no contractures, a perfectly toned and tanned body, eyes closed, mouth slightly open, with even the hint of a smile. I named this cinematic portrayal the "Sleeping Beauty phenomenon" (Figure 4.1).

DIALOGUE

Talk to Her

Friends of patients to each other	*Why are you so sure she does not hear you?*
Physician	*Because her brain is turned off.*
	Is there hope? No. I repeat, scientifically no, but if you choose to believe, go ahead.

To avoid creating nonsense, screenwriters should listen to and heed neurologists on this topic: patients in a vegetative state lack awareness, have no purposeful behavior, have marked loss of muscle bulk and severe contractures despite the best rehabilitation efforts, and are at high risk for decubitus ulcers, sepsis, and major medical complications. To be fair, nonetheless, this film shows the meticulous care given to the patients, with clean sheets being provided as well as a tracheostomy and gastrostomy. (For neurology purists, the tracheostomy is usually removed shortly after successful weaning.) It also shows the use of foot splints to help in avoiding contractures.

In the film, one of the PVS patients becomes pregnant, and the male nurse is convicted of rape. This introduces another new, complex medical problem. Pregnancy in PVS patients is less likely, and most patients stop menstrual cycles. Even in patients who were pregnant before

---

[8] The original Spanish title was *Hable **con** ella* (emphasis mine). See Fins JJ. comment on The Portrayal of Coma in Contemporary Motion Pictures. *Neurology.* 2007;68:79. The ethicist Fins argues that the Spanish preposition *con* should be translated as *with* which suggests communication. In addition, troubled by any criticism of the film's depictions of coma, he vapidly warns against "the critics' gaze."

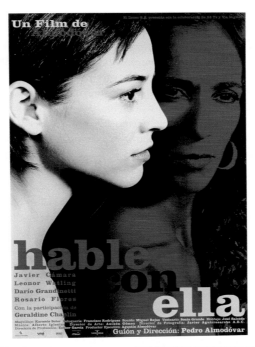

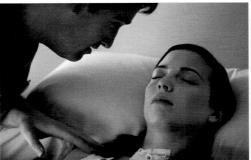
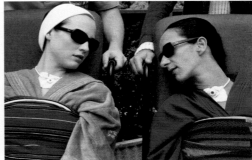

FIGURE 4.1 Film poster and actors in Actors in *Talk to Her*. (Used with permission of El Deseo Da S.L.U photo; Miguel Bracho.) Note features of "Sleeping Beauty phenomenon" and two patients in PVS with tracheostomies looking quite comfortable.

becoming vegetative, fetal loss is substantial. In this movie, for dramatic purposes, the pregnancy is brought to term, and the woman delivers a stillborn baby.[9]

A PVS is diagnosed when the patient has a severe—often devastating—brain injury with no awakening since onset. Gradually, the patient starts opening eyes ("eye open" coma), and sleep-wake cycles start. Patients may grimace but without any sign of awareness of self or what is happening at the bedside (no response to family members, no response to nursing staff or physicians). The patient just breathes, may yawn, clench the jaw, and may have some startle head movements (particularly to loud sounds) but is mute except for occasional sounds. The patient has "vegetative" symptoms, meaning an intact autonomic nervous system (blood pressure, heart rate, and respiratory function). The facial features change dramatically, and the patient becomes unrecognizable to family members if they visit weeks later.

---

[9] However, one should never say never. There has been a recent pregnancy in PVS case known as the Hacienda Healthcare sexual case. The diagnosis of PVS seemed unclear, and the case was recently settled. See Stevens M. Arizona Nursing Center Where Woman in Vegetative State Was Raped Will Close. *The New York Times*; February 7, 2019.

(A perfect cinematic example is in *The Descendants* [2011], covered in Chapter 5.) Contractures occur; decubital wounds are unavoidable and may require treatment. Patients are very vulnerable to infections. There is no evidence of suffering. Recovery is not expected after years in this situation (mostly when injury is due to prior cardiac arrest, traumatic brain injury, or both). Another, far more common state is a minimally conscious state, but this is a highly unsatisfactory term. These patients have considerable awareness once stimulated, and some recover. Patients in vegetative state show no signs of awareness of surroundings, but minimally conscious patients display inconsistent, limited awareness of self or the environment.[10]

Some films suggest reading to the patient in prolonged coma (*Rocky II*, 1979), even implying it could reduce the time in coma (*Uptown Girls*, 2003), but this is not based on fact. In the movies, some coma patients in film may shed tears. Patients in a PVS do shed tears spontaneously, but it is neither a sign of awareness nor a hint of possible improvement. Shedding tears has been used most dramatically and misleadingly in *The Past* (2013) ⫷. Although the physician forcefully argues it is not an accepted stimulus, the husband of a comatose woman tries to elicit a reaction using her perfumes. (He claims that smell is the last of the senses to disappear.) After he sprinkles himself with perfume, he leans over the patient, and she sheds a tear. She does not squeeze his hand when asked.[11] The use of perfume is notable here because it has been used in (unproven) stimulation programs (to test whether a patient would move the head to avoid the irritating stimulation of the nasal mucosa with ammonia and other noxious odors).[12]

Similarly of interest is *The Dreamlife of Angels* (1998) ⫷⫷⫷, which also depicts a comatose patient with contractures, tracheostomy, and gastrostomy remarkably well. Several patients are shown with contractures, and nurses use gastrostomy for feeding. It also shows attempts by nurses to record eye tracking and fixating on an object by the comatose patient—often a first sign of improvement. (The portrayal of the neurologist, is exemplary; see Chapter 3.)

Firelight (1997) ⫷⫷⫷ offers a reasonably good representation with eyes open, coma, and contractures. Again, however, the facial features continue to be unaffected in this movie portrayal, and the patient has a doll-like appearance.

Prognosis is a common theme in films showing PVS, and screenwriters have used offensive terms such as "the garden" (nursing home) and "vegetable" (life without activity). In *Blind Horizon* (2003) ⫷, the physician prognosticates: "50% total recovery, 35% partial, and 15% you plant him in the ground and watch him grow."

We have studied the use of coma by screenwriters in detail. Movies on coma were reviewed for cause and situation of coma, demographics of actor in coma, physician communication of coma, awakening from coma, and the role of the neurologist.[13] Some representative films are shown in Table 4.1. Because there is violence in R-rated movies, coma was typically caused by motor vehicle accidents, gunshot wounds, and other violent causes. Most actors were in their 30s to 40s. A review of 30 movies with coma portrayal showed awakening in 60% with up to 10 years of time in coma.

Successful rehabilitation after many years of coma was also shown, mostly with full physical and cognitive recovery. After awakening, the patient often indulged in murderous revenge, as seen in *Hard to Kill* (1990), *Face/Off* (1997), *Lying in Wait* (2001), and *A Man Apart* (2003). Awakening was often seen after a bizarre trigger (smoke, mosquito bite, sudden bright sunlight). *While You Were Sleeping* (1995) ⫷ shows the actor awakening during a New Year's Eve party after having been "comatose" for most of the film.

Most gratuitous is a scene in *Goodbye Lenin* (2003) ⫷, where a comatose mother awakens after eight months on a ventilator when her son enters the room to flirt with and kiss the nurse. Inexplicably, his

---

[10] Wijdicks 2022, ibid.

[11] In an interview, director Asghar Farhadi explained that his intention was to show a subtle, often unrecognized response. Although out of his wheelhouse, his concern was that unrecognized responses lead to decisions to withdraw support.

[12] Sattin D, Bruzzone MG, Ferraro S, et al. Olfactory Discrimination in Disorders of Consciousness: A New Sniff Protocol. *Brain Behav.* 2019;9:e01273.

[13] Wijdicks EF, Wijdicks CA, 2006, ibid.

TABLE 4.1 Examples of Coma in Fiction Film

Year	Title	Rated	Director	Plot	Actor Portraying Coma	Cause
1979	*Rocky II*	PG	Sylvester Stallone	Love; hope and optimism	Talia Shire	Shock
1983	*The Dead Zone*	R	David Cronenberg	Psychic	Christopher Walken	MVA
1990	*Hard to Kill*	R	Bruce Malmuth	Revenge	Steven Segal	GSW
1993	*Short Cuts*	R	Robert Altman	Loving family	Lane Cassidy	MVA
1995	*While You Were Sleeping*	PG	Jon Turteltaub	Love; loving family	Peter Gallagher	Assault
1997	*Face/Off*	R	John Woo	Revenge	Nicolas Cage	Violence
1997	*Firelight*	R	William Nicholson	End-of-life decisions; murder to be with another woman	Uncredited	Accident
1997	*Winter Sleepers*	NR	Tom Tykwer	Loss; grief	Uncredited	MVA
1998	*Seven Hours to Judgment*	R	Beau Bridges	Revenge	Uncredited	Violence
2001	*The Safety of Objects*	R	Rose Troche	End-of-life decision	Uncredited	MVA
2002	*28 Days Later*	R	Danny Boyle	Changed world; escaped killer virus	Gillian Murphy	MVA
2002	*Swim Fan*	PG-13	John Polson	Attempted murder	Monroe Mann	MVA
2003	*Kill Bill: Vol. 1*	R	Quentin Tarantino	Revenge	Uma Thurman	GSW
2003	*Blind Horizon*	R	Michael Haussman	Coma causes amnesia	Val Kilmer	GSW
2003	*A Man Apart*	R	Gary Gray	Revenge	Vin Diesel	Violence
2004	*Paparazzi*	PG-13	Paul Abascal	Revenge	Uncredited	MVA

Note: MVA: motor vehicle accident; GSW: gunshot wound; PG: parental guidance; NR: not rated; R: restricted.

mother is immediately lucid upon awakening. Other awakenings have shown a confused patient fighting with nursing staff or pulling out intravenous lines, as if awakening from a nightmare. Awakenings have also included suddenly sitting upright in bed. Sudden awakenings with stepping out of bed, pulling out catheters, walking out of the hospital in *28 Days Later* (2002) ⚔, and sudden increases in pulse rate before awakening. True to its title, in *Hard to Kill* (1990) ⚔, Steven Segal has been in coma for many years and has grown a sizable beard. During the "awakening scene," he relives the violent assault on him and his family just before he opens his eyes. His heartbeat is up; he grunts from anger, opens his eyes, and looks stunned but ready to leave the hospital.

One must conclude from these observations that screenwriters markedly deviate from currently accepted knowledge. In a 2006 study, we tried to learn how cinematic coma and recovery were perceived by the audience.[14] We compiled 22 key scenes from 17 movies to show a representative group of the lay public. These 72 viewers were asked to use statements to rate for accuracy, such as:

"I think this is how comatose patients look."

"I think the awakening shown after being in a coma for a long time can happen this way."

"After awakening from being in a coma for a long period of time, you may be able to do this."

"I believe what has been said is correct."

"If my family member were in the same situation, I possibly would remember what happened in the scene and allow it to influence any decisions that I would make."

---

[14] Wijdicks EF, Wijdicks CA. The Portrayal of Coma in Contemporary Motion Pictures. *Neurology.* 2006;66:1300–1303.

Assessment Results

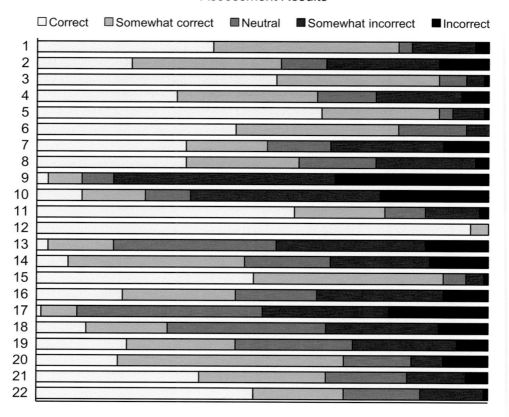

FIGURE 4.2 Study on the portrayal of coma in film. Assessment ratings of 22 movie scenes by viewers, most with no medical expertise. Our survey was skewed toward an educated audience of mature age. Most viewers identified inaccuracy of representation of coma in its appearance, awakenings, and conversations about the experience of being in a coma, with notable exceptions (neutral, somewhat agree, strongly agree) in eight scenes. The black bars are inaccuracies not recognized by the viewers, and this is a substantial minority.

The survey results are shown in Figure 4.2. Viewers were unable to identify important inaccuracies in one-third of the selected scenes, and one-third of the viewers agreed that these memories of these scenes could influence their decisions in a similar situation. This result suggests that movies have a consider-able impact on the public's perception of coma, although two-thirds did not think any of it was accurate. Similar findings were seen with a small sample of non-neurology residents, but not with neurology residents, who could identify all inaccuracies (unpublished observations.)

In summary, trivializing coma to a sleep-like state is inaccurate and potentially problematic. These films also show awakening, but never accurately, and the scenes as written are highly improbable. Seldom do directors and screenwriters use information in a meaningful way or correctly convey the major con-sequences of coma and rehabilitation. Prolonged comatose states in the movies remain misrepresented. Since the study was completed, I have noticed no change; similar mistakes continue. The clinical profile of the comatose patient in cinema has also remained unchanged; the overwhelming majority occur as a result of the assault and traumatic head injury (e.g., *Miami Vice*, 2006). A science fiction film suggested that coma leads to travel in an eerie world based on prior memories (*Coma*, 2019): "Coma? You say this is like a dream?" "It's memories; everyone comes to this place." Coma and how it feels to be in a coma continue to fascinate screenwriters, but we neurologists do not share this fascination, and we hope the audience come to recognize the absurdity.

Amnesia

Amnestic patients recall detailed autobiographical memories from their early life but have difficulty recalling detailed memories from their recent past. Some have difficulty imagining detailed future events. As noted in Chapter 2, amnesia as a neurologic sign came early in cinema. Memory difficulties have attracted screenwriters, and one can immediately imagine why. Wouldn't it be entertaining if the leading character, particularly a criminal, cannot remember what he or she has done? Many films have used this plot device, but three films stand out.

Antegrade amnesia (being unable to memorize events) is often used. This should be differentiated from dissociative amnesia, where patients recognize having lost their memories. Unplanned travel and unknown personal identity are seen in psychiatric fugues and are a result of a traumatic stressful event.[15] Such travel is often also accompanied by psychological inability to recall the past.[16]

Baxendale reviewed many films featuring amnesia and concluded, not entirely unexpectedly, that no good distinction could be made between true neurologic conditions and psychiatric manifestations.[17] Films also inaccurately suggested that memories do not disappear but are put on hold until they can be reassessed. Apart from good portrayals in *Memento* and a lesser-known movie (*Sé quien eres*, 2000) on Wernicke-Korsakov, Baxendale found a surprisingly accurate portrayal of amnesic syndromes in the character of Dory in *Finding Nemo* (2003) ◄◄◄ . It is revealed that Dory has been affected by this disability since she was very young. Dory has difficulties in retaining new information, recall, and knowing where she was going. Dory forgets Nemo's name (and calls him Chico, Bingo, and Fabio), and she cannot focus on the task at hand, which often leads to frolics. Usually, retrograde amnesia strips people of their confidence and identity, but Dory's optimism seems to inspire others. Nonetheless, her need for constant repetition frustrates the other fish.[18]

Memento (2000) ◄◄◄ , directed by Christopher Nolan, stars Guy Pearce as Lenny Shelby. Lenny has lost all ability to remember. "I can't make new memories. Everything just fades." The film is told in reverse order, is fragmented, and reflects the true condition. Fans of this complex film, after having scrutinized and combed through the scenes multiple times, are still asking questions. This adds to the confusional experience of the audience—almost experiencing the labyrinthine nature of amnesia—when film directors determine to leave their movies open to interpretation and make their audience work out the ending on their own.

DIALOGUE

Memento

Leonard   *I have to believe in a world outside my own mind. I have to believe that my actions still have meaning, even if I can't remember them. I have to believe that when my eyes are closed, the world's still there. Do I believe the world's still there? Is it still out there? Yeah. We all need mirrors to remind ourselves who we are. I am no different.*

---

[15] Bartsch T, Butler C. Transient Amnesic Syndromes. *Nat Rev Neurol.* 2013;9:86–97.

[16] Travis, in *Paris, Texas* (1984) by Wim Wenders, is a good example.

[17] Baxendale S. Memories Aren't Made of This: Amnesia at the Movies. *BMJ.* 2004;329:1480–1483.

[18] Kudos to Disney/Pixar. The 2016 sequel, *Finding Dory* expanded on this theme of otherness by introducing new sea creatures with physical disabilities but who have the ability to thrive with an impairment. It is part of their longstanding psychology themes such as the obsession with ambition in *Soul* (2020) and the relativity of success in *Cars* (2006): "they are all empty cups" (with Duc Hudson pointing at his trophies).

In short, Lenny kills an intruder who has raped and killed his wife. He gets hit on the head, causing antero-grade amnesia. Lenny makes Polaroids of places and written notes. His body has tattoos with clues to the killer of his wife. The movie also shows a different plot line (in black and white), where Leonard is introduced as an insurance investigator. He is investigating a man with anterograde amnesia but is accused of "faking it." The proof is his inability to be conditioned. It is correctly posited here that, although he cannot make memories, he is still able to develop conditioning to help him avoid potentially harmful situations. To see if he is "faking it," his wife gives him his insulin injection. She then secretly turns back the clock in the room, so it seems no time has passed, asks him again and again until he becomes comatose from the multiple injections (and never recovers). The film's dramatic proof that his condition is real is essentially correct, and this type of havoc could theoretically happen in persons with such memory loss.

Another major film on amnesia, *The Music Never Stopped* (2011) ◄◄◄◄ , directed by Jim Kohlberg and starring Lou Taylor Pucci, J.K. Simmons, and Julia Ormond, is based on an actual patient reported by Oliver Sacks in his essay "The Last Hippie" from his book *An Anthropologist on Mars: Seven Paradoxical Tales* (1995). The patient was Gabriel Sawyer, who had a large meningioma extending into the diencephalon that was destroying his optic chiasm as well as the frontal and temporal lobes. Gabriel was told by his swami that he was "an illuminate" and was becoming a saint. This interpretation delayed surgery.

After surgery, Gabriel had marked difficulty remembering events from the 1960s and nothing after 1970. He could play the guitar but was unable to generate any immediate memories. He displayed frontal syndrome in the form of "wisecracking." There was also increased word play. ("Lunch is here, it is time to cheer.") He tried to learn Braille but was unable to and could not grasp the reason for it. ("Why am I here with blind people?")

The film shows him in the hospital with an advanced brain tumor and loss of sight. The parents' con-versation with the neurosurgeon is comical in its inaccuracy. He explains that the tumor is benign, but Gabriel may be left with a major deficit after surgery. The neurosurgeon, played by Scott Adsit, points to the thalamus and incorrectly calls it the forebrain. When Gabriel's father asks, "So the tumor is in this area?" the neurosurgeon responds, irritated, "No, Mr. Sawyer, that is the tumor." Next, we see the neurosurgeon examining Gabriel after surgery. He asks him to count from 1 to 10, to which Gabriel answers, "Count me out."

The film shows him in a skilled nursing facility, where he plays "La Marseillaise" on trumpet and asks others what song it is. The film then dramatically shows that during music therapy, Gabriel sud-denly transforms from a frozen (abulic and catatonic) state to being animated and alive. (According to Oliver Sacks, his patient could not engage in a social conversation, but music elicited strong memories of lyrics and emotions.) Despite having marked anterograde amnesia, he could remember all the songs of the 1960s. When he sees a girl in the cafeteria who is named Cecilia, he sings Simon and Garfunkel's *Cecilia* ("Oh, Cecilia, you're breaking my heart") every time he sees her. Oliver Sacks met one of the Grateful Dead band members and took Gabriel to a concert, which caused Gabriel to remark that he "had the time of my life," but he forgot about it the next day. According to Sacks, Gabriel recognized most of the songs except those written after 1970; he recognized the style, though, remarking that they sounded like something the Grateful Dead might record someday. The movie mostly coalescences into a renewed connection between father and estranged son through the music of the Grateful Dead, Bob Dylan, Crosby, Stills, and Nash, and other rock stars from the "flower power" era. The movie touches on the mystery of music and emotions.

Songs or musical pieces do become encoded or hardwired in the brain and can be retrieved similarly to familiar faces. This experience may differ for a bona fide musician (or it might be more intense), but this oddity of profound amnesia—a catatonic state that nevertheless responds to favorite songs—was of major interest to Oliver Sacks.[19] The use of music in dementia is discussed in Chapter 6.

---

[19] See Sacks O. *Musicophilia: Tales of Music and the Brain.* Revised, expanded ed. New York: Vintage Books; 2008. This is yet another collection of the baffling cases of Oliver Sacks; in this one, he explores the effect of music on brain-injured patients.

One film that involves an interesting but seemingly improbable amnesia is *The Vow*[20] (2012) ◄ , starring Rachel McAdams, Channing Tatum, Sam Neill, and Jessica Lange and directed by Michael Sucsy. A traumatic head injury leaves Paige (Rachel McAdams) comatose. The film shows her still looking stunning with a few scratches and perfectly coiffed. After her surgery, we are told she is "kept" comatose using sedation. She awakens with a selective memory loss of the past five years. She does not recognize her husband, Leo (Channing Tatum), but does recognize her parents. When she meets her siblings, she recognizes them ("everyone looks older") as well as friends from high school. The rest of the plot shows her gradually becoming aware of some prior relationships but not all of them. There is a notable scene with her neurosurgeon (or neurologist), who looks at pupil reflexes and asks her about her memory and if she wants to regain her memory. The doctor warns Paige that she does not have to be afraid of remembering the accident ("Mercifully, that is rarely the case") and advises her to try to get her memory back. "I only did one psych rotation so this may be terrible advice, but I think you should try to fill the holes."

Two types of amnesia occur after traumatic head injury. Anterograde amnesia is typically impaired new learning and forgetting. Retrograde amnesia involves deficits in memory storage or retrieval. Psychogenic (functional) amnesia is not restricted to a single event (usually hours before the event) but involves a large part of the past. (It often affects young people.) This memory deficit may last for years. These patients are unable to recall information before the onset of the event, but anterograde memory is intact. Many may have a sudden loss of the ability to read, write, or use the telephone.

Memento is a correct example of amnesia, and the closest resemblance is to a real patient, Henry Molaison (also known as H.M.), who developed anterograde memory impairment after epilepsy surgery. (Although many critics have tried to link the film with his case history, the screenwriter was unaware of H.M.'s clinical course and did not base the film on his medical history.)

Henry Molaison (Figure 4.3) was treated for intractable seizures with the removal of both medial temporal lobes including important structures such as the hippocampus (space orientation and memory back-up) and amygdala (memory consolidation and human emotions). He was left with permanent amnesia, and his neuropsychologic profile was best summarized in Suzanne Corkin's book, aptly titled *Permanent Present Tense*.[21] Whenever he met someone, it was for the first time. Abundant research confirmed that he could not retain thoughts for more than 20 seconds. His motor tasks, which he had learned in the past, were intact, so he could do routine things such as cleaning the house or fixing a meal. Corkin relates that H.M., when asked, "What do you try to remember?" replied, "Well, that I don't know 'cause I do not remember what I tried." (His sense of humor remained intact.)

Corkin posits that Henry proved for the first time that a discrete medial region in the temporal lobe converts short-term memories into lasting memories. Distinctions between several forms of memory can now be made. These are *episodic memory* (remembrance of unique events), *semantic memory* (remembering facts), *declarative memory* (learning with awareness), and *procedural memory* (learning without awareness such as motor skills). Henry was dysfunctional in all except the latter. Henry could learn skills that depended on visual perception and motor abilities. He also remembered childhood events. It was "like waking from a dream," he told Corkin. "Every day is alone in itself."

Some other films deserve mention. The Hindi film *Ghajini* (2008) is considered a remake of *Memento*, which caused some controversy when Christopher Nolan was not credited. The most extreme form of global amnesia is the movie *Groundhog Day* (1990), where recall of the previous day is absent and is combined with global amnesia of everyone else in the movie. More silliness is apparent in the otherwise tremendously entertaining film *Eternal Sunshine of the Spotless Mind* (2004), where memory is erased with new technology. Another film, *50 First Dates* (2004), is discussed in Chapter 9.

---

[20] Improbable but, oddly enough, inspired by the allegedly true story of Kim and Krickitt Carpenter. (Carpenter K, Carpenter K, Wilkerson D. *The Vow: The Kim and Krickitt Carpenter Story*. Nashville, TN: B & H Group; 2000.)

[21] Corkin S. *Permanent Present Tense: The Unforgettable Life of the Amnesic Patient, H.M.* London: Allen Lane; 2013.

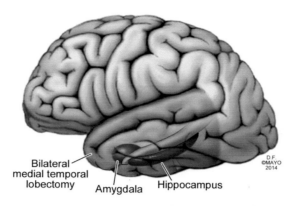

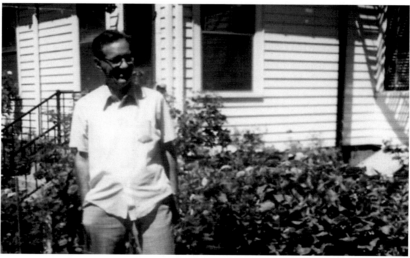

FIGURE 4.3 The major structures involved with memory are shown in the figure, and both large portions of full temporal lobe were removed. The most famous amnesiac Henry Molaison. (Used with permission from The Wylie Agency LLC.)

Screenwriters are very interested in loss of memory, and there is a large collection of fiction films that use amnesia as a plot device. For them, of course, it is a delightful gift of medicine to the arts. Very few films show the frequent presentation of selective memory difficulties, where some things are remembered and others are not. Two key films on amnesia involve dramatic cases—one based on a real patient—and this increases the entertainment value. Understanding memory deficits remains a difficult area for neurologists and neuropsychologists, and very few cases have been systematically and longitudinally examined.

Seizures

One of the most extensively analyzed films on seizures is *A Matter of Life and Death* (1946) ◄◄◄◄ , directed by the film-making duo Michael Powell and Emeric Pressburger and starring David Niven, Roger Livesey, Raymond Massey, Kim Hunter, and Marius Goring.[22] The storyline is complex and

---

[22] Powell M, Pressburger E. *A Matter of Life and Death*. Eagle-Lion Films (UK). November 1, 1946. Originally released in the United States as *Stairway to Heaven*.

fantastical. Peter, an RAF pilot and squadron leader (David Niven), miraculously survives a plane crash in the English Channel and washes ashore. He has fallen in love with an American radio operator June (Kim Hunter), whom he talked to just before the crash. Subsequently, he reunites with her, and both are deeply in love. Under normal circumstances, he would have died and appeared in heaven, but the film shows him not checking in. The story then turns to a heavenly tribunal discussing his failure to arrive in heaven and whether falling in love on earth is sufficient to postpone death.

Several scenes during the film show Peter having spells that may be interpreted as complex partial seizures. The spells are stereotyped and always begin with a smell of fried onions or with a discordant piano piece followed by visions of a "heavenly conductor" (the person sent to earth to take him back to heaven) and more complex hallucinations of a heavenly stairway to the aforementioned tribunal, where he eventually has to defend his stay on Earth.

Dr. Reeves, a neurologist, takes him home and asks Peter to signal when he feels something coming on and we see him in a spell. After he audibly sniffs to smell the fried onions, he rings a table bell. This depiction indeed is similar to our requests in epilepsy monitoring units; we ask the patient, family, or nurse to push a buzzer when they sense a weird feeling, and then we can see if there is a correlation with EEG changes. Dr. Reeves rushes in, examines Peter during a spell, and finds a pupil abnormality and a possible Babinski sign. (See also Chapter 3.) Dr. Reeves quickly diagnoses "fine vascular meningeal adhesions binding the optic nerve to the brain, the internal carotid artery, similar adhesions in chiasm and the brain." Peter is rushed into surgery and even has a spell under full anesthesia, where the key scene involves the tribunal debating whether he can stay on Earth or needs to come to heaven. (He wins his case and stays.)

DIALOGUE

A Matter of Life and Death

Dr. Reeves

He is having a series of highly organized hallucinations comparable to an experience of actual life, a combination of vision, hearing, and of ideas. To a neurologist, that compares to a direct sense of smell and taste. Once that connection is established, we know to look for the trouble.

A Matter of Life and Death has been analyzed in meticulous detail searching for every possible angle pointing to epilepsy by psychologist Diane Friedman, and she tries to make a case of complex partial seizures. (See Chapter 9 for a discussion of the fallacy of diagnosing neurologic diseases not exactly intended by the filmmaker.). One of the film's interests is the depiction of a highly unusual spell. To see the world as standing still and acutely frozen in time is a quite inventive falsehood—if anyone is frozen, it should be the patient! (Figure 4.4).[23] However, visual hallucinations as a result of an aura (a warning pre-seizure symptom) are never as complex or detailed or even include a conversation, and they never present as a full nightmare. Visual hallucinations may occur in temporal lobe seizures and could involve persons, but it is far more common the patient experiences a *Déjà Vu* aura—characterized by the realization of a familiar situation (been here before) coupled with an awareness that it "feels" very strange. Some may stare at furniture pieces in a room and feel that it just doesn't look exactly like their furniture pieces; this feeling passes in a minute or so. An illusion of being separated from your body is also known. Intense fear or discomfort with distressing body organ symptoms accompanied by thoughts of dread, being trapped, or losing control is not uncommonly heard in epilepsy clinics. Colors and shapes with flashing components are more common and some patients have been able

---

[23] Dr. Reeves's localization is way off. Although vision loss may occur, it takes some major twists and turns to connect all his symptoms with post-traumatic optochiasmatic adhesions, and I do not know how.

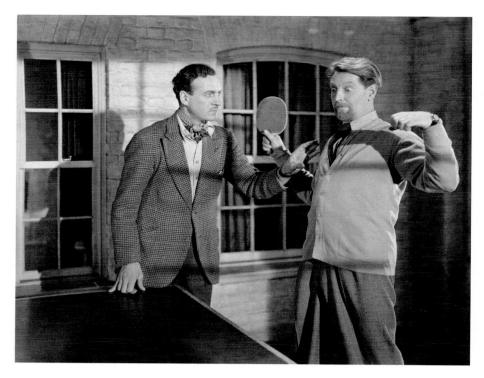

FIGURE 4.4 David Niven (Squadron Leader Peter David Carter) and Roger Livesey (Dr. Reeves) in *A Matter of Life and Death* (Everett Collection, Inc.). (Note: The patient looks at the "frozen in time" neurologist.)

to draw these vivid color lines and shapes using crayons. Ecstatic seizures (feeling of bliss or being in a nominuous place) are very uncommon in temporal lobe type seizures, but if plausible, these cases are more likely to end up in Oliver Sacks' files (Chapter 3) instead of an epilepsy clinic.

But if the premise of temporal lobe seizures in Peter is accepted—and it would be a major departure except for the smell of fried onions—no other film to my knowledge has depicted temporal lobe epilepsy in any way or form except for *The Terminal Man* (1974). (See Chapter 9 for a discussion of this film and the alleged connection between violence and temporal lobe epilepsy.) Friedman speculates that Michael Powell may have read neurology textbooks by Symonds and Purves-Steward. He may have had several interactions with neurologists. However, given the purely nonsensical dialogue and illogical neurologic exam, it is very doubtful that a neurologist reviewed the script. Dr. Reeves elicits a Babinski sign while his patient is in a postictal state. It looks professional, but this is something we do not do at all. Nonetheless, the awareness of strange odors, hallucinations, and postictal confusion may indeed point toward a temporal lobe seizure. Friedman admits she has only partial answers, and Powell's medical notes—if there were any substantial ones—were not found. In 2008, she affects surprise that no neurologist had come forward with similar claims, but one did in 1982.[24] But often in film, most

---

[24] See Friedman DB. A Matter of Fried Onions. *Seizure.* 1992;1:307–310; and Christie I, Powell M, Pressburger E. *A Matter of Life and Death.* Digitized ed. London: British Film Institute; 2008. Friedman's book *A Matter of Life and Death. The Brain Revealed by the Mind of Michael Powell* published by Author House 2008 Bloomington, Indiana, greatly expands on the idea that the original intent may have been to show complex partial seizures. Friedman interprets the storms in the film as auras. Another stretch: according to her, most of the statues on the stairway may have had epilepsy. In the absence of any proof, the evidence is circumstantial or, in her own words, "a book of informed speculation." However, this association was first reported by David Hogan from Canada. Hogan DB. Temporal Lobe Epilepsy in the Cinema. *Arch Neurol.* 1982;39:738.

TABLE 4.2   Film Depictions of Epilepsy

Post-traumatic epilepsy	*The Winning Team* (1952)
Epilepsy and violence	*Deceiver* (1997)
Epilepsy (ketogenic diet)	*First Do No Harm* (1997)
Epilepsy surgery (hemispherectomy)	*The Other Half of Me* (2001)
Side effects of anti-psychotic drugs	*Take Shelter* (2012)

neurologists (myself included) must simply shrug their shoulders, roll their eyes, laugh hard, or marvel at the inventiveness.

Other screenwriters have discovered the aura could be used as a great trope. *The Aura* (2005) ◀◀◀ features a protagonist with epilepsy. The aura is described in a lengthy scene and is used to profoundly scare the listener. It goes as follows: "There is a moment, a shift … things suddenly change; it is as if everything stops, a door opens in your head that lets things in—sounds, voices, images, smells. Smells from school, kitchen, and family. Cannot move. It is horrible and perfect." The aura is further accompanied by a screeching horror sound followed by a black screen and the protagonist awakening with a bright light shining in his eyes. The aura here creates a sense of mysticism but also a harbinger of doom.

Epilepsy in film has been well studied, and different types have even been acted out (Table 4.2). *Contagion* (2011) ◀◀◀ offers a key example with forced open eye deviation and body shaking and reveals deep research by the filmmaker into the manifestations of a generalized seizure (Figure 4.5).

One study analyzed 62 films, concluding that there were "examples of all of the ancient beliefs surrounding epilepsy such as demonic or divine possession, genius, lunacy, delinquency, and general otherness."[25] A link between epilepsy and psychiatry often implied that male characters were mad, bad, and dangerous. Female characters with seizures were exotic and vulnerable. In some films, the protagonist has seizures but rarely does a seizure disorder drive the full narrative.[26] A recent film from India, *Ek Naya Din*

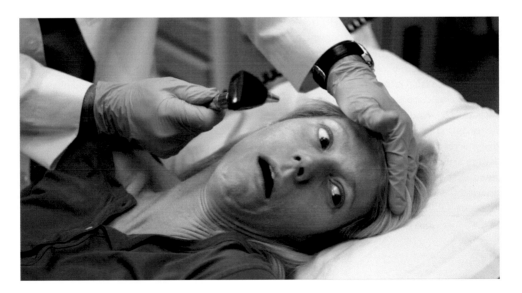

FIGURE 4.5   Gwyneth Paltrow with a seizure in *Contagion* (Photofest). (Note: Eyes open and deviated during a seizure are highly accurate.)

---

[25] Baxendale S. Epilepsy at the Movies: Possession to Presidential Assassination. *Lancet Neurol.* 2003;2:764–770.
[26] Kerson JF, Kerson TS, Kerson LA. The Depiction of Seizures in Film. *Epilepsia.* 1999;40:1163–1167.

(*A New Day*, 2013), got attention when it emphasized bad spirits in epilepsy and treatment with witch-craft. The neurologist, Misra, created this movie to improve understanding. Illiteracy and superstition are prevalent in north India and coexist with tremendous poverty.[27]

Several other films are noteworthy. In *Frankie and Johnny* (1991) , a man has a seizure in a res-taurant—"a fit or something"—and Frankie (Michelle Pfeiffer) puts him on his side during a postictal period. She sees that he wears a necklace that says epilepsy. While they are waiting for the ambulance, Johnny (Al Pacino) asks her out, but she is not interested. The man awakens rapidly and asks what hap-pened, and Frankie answers, "Nothing much. I just turned down someone."

Although initially made for TV (and therefore outside the scope of this book if we want to be legalistic), *First Do No Harm* (1997) is a movie by Jim Abrahams, who had a "similar" experience with his son, Charlie. (He is the founder of the Charlie Foundation.) The film is interesting because of its comprehensive coverage of childhood epilepsy. Meryl Streep plays a desperate mother whose son (Fred Ward) has epilepsy. The movie does not hold back and has caricatured all that may go wrong with epilepsy—arrogant neurolo-gists failing to accept ketogenic diet as a viable alternative, Stevens-Johnson syndrome from anti-epileptic drugs, paraldehyde brought in a Styrofoam cup with the cup melting away from direct drug exposure, behavior problems with anti-epileptic drugs, and even seizure on an airplane. To top it off, the movie even discusses lack of randomized trials in epilepsy treatment and thus a reason to try more experimental approaches—the "if you think this approach does not work, where is the proof of your approach" argu-ment. All is well with the child after he is started on a ketogenic diet.

A more recent film is *Electricity* (2014) , directed by Bryn Higgins and based on the acclaimed novel by Ray Robinson. For neurologists there are very recognizable moments.[28] Lily (Agyness Deyn) tries to find her estranged brother. Packed into this story are her frequent seizures. (The cause is traumatic brain injury from childhood abuse.) She tells us it feels like Alice falling down the rabbit hole. It is not difficult to show the audience the unnerving effect of epilepsy, the embarrassment of memory problems, and injury risk, but it is admirably done. The seizures come out of the blue. Drug compliance is a concern. (The neurologist in the hospital tells her there were no anti-epileptics in the blood sample.) Major portions of the film are filled with distorted sound and light, enhanced electronic house music, black-out scenes, jolts of branched electricity, and loud crashing waves, all used to convey the experience of seizures. We hear heavy breathing during her visual auras. They end with her waking up in bed (at home or in the hospital) with multiple bruises, disori-ented about time, and an occasional lip bite. The seizures do not advance the narrative except as an opportu-nity to add major visual effects. Lily is defiant, non-compliant, and verbally aggressive to the physicians who want to help her and see issues with medication reconciliation. When one physician gives her new medication and a schedule to wean the old and start the new one "in case you forget," she goes ballistic naming the large number of anti-epileptics she has been on ("carbo F … ing mezapine" as a final attempt). She yells at him, "I can give you years. I can give you dates. I can give you exact dosages. I do not forget, mate!"

Seizures are common in the movies and understandably so. Similarly, as in the real world, one is reminded that their presentation is frightening, and this opportunity for drama has been noted by screenwriters. A wide variety of causes for seizures has been depicted, but many of them occur in stress-ful situations. Obviously, seizures in film are linked to madness, perpetuating the age-old myth of a link between seizures and psychiatric disorders. This persistent cinematic association unsettles neurologists.

Headache

For filmmakers, all headaches are excruciating and ominous. Neurologists struggle to classify head-aches and identify their pathophysiology, but it is one of the most common situations in which we are consulted. The neurologist Gowers commented in his manual of diseases of the nervous system[29] in 1888

[27] Sharma DC. Indian Film on Epilepsy Busts Myths. *Lancet Neurol.* 2014;13:245.
[28] The credits acknowledge the staff of the Sutherland Royal Hospital in Sunderland, Tyne and Wear.
[29] Gowers WR. *A Manual of Diseases of the Nervous System.* Vol II. London: J & A Churchill; 1888.

that "we know almost nothing of the structures in which the pain of headache is felt or the mechanism of its production." The 20th century brought major breakthroughs such as the vascular theories based on many meticulous experiments and the neural theories associated with spreading depression.[30] In headache more than any other neurologic disease, many physicians have recounted their own migraine symptoms including the most graphic and most complete accounts of the syndrome. In his historical essay, DeJong found one of the first personal observations in 1618 by Charles Lepois, who described "winds from the west and the approach of rainstorms" as provocative factors.[31] Many therapies were tried, including many we would now abhor,[32] such as bloodletting, eels electric shocks, compression of one carotid artery, vibrating chairs or spas. Trepanation was used rarely for intolerable headache in western medicine but found its way on the screenwriter's page.

As a dramatized depiction, the film *Pi* (π) (1998) ◄◄◄◄ shows cluster headache well, and its treatment had an enduring effect on the audience. *Pi* (π) stars Sean Gullette, Mark Margolis, Ben Shenkman, and Samia Shoaib and was directed by Darren Aronofsky. Although headache does not play any role in advancing the plot, it is part of the struggle of a mathematician to find order in numbers. His assumptions are that mathematics is a language of nature and that everything can be understood through numbers. If numbers are graphed, certain patterns emerge (a philosophical concept dating back to Pythagoras).

Max Cohen, played by Sean Gullette, often discusses the nature of mathematics with Sol Robeson, played by Mark Margolis. Max is not only interested in finding a pattern in the stock market but also encounters Lenny Meyer, played by Ben Shenkman. Lenny is interested in the number 216, which represents the letters of the name of God that will open the doors to the Messianic Age. Max's headaches may be linked to having that number in his head.

The film suggests that Max's headaches started at the age of six years, when he was staring at the sun and became "blind"; his headaches are repetitive. In rapid succession, we see crosscuts of Max popping pills, screeching sounds, and hallucinations of moving doors that unlock and open to a bright light. This scene specifically mentions his medications. He uses promazine and sumatriptan followed by dihydroergotamine mesylate by subcutaneous injection. Multiple attacks are shown and include Max banging his head against a mirror to relieve the pain and injecting dihydroergotamine into the skin of his skull. Notable here is the large (nail gun–like) injector that must have been deliberately chosen by the director to add drama. The film shockingly ends with trepanning and drilling a burr hole during a severe headache attack.

The film represents cluster headache well. It shows pain on one side, on the same side as lacrimation, but it does not show ptosis or periorbital edema. It shows the repetitive nature of the pain. Most patients with cluster headaches have their attacks in the third or fifth decade. The triggers of these headaches are typically wine, nocturnal sleep with daytime naps, and strong odors such as perfume or paint. All these triggers are shown in this film.[33]

The first treatment of cluster headache is oxygen, but as mentioned in the movie, sumatriptan by subcutaneous injection can abort attack in most patients. The obsession and paranoia, as well as hallucinations, should be considered unusual in cluster headaches. *That Beautiful Somewhere* (2006) ◄ shows the leading actress (Jane McGregor) with severe migraine. We see her groping for her head and moving around, crying out in pain, and also trying to drill in her temporal lobe (similarly to in *Pi* but without trephination). For most of the movie, she wears dark-colored glasses.

Headache specialists I have consulted consider *Pi* a great movie and a teaching example of cluster headache, with its obsessional restlessness and its excruciating pain. It is the only film that markedly portrays signs and symptoms of headache in accurate detail … minus the drilling.

---

[30] Eadie MJ. *Headache: Through the Centuries.* New York: Oxford University Press; 2012.

[31] DeJong RN. Migraine: Personal Observations by Physicians Subject to the Disorder. *Ann Med Hist.* 1942;4:276–283.

[32] Koehler PJ, Boes CJ. A History of Non-Drug Treatment in Headache, Particularly Migraine. *Brain.* 2010;133:2489–2500.

[33] See Ashkenazi A, Schwedt T. Cluster Headache–Acute and Prophylactic Therapy. *Headache.* 2011;51:272–286; and Nesbitt AD, Goadsby PJ. Cluster Headache. *BMJ.* 2012;344:e2407.

Other movies use headache as an affliction associated with deranged characters and major personality disorders. A key movie is *White Heat* (1949) ⫷ , in which James Cagney plays trigger-tempered
Cody. Cody has two major headache attacks. In the backstory, we learn that he initially faked headaches
to get his mother's attention, but later the headaches become real. His headache starts abruptly, and he
falls to the floor grabbing his head. It lasts for a minute and then subsides when his mother massages his
neck. He needs some time to recover, and his mother says, "Do not let them see you like that." Once in
jail, he has a second similar attack and again gets an occipital massage. Both attacks last about a minute;
the duration on screen seems to represent the "real" duration. The headache in both attacks appears to
be very severe, as Cody falls to the ground, grimaces, and pounds his fists in the mattress. The second
attack is preceded by blurred vision, filmed from Cody's perspective. These visual disturbances do not
resemble a typical migraine zigzag scotoma, and he does not vomit.[34] The headaches are non-classifiable.
Cody's headache is linked to violent and homicidal behavior, and two psychiatrists advise him to enter a
mental institution to treat his headache. He is put in a straitjacket following a major outburst in jail after
learning that his mother has died. We also learn that his father and brother were in an insane asylum.
The headache depiction is reasonably certain to be a cluster headache, quickly subsiding with some postictal deterioration. The link to criminal behavior in this gangster movie is simply wrong.

Another interesting film depicting migraine is *Gods and Monsters* (1998) ⫷ , in which the protagonist has
a severe unilateral headache and nearly collapses, grabbing his head. We next see him lying in a chair. His
caretaker runs to him with a large assortment of pills, and he asks for luminal. A consulted physician calls it
"stroke" or "electrical activity," but he does not know how to deal with the "killing" headaches.

DIALOGUE

White Heat
Cody   *[Headache] is like a red-hot buzz saw inside my head.*
That Beautiful Somewhere
Catherine   *Pain makes you do things; makes you submit and pray for anything to stop it.*

A thunderclap headache is depicted in *Hannah Arendt* (2012). Her husband Heinrich Blucher (Axel
Milberg) collapses after a severe orbital headache. It is suggested that he has "a brain aneurysm." She
tells him, "I spoke to the doctor. He said you only have a fifty-percent chance," to which he answers,
"Don't forget the other fifty percent." He is seen in a few scenes later without any deficits, calling it "a
slight collapse."

After reviewing the characteristics of headaches in film, Vargas et al.[35] found that most actors playing headache sufferers were men with characters between the ages of 18 and 49, and nearly half of them
died from violent attacks including suicide. Many movie headaches in the movies do have an underlying
cause, with about one-third being the result of a tumor, foreign body, or toxic exposure.[36]

As it turns out, this is much ado about nothing. Headache is common in the movies, but it is only
mentioned very briefly and rarely (except for *Pi*) advances the narrative. It is briefly mentioned with
brain tumors or used incidentally (see Chapter 7 for *Rhapsody in Blue*), and its function in the plot
is seldom clear. Screenwriters may feel that evil, shady characters should have torturous headaches.

---

[34] Realism, in this case, was perhaps sacrificed to avoid offending the viewer (or the Hays Code).
[35] Vargas BB, Henry KA, Boylan LS. *Characteristics of Headache in Motion Pictures: Demographics and Outcomes of Headache Sufferers in Film.* Chicago, IL: American Headache Society; 2007.
[36] Vargas et al., 2007, ibid.

Migraine, despite its common occurrence, does not seem to interest screenwriters, perhaps because its relatively benign nature is not dramatic enough. (See Chapter 6 for a discussion about a recent documentary on migraine, which emphasizes the devastating effect it has on patients.)

Cinema and headache do link up in another interesting way. Watching 3D videos or movies can induce a headache in about one person in 10, with the chances increased in a migraine sufferer. It may be part of a poorly defined "3D vision syndrome" provoking eye soreness and blurred vision; it occurs more commonly in movies longer than two hours.[37]

Sleep Walking and Narcolepsy

An interesting chapter in neurocinema is the portrayal of sleep disorders. One should not be surprised to find the common use of dreams and night terrors, and directors have used some specific disorders. Sleepwalking, or somnambulism, is occasionally portrayed in film and often with an erotic undertone. Sleepwalking is most comically displayed in Hal Roach's *High and Dizzy* (1920) .[38] Harold Lloyd as "the boy" watches Mildred Davis as "the girl" sleepwalking on a building's ledge. She has one arm outstretched as if reaching in the dark and keeps this position throughout. He saves her from falling and places her on a bed. She caresses his face but is startled when she awakens to find him in her bedroom.

Bunuel's *Viridiana* (1961) , banned by the Spanish government due to obscenity and blasphemy, has Viridiana (a nun) dressed in a nightgown and sleepwalking, which shows off her legs. She is terribly embarrassed that her uncle did not wake her up. He suggests it is dangerous, which is another sleepwalking myth.

Sleepwalking is prominently on display in a newer film, *Side Effects* (2013) , starring Rooney Mara, Jude Law, Catherine Zeta-Jones, and Channing Tatum and directed by Steven Soderbergh. As a novelty, *Side Effects* had an associated website during the release that was eerily similar to a real advertisement until the very recognizable Jude Law shows up as psychiatrist, Dr. Banks. He asks questions about signs of depression. If all three questions are answered "yes," he looks very concerned and suggests Ablixa. If all three questions are answered "no," he still recommends a psychiatric referral. Apparently, it is hard to "escape" a psychiatrist, let alone "Ablixa."

Ablixa, a fictitious antidepressant, causes violent sleepwalking in the main character. Emily Taylor (Rooney Mara) is hopelessly depressed, possibly caused by her husband's recent release from prison after serving four years for insider trading. Emily tries to get her life back together but fails with the first social encounter. Next, she purposely drives her car into the wall of a parking garage, and hospitalization leads to therapy sessions with Dr. Jonathan Banks (Jude Law). He prescribes multiple antidepressants and, when all else fails—and after another attempt to throw herself under a train—treats her with Ablixa. The drug cures her depression but also causes sleepwalking. Despite an initial brief episode of sleepwalking, Emily refuses to stop the medication. In a subsequent sleepwalking episode, she murders her husband.

After the murder, a brief court drama ensues, but rather than presenting the difficulties with proving the relationship of violent behavior with sleepwalking, this segment ends quickly. However, it does note that consciousness provides a context for our actions and that awareness does not exist when you sleep. The film does not mention video-EEG-polysomnographic assessment and its potential value in court.

---

[37] See Danno D, Kawabata K, Tachibana H. Clinical Features of 16 Cases of Headache Which Were Provoked after Watching 3-D Videos. *Intern Med.* 2012;51:1195–1198; and Braschinsky M, Raidvee A, Sabre L, et al. 3D Cinema and Headache: The First Evidential Relation and Analysis of Involved Factors. *Front Neurol.* 2016;7:30.

[38] The origin of this absurd sleepwalking posture—outstretched arm(s), eyes closed, and sometimes marching-like walking—is not known, was not invented in Hollywood, and may have originated in German expressionist films from the Weimar period. The first known appearance is in Murnau's *Nosferatu* (1922), when Greta Schröder as Ellen Hutter walks on a balcony ledge with both arms outstretched. Subsequently, it made its way into many art forms. The unrealistic posture of outstretched arms and eyes closed was found in 20% of movies and in 79% of cartoons. (See Dalloz MA, Kovarski K, Tamazyan R, Arnulf I. From Burlesque to Horror: A Century of Sleepwalking on the Silver Screen. *Sleep Med.* 2021;85:172–183.

The case quickly goes to a plea bargain, case closed. Meanwhile, Dr. Banks's psychiatry practice suffers, his marriage almost falls apart, and he is grilled in a deposition asking about his workload and whether he can handle it. His colleague psychiatrists threaten to ostracize him for losing patients.

The film has other not-so-subtle themes and shows psychiatrists talking about medication options (the "try-this-in-your-patient-because-it-worked-well-in-mine" argument) and cavalierly prescribing for family members. (He gives his wife a beta-blocker, and she jokes that there are advantages of having a husband who can provide medication.) It further caricaturizes a lavish lifestyle of specialists, among other unsympathetic portrayals.

The film claims that antidepressants cause violent behaviors during sleep, an exceedingly uncommon side effect. Violent behaviors during sleep are well known and may have dramatic implications including homicide, non-fatal assaults but also sexual misconduct. Sleepwalking is usually benign in children, but in adults, it can become quite harmful, with not only destruction of property, but also serious injury to bed partners or others. Sexsomnia is a form of parasomnia characterized by atypical and often violent or injurious sexual behavior during sleep. The American Academy of Sleep Medicine has clear criteria for somnambulism that include persistence of sleep or impaired judgment during ambulation and a disturbance not better explained by other disorders, drug use, or substance-use disorder. A leading textbook of sleep medicine mentions that sleep specialists are increasingly asked to evaluate potential court cases where violent behavior might be the result of a sleep disorder.[39] Connecting violence with an underlying sleep disorder is far more difficult, although the literature suggests some criteria such as (1) previous episodes and documented sleep disorder, (2) arousal stimulus, (3) no attempt to escape, (4) amnesia for the event, and (5) precipitating factors such as recent sleep deprivation and newly introduced medication.[40]

In *Side Effects*, neurologists may see a grain of truth, and the bland emotion with which Emily commits the murder is very well portrayed. This film is a good example of how psychiatry and neurology may intersect and how sleepwalking-associated murder is linked with real astonishment in the perpetrator.

Rooney Mara plays a very convincing sleepwalker. Sleepwalking shows her putting on music and setting a table (a common occurrence in real-life situations) and waking up her husband. She walks and acts like an automaton. Her eyes-open blank look while performing some detailed tasks is well depicted.[41] In the key scene, she ends up committing a murder.[42] *Side Effects* is one of those films in which nobody is what they seem. *Side Effects* highlights an interesting and disturbing phenomenon. That makes the film worth watching, but ultimately, *Side Effects* is a thriller—with greed and conceit as a leading motif.

DIALOGUE

Side Effects

Attorney	*What you're saying is that to have intent you must also have consciousness.*
Dr. Banks	*Consciousness provides a context or meaning for our actions. If that part of you does not exist, then basically we are functioning much like an insect, where you just respond instinctively without a thought what your actions mean.*
Attorney	*That part "provides meaning to action" …does that exist when we are asleep?*
Dr. Banks	*No.*

---

[39] Kryger MH, Roth T, Dement WC. *Principles and Practice of Sleep Medicine.* 7th ed. Philadelphia: Saunders; 2021.

[40] Siclari F, Khatami R, Urbaniok F, et al. Violence in Sleep. *Brain.* 2010;133:3494–3509.

[41] See Sutcliffe JG, de Lecea L. Not Asleep, Not Quite Awake. *Nat Med.* 2004;10:673–667; and Zadra A, Desautels A, Petit D, Montplaisir J. Somnambulism: Clinical Aspects and Pathophysiological Hypotheses. *Lancet Neurol.* 2013;12:285–294.

[42] No spoiler is intended here; the crime is already implied in the first minute of the film and prominently present in the trailer.

Sleepwalking is not the only aspect of sleep disorders depicted in film. Dreams and nightmares are omnipresent in cinema. Dreams are often effectively used to create a certain mood, to add a surprising twist, or to unveil a suppressed memory. Even awakening from a terrifying dream only to find it playing out in reality is used with much effect in *Take Shelter* (2011). The most phantasmagorical depiction of dreams is in *Inception* (2010), showing a dream within a dream—within a dream.

Nightmares have been effectively used in the classics of cinema, and there are numerous examples including most memorably the dream sequence featuring Dali-designed, psychoanalytic symbols in *Spellbound* (1945). Particularly gripping for physicians is the unsettling nightmarish examination of Professor Isak Borg in the Ingmar Bergman-directed *Wild Strawberries* (1957). In one of his frequent dreams, he must retake a bacteriology exam but cannot see what is under the microscope. In the dream, he not only fails but is also graded as incompetent—a grade that ends his medical studies.

Other common sleep disorders depicted in film are narcolepsy and insomnia. Insomnia is characteristically defined as difficulty initiating sleep and inability to have a restorative sleep. As a result, it may increase the risk of daytime accidents and a later risk of depressive illness. The twilight state with lack of sleep has been used repeatedly but with little insight on why it occurs and its consequences. *Insomnia* (2002) uses lack of sleep and exhaustion because of perpetual daylight in Alaska as a plot device.

The Machinist (2004) ◄ takes the problems with insomnia to truly absurd levels. The main character in this film (played by Christian Bale) is almost moribundly skinny from lack (a full year!) of sleep. Sleep deprivation also causes his paranoid behavior.

Narcolepsy and narcoleptic hallucinations are well depicted in *My Own Private Idaho* (1991) ◄◄◄ , directed by Gus Van Sant. River Phoenix plays a gay street hustler with multiple cataleptic attacks. Here, the narcoleptic attacks are triggered by anything that reminds him of his mother and his abandonment as a child. Most hallucinations here are vivid prior childhood memories, presented as old Super-8 films. Most narcoleptic hallucinations are simple acoustic (sound or melody) or simple visual (objects or circles). Hallucination of a person may occur, too, and in this film, it is often the face of his mother. These hallucinations are then followed by quivering eyelids and prolonged unconsciousness. Cataleptic attacks are usually brief but may last for 30 minutes; therefore, the prolonged attacks in this film are incorrectly represented. Here, they seem to be a combination of long cataleptic attacks in combination with signs of sleep paralysis.

DIALOGUE

My Own Private Idaho

Friends   *I am surprised he can even exist like this on narcolepsy.*

                                     He is not dead. He is just passed out, and it is a condition.

In other situations, narcoleptic patients may be unable to move, speak, or open their eyes while falling asleep or coming out of sleep, but this lasts only a few minutes. For many patients with cataplexy, the most frightening aspect of the attack is remaining fully conscious with a paralyzed body. The International Classification of Sleep Disorders includes two forms: narcolepsy with cataplexy and narcolepsy without cataplexy.[43] Cataplexy is also shown in an exaggerated manner in the film *Deuce Bigelow* (1999) ◄ , with an actress dropping to the ground like a stone in contrast to the actual typical slow loss of muscle tone.

A reasonably good depiction of cataplexy is in the more recent film *Ode to Joy* (2019) ◄◄◄ , starring Martin Freeman and Morena Baccarin and directed by Jason Winer. The attacks show not only knee-buckling and falling to the ground but also absurdly rigid tumbling backward. Unconsciousness is inaccurate. Retaining consciousness distinguishes catalepsy from syncope. As expected, strong, happy emotions

[43] Bassetti CLA, Kallweit U, Vignatelli L, et al. European Guideline and Expert Statements on the Management of Narcolepsy in Adults and Children. *Eur J Neurol.* 2021 Sep;28(9):2815–2830.

trigger catalepsy; these include exchanging vows, intimacy, and seeing babies and puppies. (The inventive movie tagline is "He has never been happier. And that is the problem.") Other symptoms of cataplexy are not depicted, but that is an understandable choice for a comedy. The filmmaker may not know what to do with excessive daytime sleepiness, hallucinations both hypnagogic (before falling asleep) and hypnopompic (with awakening). There is often a feeling of weightlessness. In one hospital scene, with everyone laughing, Charlie, the patient, tells them "it's not funny," and this addition by the screenwriter is astute. Many bystanders find the disorder amusing, which is annoying and insensitive to those affected by the disease.

Other parasomnias have not found the page of the script writer with one notable exception. By creating fright and anxiety, *Memoria* (2021) ◄◄◄ uses the (harmless) exploding head syndrome to great cinematic effect. The strange (rumble) sounds she (Tilda Swinton) hears serve as the ticking of a doomsday clock, and she hears it not only in the morning but throughout the day. She searches for its origin in Colombia, not Colombia's tropics, which are full of eerie diegetic sounds. This syndrome, actually experienced by the Thai filmmaker Apichatpong Weerasethakul, is characterized by a loud bang during the transition of sleep to wakefulness, and the episodes can repeat even in one night. Antidepressants have helped patients, but it can resolve spontaneously. Weerasethakul was clearly fascinated by the strange nature of these sounds and effectively runs with the idea that it could become a larger story of sensuous experiences. (It won the 2021 Cannes Jury Prize.)

Normally, sleep should provide rest. When most of us have a dream, it does not make much sense but, alas, not in the movies. For screenwriters, there are good reasons to use dream sequences and sleep disorders because they provide a good storytelling device, particularly an ethereal dream or night terrors. With the release of *Side Effects,* sleepwalking is now correctly on display—although in its most severe and exceedingly rare form.

Neurologic Disorders

Fictional feature films have also portrayed a neurologic illness with considerable detail in onset, care, and clinical course. Outcomes might include progression or recovery, and endings were unpredictable, some glib, some shocking, and in a mixture of genres. It is remarkable that many common neurologic disorders had a cinematic treatment and even more remarkable that they appeared mostly since the 1980s. Before, neurologic depictions of major neurologic disorders were mainly traumatic spine injury (*Stella Maris, Pollyanna,* and *The Men*), brain tumors (*Dark Victory* and *Rhapsody in Blue*), and epidemics such as poliomyelitis (*Leave Her to Heaven* and *The Five Pennies*). The reason is not clear, but the movie moguls must have thought that watching neurologic disease might be profitable—a motive we should never forget when reconstructing the history of neurology in film. Changes in censorship and cultural changes may have been a factor. Medical education films have been around since the invention of the camera, but now medical themes have jumped over to fiction films, the so-called "entertainment industry." One observation is that dementia and social deprivation have inspired many recent films. It is undoubtedly the result of increased longevity, age-related diseases, and ageism in the form of negative stereotypes.

Traumatic Brain Injury

Concerned about misinformation, the neurosurgeon William Mosberg wrote, "Of particular concern to neurosurgeons is the popular portrayal of a blow to the head is as effective and safe as a carefully administered anesthetic rather than being frequently a cause of serious injury or death." But informing (or kindly coercing) the movie industry, as he subsequently suggests, is futile.[44] A slow-moving train has been long in arriving. Silent film and slapstick movies were packed with head injury but never with long-standing consequences. After the 1960s revolution in cinema and the explosion of world cinema, plots became more brutally graphic, and violence had its own starring role. Westerns, with bar-fight scenes and people getting hit on the head by a poker (or a chair or a bar stool) are common, but shootouts and gunfights are also a rich Hollywood tradition. The body is riddled with bullets, and many do not make

---

[44] Mosberg WH, Jr. Trauma, Television, Movies, and Misinformation. *Neurosurgery.* 1981;8:756–758.

it far. Graphic gunshots to the head in film came much later. With multiple gunshots to the head, the protagonist (e.g., Woody Harris as Ace in *Paid in Full* [2002]) still manages to survive.[45] There is no shortage of trauma and gunshots in the entertainment industry—no poetic realism here. Head injuries occur often in the movies, but it is remarkable that the effects of traumatic brain injury are rarely shown. More broadly, it is impossible to review all films on traumatic head injury; many do not offer details or background information, and we are left with a fully wrapped trauma patient in a hospital bed. Readers of this book who are looking for accuracy are better off viewing *The Crash Reel* (2013), discussed in detail in Chapter 6.

It took nearly a decade for cinema to get more serious with it.[46] *Regarding Henry* (1991) ⚑ stars Harrison Ford, Annette Bening, and Bill Nunn and was directed by Mike Nichols. It is considered one of the most recognizable movies about the long-term effects of severe traumatic brain injury (TBI). This movie is about a callous, arrogant attorney who gets shot in the head while getting cigarettes late at night. He is resuscitated after blood loss, causing additional anoxic injury. (The movie surprisingly suggests that he could do well if it only had been a gunshot to the right side of the brain.) In several scenes, we see him in extended coma following a neurosurgical procedure (Figure 4.6). His prognosis is uncertain. Then he suddenly opens his eyes but does not fixate and remains mute.[47]

DIALOGUE

Regarding Henry

Colleague attorney   *… and went off the side of the road. The doctor says forget it, no change. Three months later, he beat me in tennis, swear to God, you never know … you never know.*

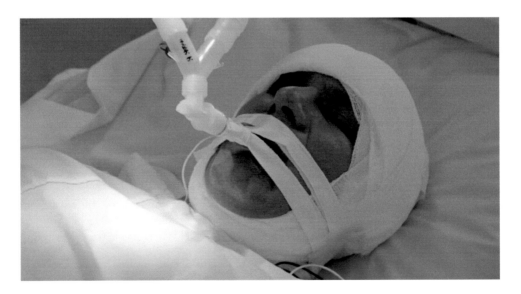

FIGURE 4.6   Harrison Ford in *Regarding Henry* (Photofest).

[45] Aarabi B, Tofighi B, Kufera JA, Hadley J, Ahn ES, Cooper C, et al. Predictors of Outcome in Civilian Gunshot Wounds to the Head. *J Neurosurg.* 2014;120:1138–1146.

[46] Azouvi P, Vallat-Azouvi C, Belmont A. Cognitive Deficits after Traumatic Coma. *Prog Brain Res.* 2009;177:89–110.

[47] As an aside, the head wrap and fixation of the breathing tube is amusing. When it is finally removed, he has perfectly coifed hair rather than the large shaven area needed to allow brain surgery.

The film effectively depicts the long, painful rehabilitation and recovery from traumatic brain injury. ("It is going to be a long, tough rehabilitation." "The brain is very mysterious." "In some ways, he is starting from scratch here.") After he seems to be improving and returns home, the film shows him markedly changed and awkward. In one scene, Henry is wandering the street buying a hot dog (he does not know what "kraut" is), answering a phone in a random phone booth, watching an X-rated movie, and buying a puppy—all in one afternoon.

Regarding Henry is, of course, about redemption—learning to start anew, being a better person with a "clean slate" after prolonged coma. Initially, the personality changes after such an injury depicted here are very real. Frontal lobe injuries result in major problems in mood (the flat mimicry of Harrison Ford is generally accurate), difficulty understanding complete conversations, and loss of verbal fluency. Henry also shows impulsivity and disinhibition, which are common after these types of injuries. However, the "clean slate" and, especially, the change to a lovable person in this film is far less likely. Most patients remain easily irritable, or their prior personality flaws become accentuated. These types of brain injuries do not improve the personality; persons are changed forever, plans are thwarted, and many must cope with major attentional deficits and emotional lability.

Another notable film—at least for a couple of opening scenes—is *The Lookout* (2007) ◄◄◄ , which stars Joseph Gordon-Levitt, Jeff Daniels, and Matthew Goode and was written and directed by Scott Frank. This film shows some interesting aspects about the long-term consequences of TBI. Chris (Joseph Gordon-Levitt) is injured in a motor vehicle accident (MVA), and we see him later explaining his difficulty with "sequencing"—that is, putting things he does during the day in order. He cannot remember names. He writes down exactly how his day is planned and who he meets and then follows this routine. He meets his female case manager, and there are some sexual innuendos. ("Did you have these thoughts before head injury?") There are yellow stickers everywhere, multiple notebooks, and drawers with names for clothing. He also becomes unhinged and has a "frontal" behavior. He shares a room with a jokester blind man (Jeff Daniels), whom he can consult if he forgets how to open a can. The movie turns into a caper involving a bank heist, and there is a little further explanation of his behavior. One of the reasons the screenwriter wrote this character is that Chris seems subdued and thus oblivious to his surroundings. *The Lookout* is a generally accurate representation of the "forgetfulness" of patients with moderate TBI. The inability to organize the day ("sequencing") does occur, and the use of Post-it notes on telephones as a reminder to call someone is a credible behavior. Many patients work with compensatory strategies, and cognitive rehabilitation may improve the executive aspects of attention and everyday functioning.[48] Strategic memory training has also been developed and includes notebooks and electronic memory aids that send reminders to compensate for deficits.[49]

Trauma (2004), ◄ also concentrates on "recovery" from an MVA. Colin Firth is briefly comatose but awakens. He has full flashbacks of the entire accident when looking at pictures of his wife (who died in the accident), feels people are looking at him, startles easily, and hallucinates. The psychologist or psychiatrist (not credited) explains these episodes. ("It is not uncommon, especially when you are tired … that it [the brain] translates sounds or sights into images of that.") He visits old friends, who tell him,

---

[48] See Cicerone KD, Langenbahn DM, Braden C, Malec JF, Kalmar K, Fraas M, et al. Evidence-Based Cognitive Rehabilitation: Updated Review of the Literature from 2003 through 2008. *Arch Phys Med Rehabil.* 2011;92:519–530; and Lewis FD, Horn GJ. Traumatic Brain Injury: Analysis of Functional Deficits and Posthospital Rehabilitation Outcomes. *J Spec Oper Med.* 2013;13:56–61.

[49] See Powell LE, Glang A, Ettel D, Todis B, Sohlberg MM, Albin R. Systematic Instruction for Individuals with Acquired Brain Injury: Results of a Randomised Controlled Trial. *Neuropsychol Rehabil.* 2012;22:85–112; and Powell LE, Glang A, Pinkelman S, Albin R, Harwick R, Ettel D, et al. Systematic Instruction of Assistive Technology for Cognition (ATC) in an Employment Setting Following Acquired Brain Injury: A Single Case, Experimental Study. *NeuroRehabilitation.* 2015;37:437–447.

"Get on with your life." The film shows a post-traumatic stress disorder well,[50] but soon it becomes clear that the film belongs more in the horror genre.

A similar theme returns in *Every 21 Seconds* (2017) ◄◄◄ but shows the consequences of a severe traumatic head injury much more profoundly. (The title refers to the statistic that someone is affected by a traumatic brain injury every 21 seconds.) It is based on a true story and a book by Brain Sweeny, who is portrayed by Shannon Brown. After becoming intoxicated and starting a bar fight, he is first hospitalized in a Green Bay hospital with a "hangover," which then worsens to "brain swelling." His wife is frantic and does not trust anyone there anymore. He transfers to Chicago, where he is seen by Dr. Synkowski played by Jim O'Heir. Although unusual for a celluloid surgeon, Dr. Synkowski is a compassionate and considerate neurosurgeon who guides the family through this ordeal very well ("for starters, we know the difference between hangovers and traumatic brain injuries"). He suggests the removal of a frontal contusion, which leads to considerable upset with the family. ("So then what if you do it [and] he turns into 'one flew over the cuckoo's nest' or something?") It shows a long and arduous rehabilitation. It superbly depicts a family suddenly confronted with a different man and its impact on his family—one man potentially pulling a young family into the abyss. ("He goes from zero to nuclear in a matter of seconds and usually without warning.")

However, another more recent film requires attention; it is one of the first movies to show the early and late effects of a subdural hematoma. *The Meyerowitz Stories (New and Selected)* (2017) ◄◄◄ , written and directed by Noah Baumbach, has an important teachable segment. Dustin Hoffman has a fall and, while managed in the ICU, suddenly and additionally develops aphasia and is treated for seizures with pentobarbital. It is an accurate scene with a remarkably accurate clinical course and management.

At the heart of these questions about the consequences of traumatic brain injury lies the further issue of chronic form of traumatic brain injury and its association with contact sports. We already have a key film to watch. *Concussion* (2015) ◄◄◄◄ , directed by Peter Landesman and starring Will Smith as the neuropathologist Dr. Bennet Omalu, is an important film about sports-related concussions and the recent interest in chronic traumatic encephalopathy (CTE). Omalu's slides show amyloid plaques and tau-positive threads in NFL football players. Omalu explains that gannets, woodpeckers, and rams have internal shock absorbers, adding, "God did not intend for us to play football." Neurologists may know, for example, that punch-drunk syndrome was first described by the British neurologist McDonald Critchley in a 1949 book as the "chronic traumatic encephalopathy of boxers."[51] James W. Geddes found tau neuropil threads in the depth of sulci in 1999. CTE is now being studied by several academic institutions in the United States, most notably by Boston University's Center for the Study of Traumatic Encephalopathy. This comprehensive work can be attributed to neuropathologist Ann McKee at the New England Veterans Administration Medical Centers in Boston.[52] Omalu's report of CTE in National Football League (NFL) player, coauthored by neurologist Steven DeKoskey and neurosurgeon Julian Bailes, was first published in the journal *Neurosurgery* in 2005.[53]

Concussion makes very effective use of sound-enhanced helmets crashing into each other, including NFL footage, in semi-documentary style clips showing kids playing rough. It must have a disturbing

---

[50] See Fleminger S. Long-Term Psychiatric Disorders after Traumatic Brain Injury. *Eur J Anaesthesiol Suppl*. 2008;42:123–130; Warriner EM, Velikonja D. Psychiatric Disturbances after Traumatic Brain Injury: Neurobehavioral and Personality Changes. *Curr Psychiatry Rep*. 2006;8:73–80; and Stuss DT. Traumatic Brain Injury: Relation to Executive Dysfunction and the Frontal Lobes. *Curr Opin Neurol*. 2011;24:584–589.

[51] Cantu RC, Bernick C. History of Chronic Traumatic Encephalopathy. *Semin Neurol*. 2020;40:353–358.

[52] McKee AC, Abdolmohammadi B, Stein TD. The Neuropathology of Chronic Traumatic Encephalopathy. *Handb Clin Neurol*. 2018;158:297–307.

[53] Omalu BI, DeKosky ST, Minster RL, Kamboh MI, Hamilton RL, Wecht CH. Chronic Traumatic Encephalopathy in a National Football League Player. *Neurosurgery*. 2005;57:128–134; discussion 128–134.

effect on viewers. In another scene, Omalu is told by a team doctor that he will face resistance from the NFL, a major multi-billion-dollar organization, which will cast doubt on his origin and immigration status. Basically, it is a David vs. Goliath story from screenplay writer and director Peter Landesman, pitting the Nigerian pathologist Omalu against the "monster" (Goliath) that is the NFL.[54] Any person will start to feel very uncomfortable here, and neurologists will shrug their shoulders in disbelief. Why has it come to this with these modern gladiators? The camera's frequent focus on screaming, fist-pumping fans after a slobber-knocker speaks volumes—a case in point.

Omalu maintains a visible presence through lectures, although his research has taken a back seat. Omalu has repeatedly clashed with the Boston group on criteria, and this group has clearly become the leading research group. Ann McKee was part of an expert panel of 20 clinician-scientists who published a consensus statement for traumatic encephalopathy syndrome underwritten by the National Institute of Neurologic Disorders and Stroke.[55] The statement concluded with: "A provisional level of certainty for CTE pathology is determined based on specific repeated head impact exposure thresholds, core clinical features, functional status, and additional supportive features, including delayed onset, motor signs, and psychiatric features." Again, Omalu countered aggressively arguing for much wider criteria.[56]

Stroke

Stroke has been underrepresented in film, which is puzzling given its increasing incidence.[57] Some films—*Legends of the Fall* (1994) and *Flawless* (1999)—explore stroke, but they do not deal with the human toll on relationships. Moreover, these two films show stroke portrayed in a curious way by two world-class actors. Robert De Niro plays a character with marked dysarthria and crooked smile in *Flawless* (1999) ◄ , and Anthony Hopkins plays a character who suffers a stroke in *Legends of the Fall* (1994) ◄ . Hopkins contorts his face to one side, moans and groans, but nevertheless can write full words on a chalkboard hanging on his neck. (It is closest to an anomic aphasia but otherwise unclassifiable.) He is also able, in the climactic shootout scene, to kill everyone using his paralyzed side—what a delightful irony!

In 1996, after suffering a severe stroke at 79, which impaired his ability to speak, Kirk Douglas underwent years of speech therapy. He made *Diamonds* in 1999, in which he played an old prizefighter recovering from a stroke. There is nothing acted with his marked dysarthria. In *St. Vincent* (2014), Bill Murray capably demonstrates aphasia with halting speech and neologisms—something that other renowned actors have not been able to do. In *Chappaquiddick* (2017), Bruce Dern plays Joseph P. Kennedy, Sr., who, at the time, had survived a major stroke with severe residual aphasia and was wheelchair bound. In his portrayal, he looks angry and accusatory with a pulled lip to mimic facial paralysis, mostly grunts. Despite being rendered speechless, when confronted with his son Ted after the tragic accident, who is trying to say he has it all under control, Joe is able to give a written note to his caregiver ("you lost my confidence; do as I say and never lose it again") and subsequently mumbles out a perfect damning

[54] See Martin M. *Doctor Behind "Concussion" Wanted to "Enhance the Lives" of Football Players*. National Public Radio (United States). December 27, 2015. In this National Public Radio interview, Omalu stated he personally felt the NFL committees insinuated he was a nobody practicing voodoo.

[55] Katz DI, Bernick C, Dodick DW, Mez J, Mariani ML, Adler CH, et al. National Institute of Neurological Disorders and Stroke Consensus Diagnostic Criteria for Traumatic Encephalopathy Syndrome. *Neurology.* 2021;96:848–863.

[56] Omalu B, Hammers J. Letter: Traumatic Encephalopathy Syndrome [TES] Is Not Chronic Traumatic Encephalopathy [CTE]: CTE Is Only a Subtype of TES. *Neurosurgery.* 2021; 89:E205-E206.

[57] The global prevalence rate is about 5 per 1000 person-years, corresponding to 33 million people living after a stroke. There is an increase in stroke among younger people. See Kissela BM, Khoury JC, Alwell K, Moomaw CJ, Woo D, Adeoye O, et al. Age at Stroke: Temporal Trends in Stroke Incidence in a Large, Biracial Population. *Neurology.* 2012;79:1781–1787; and Johnston SC, Mendis S, Mathers CD. Global Variation in Stroke Burden and Mortality: Estimates from Monitoring, Surveillance, and Modelling. *Lancet Neurol.* 2009;8:345–354.

sentence: "you will never be great." Bruce Dern's portrayal of a stroke is an example of "it looks like a duck, swims like a duck, quacks like a duck so it must be a duck" intent, and perfectly acceptable, so we need to put the major inaccuracies somewhat aside.[58]

The film director Michael Haneke, a luminary of cinema, must have sensed an opportunity when he made his film on stroke. *Amour* is extreme, as you would expect from a director who specializes in brutality. He expects his audience to be sickened and have nightmares. Many of us unfortunately can identify with his characters. Haneke forces us to not only watch the scenes but also to witness the events and feel the heaviness of compromising situations. Arguably, he does this by manipulating the audience. His inspiration for *Amour* was autobiographical: the suffering of a 92-year-old disabled aunt who asked him to help her commit suicide. He said he refused: "I am your legal heir, and I'd go to jail." She tried unsuccessfully to kill herself without his help and said, "Why have you done this to me?" (Two years later, she was successful.[59])

For me, *Amour* belongs at the top of the pantheon of neurocinema because it touches on everything that we as healthcare professionals encounter but often do not recognize or manage enough. *Amour* (2012) ◄◄◄◄ , stars Jean-Louis Trintignant, Emmanuelle Riva, and Isabelle Huppert. It received Palme d'Or Award at Cannes Film Festival, César Award for Best Film, Academy Award for Best Foreign Language Film, among the many US and international nominations. This is a multi-layered film about the life-changing effects of a stroke in the nearest and dearest. *Amour* changes one's outlook on the topic. *Amour* is a character study of two highly cultivated octogenarian piano teachers, Anne (Emmanuelle Riva) and Georges (Jean-Louis Trintignant), and their daughter Eva (Isabelle Huppert), played phenomenally by three icons of French cinema. The film is staged as classic theater and filled with emotional dialogue mixed with Schubert's impromptus. Anne suddenly develops neurologic symptoms, is devastated by a stroke, and deteriorates. Georges is now faced with the care of his wife. Initially, this seems not too much of a chore, but soon the care becomes increasingly complex.

Amour offers some clues on Anne's condition, but there is little to allow a detailed neurologic assessment. In an indelible scene, the sudden speech arrest and stare—with no recollection—are dramatic (Figure 4.7) and closest to what appears to be a complex partial seizure. She subsequently has difficulty pouring tea with her right hand. A major blockage in her carotid artery is found, followed by vascular surgery (endarterectomy), and she is left with profound right-sided weakness but no speech impediment. She is wheelchair bound. Before surgery, they have been told she could have a 5% chance of complications, but apparently, she does not belong to the supposedly 95% risk-free surgical group. There is no doctor–patient conversation about the complications, which seem to be treated as a matter of fact and just bad luck—a classic Haneke theme.

Soon after this surgery, Anne experiences another, far more devastating stroke. This should give pause to any neurologist. Stroke specialists—assuming the first presentation was a stroke and not a seizure or an unclear spell with asymptomatic carotid disease—may certainly come away with some reservations if (at least in this film) the result is much worse than before and quickly leads to another stroke. Carotid endarterectomy has been performed in octogenarians, and vascular surgeons have reported no increase in post-operative mortality or stroke when compared with "younger" patients. Carotid endarterectomy may be justified knowing the average life span of a woman of 85 years is still about 5 years; thus, there might be potential for benefit. All of this may not be terribly relevant to the main plotline of the movie, but it could prompt discussion about medical and surgical decisions in the vulnerable elderly population. Coercion into questionable surgery after a questionable event with eventually poor results could easily be another frightening

---

[58] The timing or veracity of the line can be questioned, and allegedly, the only word Joe said was "alibi." Sydney L. Nice People—Bruce Dern, Michael Kelly—Who Play Ruthless People Sample the Wares at Emmy Salon. Roger Friedman's Showbiz*411: Showbiz411.com; 2017.

[59] Shone T. Vulture: Michael Haneke Goes Cruelty-Free with *Amour*. *New York Magazine*. December 17, 2012.

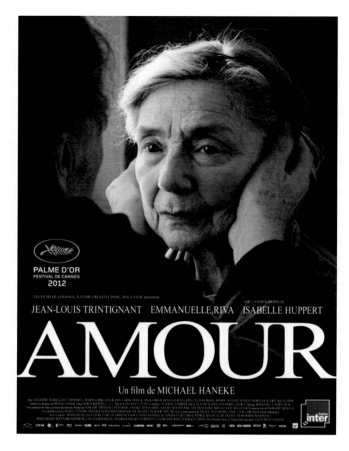

FIGURE 4.7 Film poster of Amour showing the key scene of Anne's sudden stare associated with speech arrest. (Used with permission of El Deseo Da S.L.U. photo; Miguel Bracho.)

theme for Haneke. Emmanuelle Riva's portrayal of a stroke victim is unsurpassed, and there is truly no better representation on film. Georges, played just as convincingly by Jean-Louis Trintignant, nurtures her to the best of his ability, although he is hampered by his own frailty. He provides for all transfers, performs passive range of motion, and even provides melodic intonation therapy. There is some humor in this part of the film, and it is very touching to see both Anne and Georges try to make

DIALOGUE

Amour

Georges	*What can I say? The carotid artery was blocked. They did an ultrasound scan, two in fact, and they said they had to operate on her. She was confused and scared.... They said the risk was very low and that if they didn't operate, she'd be certain to have a serious stroke.*
Eva	*And what do they say now?*
Georges	*Just that it didn't go well. It's one of the 5% that go wrong.*

the best of the situation. Together they look at photos from earlier times, eliciting Anne's response, "It is beautiful … this long life."

But now, they seem imprisoned in their Paris apartment. The only contact with the outside world is a concerned neighbor (and a pigeon). Professional support at this stage would have been expected, but Georges has little except for a biweekly visit with a family doctor, who tells Georges that admission to the hospital after the second stroke would have little use and staying home would spare her exhausting, futile tests. Also, Anne told him clearly that she would never want to be hospitalized again. She rejects any form of sympathy and gets visibly irritated when the topic comes up. Georges displays repressed pain, and by the time his exhaustion becomes visible, he fires a private nurse. He tells his alienated daughter, "None of this deserves to be shown."

A major element of the film is not only the loneliness but also the desire to be left alone, even if assistance is offered. This might be one of the main lingering themes for neurologists to consider: How do we organize care for stroke patients after they are dismissed from the hospital, and can we help to preserve their dignity? Do we appreciate the spouse's ordeal, and should we help?

Amour is not specifically about how society deals with the problems or infirmities of the elderly, but the film could still start that discussion. All of this cannot be waved away as if it could only happen in France (or Europe) because it can happen to anyone anywhere. In a very dramatic way, the film shows the familiar, yet often unrecognized, problems of denial and burnout in a caregiver. At the end of life, the ultimate sign of love may be to alleviate pain and suffering, which the movie shockingly portrays after Anne refuses fluids and frequently cries out in pain. Is this the crime of passion of advanced age?

Amour shows us the cruel change in a loving relationship brought about by illness. It is the realization that genuine, deeply rooted love for each other is the only thing we have, and it may be suddenly taken away for no good reason, just at random and unannounced. It also sheds a harsh light on the major problems with the home care of a neurologically disabled patient; I cringed each time Anne with her swallowing difficulties was given water and coughed. The lack of adequate neuro-palliation is very apparent and a warning.

A similar theme has recently been explored in the film *A Simple Life* (2012) ◄◄◄ , this time in Hong Kong. Ah Tao (played by Deanie Ip) suffers a non-dominant hemispheric stroke. She suddenly develops a (well-portrayed) left-sided hemiparesis and dysarthria. She will not allow her "master" (as she calls him), Roger (Andy Lau), to care for her, and she asks to go to a nursing home. Her main motivation is that she knows a second stroke is coming and that the end is near. Roger now feels responsible for her well-being (Ah Tao worked 60 years for his family), and his normal daily routine changes, visiting her frequently and just trying not to neglect her. Ah Tao tries to hold on to her dignity. The film has been somewhat overshadowed by the grandeur of *Amour*, but this work is equally important in depicting a new reality after a major stroke. There is full recovery, and the film does emphasize changing relationships and compassion, but it does not provide any more insight in the management of a stroke. The title refers to a simple life, and that is what is shown.

Equally memorable (discussed in the next section) is *The Diving Bell and the Butterfly* (2007), which is an extreme manifestation of an acute clot in the basilar artery. *Run & Jump* (2014) ◄ depicts bilateral frontal lobe infarcts, which the director has chosen as the origin of behavioral problems. The family's means of coping with the situation is insufficiently developed. In his portrayal, Conor (Edward MacLiam) seems more surly than abulic, more hesitant than aphasic, and more childish than inappropriate, but then, again, how do you play such an extremely rare and far more serious condition? In these films, other than showing a turn for the worse, dealing with adversity, and suddenly being hit by a major handicap, there is no further insight or explanation about stroke in the screenplay.

Observing the rapid neurologic decline of a loved one after stroke is unfathomable. These films focus on one major aspect of humanity—the desire to engage in and maintain loving relationships when such an ordeal strikes. *Amour* forces the viewer to ask these questions: Are we doing enough to prevent this isolation in couples? How might we better help them accept the reality? What are the consequences of certain medical care choices?[60] *Amour* and *A Simple Life* do not answer these questions—they do not have to do that—but they will force the viewers to think about them—for quite some time.

Locked-in Syndrome

Locked-in syndrome can have multiple causes, but a brainstem infarct is the most common.[61] The syndrome is complex and unique but utterly devastating. It became front and center after the release of the film *The Diving Bell and the Butterfly,* which is based on an autobiography "written" (blinked) by Jean-Dominique Bauby (*Le Scaphandre et Le Papillon*).[62] *The Diving Bell and the Butterfly* (2007) ◄◄◄◄ stars Mathieu Amalric, Emmanuelle Seigner. Marie-Josee Croze, Anne Consigny, and Max von Sydow and was directed by Julian Schnabel. Bauby, as played by Mathieu Amalric, was editor-in-chief of the fashion magazine *Elle* when he had a stroke at age 43. The cause is unknown, but in this age group, it most likely was a vertebral artery dissection with basilar artery occlusion (or, less likely, a pontine hemorrhage from an arteriovenous malformation). The locked-in syndrome makes it impossible for the patient to move, and only eye movement (eyelid blinking and up-and-down eye movements) are possible. There is no effective swallowing, and patients initially need assistance with ventilation. Vision, hearing, and feeling are all preserved. Here the mind is truly locked in a non-functioning body.

The American director, Julian Schnabel, appropriately decided to make the movie in French. In an interview with Charlie Rose,[63] Schnabel explained that he made the movie after his father died, as a self-help device to help himself deal with his own inevitable death. The film is accurate and unique in showing what Jean-Dominique would have seen in this condition. On the screen, Jean-Dominique's visual field is shown through the lens of the camera. Blinking is imitated by having the cinematographer move objects in front of the camera. His thoughts are the main narrative in the film. The camera shows double vision, difficulty focusing, and a constricted keyhole visual field, which would be quite correct if—in the setting of a basilar artery occlusion—the posterior occipital fields were involved. It also mostly shows his limited eye movements, although the camera does move vertically and horizontally and scans the room. (In locked-in syndrome, only vertical eye movements are possible, which then produce double vision.) Nonetheless, it remains highly speculative what patients see and notice in the acute phase. The rehabilitation and extreme effort of a speech therapist to communicate with him are notable and mostly correct. Standard orientation questions are asked ("Are we in Paris?" and "Does wood float?"). In patients with locked-in syndrome, establishing communication is, however, far more difficult in the early post-stroke phase, although later computer-assisted communication can be very effective.[64]

The film clearly shows an important technique of communicating, starting with the alphabet, using the most used letters (all attempts start with the letter E). Jean-Dominique was able to dictate a full work (Figure 4.8) but died soon after its publication. Jean-Dominique felt like he was living in a diving bell and could use his memory and imagination to go to past worlds. "My cocoon becomes less oppressive, and my mind takes flight like a butterfly."

The movie includes a forceful scene when he dictates, "I want to die," prompting a negative, overly dramatized reaction by the speech therapist, but according to the real transcriber, this was never mentioned (nor was she present during his demise, in contrast to what was shown in the film). Bauby's case is unique, and his book has given us unprecedented detail into the condition.

---

[60] Cecil R, Thompson K, Parahoo K, McCaughan E. Towards an Understanding of the Lives of Families Affected by Stroke: A Qualitative Study of Home Carers. *J Adv Nurs.* 2013;69:1761–1770.

[61] Goldberg C, Topp S, Hopkins C. The Locked-in Syndrome: Posterior Stroke in the ED. *Am J Emerg Med.* 2013;31:1294. e1291–e1293.

[62] Burki T. In the Blink of an Eye. *Lancet Neurol.* 2008;7:127.

[63] Rose C. Painter and filmmaker Julian Schnabel introduces the film, *"The Diving Bell and the Butterfly,"* in which main character suffers from "locked-in syndrome." January 31, 2008.

[64] Phipps E. A View from the Inside: The Diving Bell and the Butterfly. *J Head Trauma Rehabil.* 1999;14:89–90; and De Massari D, Ruf CA, Furdea A, Matuz T, van der Heiden L, Halder S, et al. Brain Communication in the Locked-in State. *Brain.* 2013;136:1989–2000.

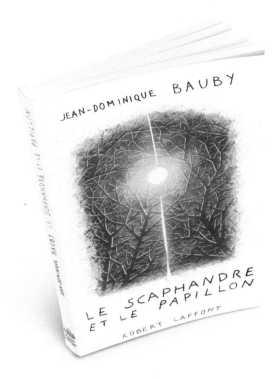

FIGURE 4.8 First edition of Bauby's book (also shown at the end of the film). Bauby blinked more than 200,000 times to produce this 137-page book describing his desolate state before he died. (Used with permission of Robert Laffont.)

Bauby's care was complicated and with complications.[65] Improved communication and meticulous care may lead to some prolongation of survival and even acceptable quality of life.

One of the existential fears is being trapped in one's own body and being misdiagnosed as comatose. In 1844, Alexandre Dumas described such a state in the fictional character of Monsieur Noirtier, who was in this condition for more than six years and was described as a "corpse with living eyes." Ironically, as an aside, Jean-Dominique noted in his book that he wanted to write a book based on Dumas's *The Count of Monte Cristo* before this ordeal.

DIALOGUE

The Diving Bell and the Butterfly

Dr. Lepage (neurologist)	*It won't comfort you to know that your condition is extremely rare …. We simply do not know the cause …. I'm afraid it's just one of those things.*
	In the past, we would have said you'd had a massive stroke. You would very probably have died. But now we have such improved resuscitation techniques that we're able to prolong life.
Bauby	*I do want to die. I really do.*

---

[65] At some point, a divine intervention through a pilgrimage to Lourdes was considered. See Chapter 6 and footnote.

An equally insightful book is by historian Tony Judt, *The Memory Chalet*,[66] where he describes his decline from amyotrophic lateral sclerosis (ALS) and becoming locked in. His book is, in his own words, "nostalgic recollections of happier days." His description evokes a major deafferentation syndrome that spares hearing, vertical eye movement, blinking sensation, and pain perception ". . . and there I lie; trussed, myopic and motionless like a modern-day mummy alone in my corporeal prison accompanied for the rest of the night only by my thoughts."

The Diving Bell and the Butterfly is an iconic film in this collection and should be required viewing for any medical professional. There are lessons to be learned about how best to communicate with patients, the power of communicating with respiratory therapists, and the tremendous challenge of rehabilitation.[67] It has rarely been transient, but patients with so-called *locked-in syndrome plus* (some arm preservation and some more bulbar function) can improve dramatically over time. The film correctly identifies improvement of oropharyngeal function as a potential prelude to recovery of speech. Paralysis almost always remains profound, as does the imbalance, creating major rehabilitation difficulties. Late recovery has not been reported, but patients may remain cognitively intact. Some improvements may occur, such as movement of fingers, which allows better signaling. Many of these patients die from pulmonary complication, which seems to have been Bauby's fate as well, but some, through a feat of great willpower, have survived for decades.

Alzheimer's Dementia

We have come to one of the most common neurologic degenerative brain disorders. Fiction features and documentaries on ungraceful aging and dementia are increasing in numbers, which almost justifies a separate book. Many films unfortunately present dementia as a consequence of old age (*On Golden Pond* [1981], *Agnes of God* [1985]). Some famous actors now are playing themselves as frail octogenarians and act as if normal situations are often too much. (See Jeanne Moreau in *Gebo and the Shadow* [2012] and Jean-Louis Trintignant in *Amour* [2012].) Early cinema featured nothing equivalent; the old were just very old, had difficulties with their offspring, pondered disappointments, were full of regret, and then they died. In *Tokyo Story* (1953), we hear one elderly character say, "Isn't life disappointing?" and after she dies: "If I had known things would come to this, I'd have been kinder to her while she was alive."[68] In modern cinema, it is also increasingly less common to see wellness in a venerable age—a sharp mind and freedom from decrepit joints.

And then there is dementia. There are some remarkable films portraying dementia in the elderly but also with young-age onset using the anticipation of grief and change in a loving relationship most recently in *Supernova* (2021) ◄◄◄ . We had to wait until recently to see the ultimate perfection with the release of *The Father*. But this was also the year in which we were continually annoyed by filmmakers who used patients with dementia as insane, slowly creeping creatures prone to random aggression—haunting tropes so commonly used in the Horror category (*Relic* [2020], ◄).

The Father (2020) ◄◄◄◄ stars Sir Anthony Hopkins and Olivia Colman and was directed by Florian Zeller. Anthony (played by Oscar- and BAFTA-winning Sir Anthony Hopkins) is a retired engineer living in a London luxury flat that he thinks is his own. He seems quite content, whistling operatic arias and listening to music on his headphone. He has maintained a regal attitude and is well groomed. But mystifying things happen in his flat. Unfamiliar people identify themselves as living in his flat, and then they disappear. Then the flat is changing: "where are these from?" pointing at chairs,

[66] Judt T. *The Memory Chalet*. 1st ed. London: Penguin Press; 2010.

[67] See Snoeys L, Vanhoof G, Manders E. Living with Locked-in Syndrome: An Explorative Study on Health Care Situation, Communication and Quality of Life. *Disabil Rehabil*. 2013;35:713–718; and Farr E, Altonji K, Harvey RL. Locked-in Syndrome: Practical Rehabilitation Management. *PMR*. 2021. Jan 19. Online ahead of print.

[68] Next to Ozu's moving and cruel classic, *Tokyo Story,* is McCarey's 1937 *Make Way for Tomorrow*. Orson Wells said, "*Make Way for Tomorrow* is the saddest film ever made and would make a stone cry. Nobody went." see Peter Bogdanovich on *Make Way for Tomorrow*, Criterion May 2015.

and now also the painting by his favorite daughter Lucy seems to have disappeared. He thinks he is losing all his valuables. "Everyone's just helping themselves ... if this goes on much longer, I will be stark naked." But there is more than meets the eye. We soon find out he accused his caregiver of stealing, and he was taken into his daughter's flat—Anne, brilliantly portrayed by Olivia Colman. Gradually, we see that he has great difficulty remembering names and chatters incessantly. (The brilliantly written script makes this slowly and incrementally apparent.) But he does not see any problems: "Take a good look at me. I can still manage on my own." Actually, he cannot, and with every new surprise or situation that he cannot comprehend, he retreats to his bedroom for comfort. A more immediate threat looms when Anne announces she is moving permanently to Paris. He is visibly shaken. "You are abandoning me ... What is going to become of me? ... The rats are leaving the ship."

The Father by the French playwright Florian Zeller (translated by Christopher Hampton) originated as a much-awarded play (*Le Père* and later *The Father* at London's West End and Broadway). The protagonist's name changed from Claude to André to Anthony. All action in the film occurs in the poorly lit apartment, which is ideal for sundowning. Zeller posits that dementia causes every day to be filled with sudden surprises and shocks but never explains it to the perplexed, disoriented viewer as he leads us into Anthony's discombobulated world. Is he plagued by hallucinations of strangers? At the doctor's office, Anne denies any intention of moving to Paris ("there has never been any question of me living in Paris"), making it most likely another paranoid delusion.

Hopkins is an estimable actor in what may be his best role since the forensic psychiatrist Hannibal Lecter. (He may even be compared to other ailing elders and paterfamilias including King Lear.) Hopkins reveals Anthony as a multi-faceted character. We see his charm when he meets his caregiver Laura (Amanda Peet) and tells her (to Anne's astonishment) that he used to be a tap dancer; she is very amused when he demonstrates his chops. Later, when she gives him his medication ("[This is] your little blue pill, it is a pretty color is it not?"), he becomes visibly irritated and fully cognizant of being patronized. ("Are you a nun? Why do you speak to me as if I am retarded?" "Thing is, I am very intelligent [and] you need to bear that in mind ... It is true I am very intelligent; sometimes I even surprise myself.")

Zeller achieves the feeling of descending into a strange, spatially disoriented world by jumbling the chronology and repeating scenes with slightly different setups in each one and maintaining the dialogue but also by having different actors play the same character. Filmmakers have typically used other tropes to show dementia in the early stages, such as vacant stares, detachment, hoarding, and loss of decorum. And they certainly do not want to leave the house (see Chapter 6). Anthony is very much the same: "Let me be absolutely clear; I am not leaving my flat."

There is a poignant dream sequence at the end of the film, where he opens a door to a hospital room and sees his other daughter before she died after a severe polytrauma. The next morning, he walks confusedly to the same door only to discover it is a storage room. Anthony seems to grasp this is reality and not a dream, but he is not sure. He deals with contradictions but seems unable to find his path. (Anthony Hopkins' facial mimicry in this scene demonstrates how stupendously effective he can be as an actor.) He occasionally looks out sadly from a window to the real world passing him by (Figure 4.9), but he stays in his flat for most of the film. Even a brief doctor visit seems to take place in his apartment complex, and this all adds to his perception of the world closing in.

The Father also deftly shows the misunderstandings (and risk of elder abuse) by outsiders. Anne's husband Paul (Rufus Sewell in a perfect cameo) is very doubtful: "Sometimes I think you are doing it deliberately." He is visibly irritated about having Anthony stay in their flat, which is clearly straining Anne and Paul's marriage, and wants him to go to a nursing home. Paul is verbally (and possibly also physically) aggressive to Anthony and reminds him they canceled their holiday because of his row with a caregiver. With sarcastic amusement, he asks, "Are you satisfied? You have a daughter that looks properly after you; you are lucky." In the last scene, Anthony says, "I'm losing all my leaves." and he ends up emotionally labile and deteriorated to the point of necessitating constant monitoring in a nursing home.

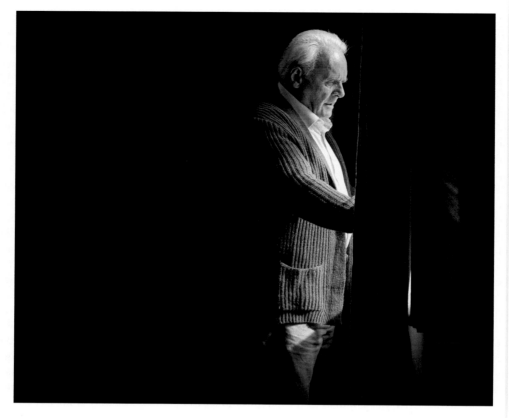

FIGURE 4.9 Anthony (Anthony Hopkins in *The Father*) confused in "his" dark flat (Photofest).

It is a remarkably penetrating film and much better than a prior version, *Floride* (2005) ◄◄◄ . Although also based on the play *Le Pere*, the screenplay of *Floride*, directed by Phillipe Le Guay and starring Jean Rochefort and Sandrine Kiberlain, is considerably different. The protagonist (Jean Rochefort) lives in a country mansion and is a retired CEO of a paper mill. His dementia becomes quickly evident after he has forgotten time and dates and has spent large amounts of money on antiques and useless bric-a-brac. Hoarding in his house is evident. Sexual innuendo is everywhere. His favorite daughter is in Miami, Florida, and at the end of the film, he is seen flying to her place. (This turns out to be a hallucination.) Upon arrival, he is guided through a door that transports him back to his nursing home. Such delusion is where the two films overlap, but the screenplays could not be more different. *The Father* is far closer to the play.

Another recent film is *Still Alice* (2014) ◄◄◄◄ starring Julianne Moore, who won an Oscar and numerous other awards, and directed by Richard Glatzer. "I am sorry I forgot I have Alzheimer's ... I wished I had cancer." In a major speech at Alzheimer's Association, she explains her experiences: "we become a comic ... Live in the moment I tell myself." Alice is a 50-year-old professor of linguistics who develops cognitive impairment. After the diagnosis, she is seen frantically testing word recall using all means possible—an unusual behavior that may perhaps be expected with her expertise. She uses a highlighter to highlight sentences she just said (a common device of patients). Normally, this early variant results in rapidly burdening effects on work and income—but Alice's world is privileged, and she seems to hold on to her job. Her family's response is unfriendly, initially detached, with many recriminations. Earlier screenplays on dementia often shortsightedly show deteriorating, angry high-functioning, intellectuals.

Still Alice is based on a well-researched fiction book and, through the Alzheimer's Association, whose banner appears in the film, Julianne Moore spoke with women who had been diagnosed with the disease. The film stops at the early stage and does not venture into the later realities. Julianne Moore registers either an anxious, showy disorientation or absent-mindedness. "I am defined by my intellect and afraid to lose it." Also, sudden, seconds-long blackouts and speech arrest are early signs. She tests herself by writing complex words on a blackboard that she can remember easily. She visits a nursing home and then saves a suicide video to use later. The film is a bit unusual but not improbable and of interest.[69]

Several notable films have appeared over the last two decades. *A Song for Martin* (En Sang for Martin, 2001) ⃰⃰⃰⃰ stars Sven Wollter, Viveka Seldahl, and Reine Brynolfsson and was directed by Bille August. The protagonist, an orchestra director and composer, first forgets the name of his manager, then confuses the name of his wife with his ex-wife, and, in a poignant scene, has a major derealization episode in the bedroom. He asks his wife to look up signs of cerebral hemorrhage, but because he has no paralysis, they conclude it must be something else. He has marked difficulties remembering that night and, in his confusion, tries hard to get all the details right. The general physician concludes it is over-exertion and tells him to slow down. The relentless deterioration is shown with him suddenly forgetting the score while directing the orchestra, and embarrassingly, he is led away. He demonstrates aggressive outbursts and accusatory behavior and urinates in a plant container in a restaurant. His wife lovingly copes with his decline but never leaves him alone until institutionalization. The film is a carefully scripted, accurate depiction of all phases of Alzheimer's disease. The protagonist shows the dazed and confused behavior and finally emptying of the mind.

A Song for Martin also discusses early management, and the neurologist argues against memantine (NMDA antagonist) and cholinesterase inhibitors (donepezil or rivastigmine) in the early phase, but this would be more easily prescribed in the United States. The neurologist also wrongly mentions reduced cerebral blood flow in explaining Alzheimer's disease, which is an antiquated theory ("cerebrovascular insufficiency"). In clinical practice, unfortunately, some patients are still prescribed vasodilators with no measurable effect.

The film arguably presents the phases of Alzheimer's disease in a somewhat reversed format. The neurologist diagnoses "incipient Alzheimer's" (now called mild cognitive impairment) when Martin suddenly loses track of an entire musical score. The inability to continue while the orchestra is playing is likely seen more often in advanced Alzheimer's disease but is used here—I am sure—to obtain a major dramatic effect. Sudden episodes of complete derealization while looking in the mirror are another highly unusual presentation. Alzheimer's disease is slowly progressive, but forgetting names is an early sign. The film is correct in associating name forgetting with work situations and not the more benign name forgetting in social situations. Misplacing objects and the inability to find one's way back home are also early signs of Alzheimer's disease. Nonetheless, early-onset Alzheimer's disease may present with behavioral or executive dysfunction in one-third of the patients.[70]

Away from Her (2006) ⃰⃰⃰⃰ stars Julie Christie, Gordon Pinsent, Olympia Dukakis, and Michael Murphy and was directed by Sarah Polley. It is of particular interest because it focuses more on the social conundrum facing spouses.[71] There is progression of Alzheimer's disease and particularly of interest due to the husband's reaction to and final acceptance of his wife's dementia. The film starts with Grant explaining, "I never wanted to be away from her. She had the spark of life." Fiona (Julie Christie) finds out that her memory is failing when she is cross-country skiing and cannot remember where she is. Her husband, Grant (Gordon Pinsent), notices that she put a frying pan in the freezer. Fiona shows a failing memory and the embarrassment and

[69] Balasa M, Gelpi E, Antonell A, Rey MJ, Sanchez-Valle R, Molinuevo JL, et al. Clinical Features and APOE Genotype of Pathologically Proven Early-Onset Alzheimer Disease. *Neurology*. 2011;76:1720–1725.

[70] Scheltens P, De Strooper B, Kivipelto M, Holstege H, Chetelat G, Teunissen CE, et al. Alzheimer's Disease. *Lancet*. 2021;397:1577–1590.

[71] Macip S. Love's Memories Lost. *Lancet Neurol*. 2007;6:675.

denial that often accompany these episodes in a very accurate way. Fiona does not know when they bought the cottage, has difficulty finding her coat, and seems to be very aware of her evolving deficit. In fact, she reads a book on Alzheimer's disease and, specifically, a chapter on caregivers' burden and how they may have to cope with accusatory behavior ("sounds like a regular marriage").

We are told Fiona is young; indeed, she may be in her mid-60s after marrying early and 45 years of marriage. When she starts wandering, her husband drives through the neighborhood and eventually finds her shivering on a bridge. They both seem to realize the time has come for her to go to assisted living. Here she meets another man and becomes his caregiver. (The nursing-home staff is not surprised; this happens often.) Her husband visits often, but her answers are platitudes, and she is unaware of his presence. However, she remains composed and does not lose her decorum ("she is a lady"). Most interestingly and accurately portrayed is the part when Grant wonders if she is putting on a charade ("some kind of punishment") by not recognizing him as her husband but then having periods of lucidity. She progresses, stays in bed for weeks, and then must be moved to another section where the more severely affected people reside ("the second floor"). The movie is based on a short story by Alice Munro.

DIALOGUE

Away from Her

Fiona   *Once the idea is gone, everything is gone. I just wander around trying to figure out what it is that was so important earlier.*

Husband   *She is in her own world. Perhaps that is what she always wanted.*

One of the most deceptive in its depiction of dementia is the love story in *The Notebook* (2004) ◄ . The film starts with an older couple, James Garner (Duke) and Gena Rowlands (Allie). Allie has advanced Alzheimer's disease, and there are multiple flashbacks to their complicated romance. She does not recognize her children. The children tell Duke to come home, but he wants to be with "his sweetheart." He reads her a story she likes very much, but she does not recognize that it is her own life story. ("It is a good story. I heard it before, perhaps more than once?") Suddenly, in a moment of lucidity, all becomes clear, and she remembers everything—but only briefly—and immediately snaps into agitated, angry behavior. Other moments of lucidity occur despite a more progressive decline. At one point, she asks, "What will happen when I cannot remember anything anymore?" to which he answers, "I'll be here." The film points toward a common theme of caregivers hoping for a single moment when there is full recollection, but it is misleading in suggesting that emotional bonding could lead to such a lucky moment. Terminal lucidity exists, but it is exceptional.

The general public may not have seen many films on dementia. A paper by Asai discusses ten films from Japanese cinema.[72] This paper emphasizes the difficulty of telling patients they have Alzheimer's and the anger it can cause in spouses. Despair, disbelief, anger toward the spouse, suicide attempts, and care of a severely disabled husband (played by Ken Watanabe) are shown in *Memories of Tomorrow* (2006) ◄◄ , a popular movie in Japan. His method of coping with Alzheimer's is difficult to watch; he somewhat overplays the frustration faced by early Alzheimer's (his anger is dramatic). The age of onset here is late 40s in a business executive, further adding to the drama.

Memories of Tomorrow has some recognizable themes (dementia in a highly functioning person) and some new ones. It uses early-onset Alzheimer's as a theme—a highly uncommon scenario. The onset of

---

[72] Asai A, Sato Y, Fukuyama M. An Ethical and Social Examination of Dementia as Depicted in Japanese Film. *Med Humanit.* 2009;35:39–42.

dementia is introduced when a wife notices her husband missing an exit while driving and then notic-ing that he has bought many shampoo bottles—more than needed—which prompts her to seek medi-cal advice. We see him deteriorating, not being able to find his office and running frantically through Tokyo. We see him unable to find his wife in a restaurant, accusing her of infidelity, unable to speak at his daughter's wedding, and eventually retiring to a serene home in the woods. In the final scenes, he watches sunsets while being vegetative in a wheelchair. The film moved many viewers in Japan.

Other lesser films have used dementia as a theme but without further insight. *Firefly Dreams* (2001) is about a self-absorbed teenager taking care of a person with Alzheimer's disease. The Hindi films *Black* (2005) and *I Did Not Kill Gandhi* (2005) have depicted Alzheimer's without much distortion of medi-cal facts. In *U Me Aur Hum* (*You, Me and Us*, 2008), the pregnant protagonist suffers from early-onset dementia, but the portrayal is theatrical and does not provide any additional insight.

Several other films have depicted certain aspects of Alzheimer's disease quite well. *Small World* (2010) ⫷ is Bruno Chiche's French-language adaptation of the Austrian bestseller by Martin Suter. (The French title, *Je n'ai rien oublié* or "I have not forgotten anything," is a far more specific title). This well-structured story uses the fact that although Alzheimer's patients lose track of the present, childhood memories return to them vividly, which here might inadvertently uncover a dark family secret.

In the celebrated film *Nebraska* (2013) ⫷⫷ , the leading character with dementia, Woody (played by Bruce Dern), shows the urge to wander but also shows detachment, and he answers many questions about the past with "I don't remember." He is determined to claim prize money from a million-dollar sweepstakes he is convinced he has won. His son David (Will Forte) decides to play along and drive from Montana to Nebraska to cash it in. The film is of interest because it shows the futility of such a decision (his father falls and ends up in the hospital to get stitches) and how little impact it has on the son-and-father relationship despite an admirable, well-intentioned attempt.

These acts of kindness are also seen in the more recent film, *Falling* (2020) ⫷ , which is about very complex, toxic family dynamics, child abuse, adultery, divorce, and an unrelenting agitated protago-nist Willis (Lance Hendriksen) with advanced dementia. The old man's ceaseless raging is loaded with smutty, misogynistic, racist, and homophobic yells against his son, who was in the military ("Being a fairy outweighs whatever you think you have done for your country" and "California is for flag burners"). He bombards his son John with insults throughout the film and never seems to stop. Willis is unhappy, and John accepts what is coming to him most of the time, but sometimes it gets to him and says sarcastically "Every once in a while, you still surprise me." It is unclear what the film is trying to say—be prepared for the devil to come out when the natural inhibitions come loose with advanced dementia? Viggo Mortensen, who wrote and directed the film, unfortunately, has a high prevalence of dementia in his family. One notable theme is how to maintain some sort of communication with persistent kindness when communication has always been virtually impos-sible and now made worse by dementia.[73]

Finally, I would be remiss if I do not briefly mention *Iron Lady* (2011), which depicts Margaret Thatcher's visual and auditory hallucinations at the very end of the film.

Dementia is often accurately depicted in film and usually involves early but not terminal care. The portrayal often involves disorientation and wandering but rarely combative behavior. It emphasizes the inability of Alzheimer's patients to recognize themselves, their actions, and their spouses. The fiction films can be seen together with the documentaries discussed in Chapter 5.

Parkinson's Disease

A Late Quartet (2012) ⫷⫷⫷ stars Christopher Walken, Philip Seymour Hoffman, and Catherine Keener and was directed by Yaron Zilberman. How Parkinson's disease can affect someone's life

---

[73] The inclusion of horror-film director Davis Cronenberg as a proctologist detracts from the movie's seriousness.

and musical ability over time is the major theme here. The film deals with the consequences of early diagnosis of Parkinson's disease in a closely knit string quartet celebrating its 25th anniversary.

DIALOGUE

A Late Quartet

Neurologist	*Well, based on the examination that we just ran and the complaints you've described to me, it's my opinion that you are experiencing the early symptoms of Parkinson's disease.*
Patient	*From this... from what we just did, you can tell that?*
Neurologist	*Yes, I am afraid I can, but we should still run a blood test and have the MRI.*
Patient	*Wow.*

The representation of Parkinson's disease in this film is very accurate because the director asked neurologists, Stanley Fahn and Lewis Rowland, among others, for advice. Christopher Walken plays Peter, the cellist and founder of the quartet. During a practice session, he is suddenly unable to move his left hand and fingers well enough (Figure 4.9) to produce a colorful vibrato (oddly enough, primarily an oscillating movement of the wrist). The female neurologist is played by Madhur Jaffrey, who is compassionate and instructs him to make rapid hand-opening and -closing movements, to stand up and walk a few steps, and to turn around. He shows left-sided hypokinesis, with no instability in arm swing, gait, or balance.

The consequences are substantial, and Peter knows that he should be replaced despite being treated with medication. "I may be able to play one season, but then it will be over." All of them are aware that their season choice—Beethoven's *Late String Quartet Opus 131 in C-Minor*, with its 40 minutes of uninterrupted playing—requires perfectly functioning basal ganglia.

Christopher Walken may be the most ideal actor to play Peter, and he truly shows the appearance of hypokinesis and lack of mimicry. (Playing a subdued and monotonous character is one of Walken's trademarks and comes to good use; Figure 4.10.) As befits a serious film, it also shows a Parkinson's rehabilitation group (the Brooklyn Parkinson's group, known for dance therapy), which emphasizes that "in Parkinson's disease everything gets small ... everything contracts and

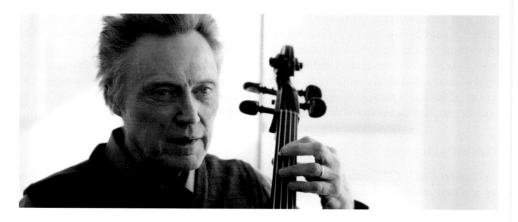

FIGURE 4.10 Christopher Walken in *The Late Quartet* (Everett Collection, Inc.).

closes in," and the goal is to "push those boundaries out." After treatment, Peter has a brief visual hallucination where he sees his late wife (a mezzo-soprano) singing, and there is an episode where he contemplates suicide—all familiar issues in the long-term management of Parkinson's disease.

Suddenly, and much to his surprise, he discovers during a teaching class that he can play very well ("the medication is working"), and he rallies his quartet members to practice again. However, while he was resting and taking a break, the supposedly coherent and civilized quartet has fallen apart due to marital problems and extramarital flings. The quartet suffers a cathartic explosion during a practice session. Nevertheless, they reconvene and start the new season. During the performance, Peter realizes that he cannot play the *Presto* fifth movement, and he suddenly stops and, after a moving speech, introduces a replacement cellist.

The film shows the enormous impact a tiny change in motor function can bring about—common knowledge for all neurologists first diagnosing a neurodegenerative disease. When professional musicians develop Parkinson's disease, it is often the end of a career and, sadly, early in the process. Inability to make rapid fingering shifts results in loss of tempo; additionally, long passages of music requiring close harmonization with other musicians are quite challenging. While many other patients with Parkinson's disease are successfully treated and lead valuable lives, the demands on a musician, playing complex musical parts and memorizing transitions, may become too challenging both physically as well as mentally if cognition becomes impaired in later stages. In these situations, successfully treating the movement disorder in tremor-dominant asymmetric Parkinson's disease may not resolve the issue completely. It is also likely much different than the treatment of focal dystonia—a disorder commonly found in musicians.

Musicians and composers may have a major illness, just like anyone else, but there is some fascination about how it can affect their creativity.[74] Systemic and neurologic illnesses have been carefully studied in many classical composers, with a considerable presence of venereal disease.[75] Parkinson's disease is not well known in famous contemporary musicians or composers. Johnny Cash was diagnosed with Parkinson's disease and then, allegedly, multiple system atrophy. The latter diagnosis may have spared his cognitive abilities and even enabled him to record landmark albums before his final months (i.e., the legendary *American Recordings*). Most rock-and-roll musicians—with some taking a variety of potentially damaging drugs—seem to have been spared from nigrostriatal injury.

A much less convincing film is *Love & Other Drugs* (2010) ◄, which stars Anne Hathaway and Jake Gyllenhaal and was directed by Edward Zwick. Hathaway plays a patient (Maggie) with young-onset Parkinson's. Her representation—tapping fingers that nonsensically mimic resting tremor—is all we see. She also tries to open a pillbox during a tremor, possibly simulating abnormal finger-eye coordination as an early sign, but again with unusual trembling. This film offers no insight into the daily challenges and fatigue. The film shows a self-help meeting of (real) Parkinson's patients, but it is characterized by juvenile jokes. However, there is one key scene where the husband of a patient with advanced Parkinson's disease is asked if he has any advice. He tells Maggie's boyfriend, "My advice is to go upstairs, pack up your bags, leave a nice note, and find yourself a healthy woman." In another key scene, Maggie points out a reasonable list of other diagnoses that have been considered—in her case, essential tremor, Wilson's disease, multiple system atrophy, progressive supranuclear palsy, obscure dystonia, and surprisingly, neurosyphilis. She also mentions a "scary 6-month brain-tumor week," but in the end, "it turned out to be old-fashioned Parkinson's disease." The film has some good to say about acceptance of Parkinson's disease, but there is little to advance the knowledge of living with Parkinson's disease, and much of it is dismissive and contrived.

[74] Bogousslavsky J, Boller F, eds. *Neurological Disorders in Famous Artists*. Basel, Switzerland: Karger; 2005.
[75] Neumayr A. *Music and Medicine*. Lansing, MI: Medi-Ed Pr; 1994.

Early Parkinson's disease (called Stage I in this film and likely referring to the Hoehn and Yahr scale indicating unilateral disease) has other features, typically difficulty with slow movement, hesitation, and difficulty standing up; less mimicry or "poker face"; and less gesticulation with speech. Tremor occurs when the hand is at rest in a lap, and the voice becomes soft and monotone. Voice and face akinesia occur first, followed by rigidity, gait abnormalities, limb bradykinesia, and finally tremor. In young-onset Parkinson's disease, postural reflexes are often preserved. We see none of this in Maggie, even when she is shown to be off medication.[76]

Music and Parkinson's disease are closely connected, generally in a good way. Patients with Parkinson's disease may successfully use musical rhythms for gait initiation, and the enjoyment of music—hearing a favorite musical piece or song—not only may remain present for quite some time but could potentially also lift them up physically. However, slowing of motor function hampers musicians. During his farewell speech in *A Late Quartet*, Peter explains that he cannot keep up and he cannot play the piece in one uninterrupted session *(attacca):* "It is Beethoven's fault."

Brain Tumor

Two key films—dramatically different in approach and accuracy—deserve detailed discussion. *Dark Victory* (1939) ⚔ stars Bette Davis, George Brent, Humphrey Bogart, Geraldine Fitzgerald, and Ronald Reagan and was directed by Edmund Goulding. *Dark Victory* premiered on March 7, 1939, but the plot was not revealed until opening night. Ed Sikov—Bette Davis's biographer—wrote that filming *Dark Victory* was "nerve wracking for Bette, almost to the point of debilitation."[77] The subject matter was just too much for her, and she sobbed constantly during the filming of the last scene.

Dark Victory is a farce when it comes to neurologic manifestations of a brain tumor.[78] The protagonist gets headaches after some sort of aggravation, develops sudden double vision, and falls off a horse but still refuses to see a doctor. ("He will say it is a hangover and I am smoking too many cigarettes.") She then notices burns on her right hand. She sees a neurosurgeon Dr. Steele (George Brent), who examines her (see Chapter 3 for details) and subsequently consults three other physicians and advises her to proceed with surgery for brain tumor. When he discovers that the tumor is malignant, he still tells her that there will be "complete surgical recovery."

DIALOGUE

Dark Victory

Neurosurgeon	*Technically it is called glioma.*
Patient	*Sounds like a plant.*
Neurosurgeon	*Yes, it is like a plant—a parasitic one.*
Friend	*How will it come?*
Neurosurgeon	*Peacefully, God's last small mercy.*

Dark Victory, which, I suspect, is known by few neurologists as a major motion picture on the presentation of a brain tumor, is bold because it addresses the dilemma of how to discuss the diagnosis.

---

[76] Postuma RB, Lang AE, Gagnon JF, Pelletier A, Montplaisir JY. How Does Parkinsonism Start? Prodromal Parkinsonism Motor Changes in Idiopathic REM Sleep Behaviour Disorder. *Brain.* 2012;135:1860–1870.

[77] Sikov E. *Dark Victory: The Life of Bette Davis.* 1st ed. New York: Henry Holt and Company; 2007.

[78] For a more detailed analysis, see Wijdicks EFM. "Dark Victory" (Prognosis Negative): The Beginnings of Neurology on Screen. *Neurology.* 2016;86:1433–1436.

Clinical presentation of a malignant brain tumor can be non-distinctive. It is usually of recent onset over days rather than months and may be a change in pattern in a patient with prior headaches. Nausea and vomiting are common (but rarely seen in film). Seizures are presenting symptoms in up to 40% of patients and are often focal rather than generalized. Personality changes are also common.[79]

After surgery, she demonstrates good walking (even demonstrates walking backward and tests her own reflexes). When her brain tumor recurs, it presents as diminished vision ("getting dark," hence the title), becoming blind. It all happens within minutes. She says goodbye to her dogs, unsteadily climbs the stairs, goes to bed, and dies peacefully. *Dark Victory* contains scenes in which doctors give misleading information and a highly unusual clinical presentation. Nothing can even be attributed to the Zeitgeist of the times. From a historical perspective, *Dark Victory* conjures several important issues, which make it potentially interesting for neurologists. Bette Davis' cinematic portrayal of the vicissitudes of living with a brain tumor (and not knowing it) is close to the reality of denial and a persistent hope for a cure. Her pressured speech may signal the general anxiety she feels. *Dark Victory* depicts progressive, rapidly fatal neurologic disease but also depicts a doctor withholding information from the patient. The film was included at #32 in AFI's 100 Years ... 100 Passions[80] and considered by many critics to be a major poignant work at the time. It is a prime example of how the interpretation of a film—the neurology message and cinematic message—can be so different.

The topic would not re-emerge until 1984 with the film *Garbo Talks*, which tells the story of a terminally ill woman (Anne Bancroft) with a dying wish to meet the recluse Greta Garbo. This is a "bucket list" movie in which everyone finds peace in the end.

A much better film is the autobiographical *Declaration of War* (*La Guerre est déclarée*, 2011) starring Valérie Donzelli, Jérémie Elkaïm, César Desseix, and Gabriel Elkaïm, directed by Valérie Donzelli and written by Valérie Donzelli and Jérémie Elkaïm. The writers and their children play the lead roles. It was even filmed in the same hospital where the actual events occurred. The film is, therefore—albeit somewhat fictionalized—reasonably precise, certainly when it comes to the medical and neurologic aspects. Romeo and Juliette are their fictional names, and their child (Adam) does not seem to thrive at the age of three and then has difficulty walking and vomits. A facial asymmetry is noticed. This leads to multiple visits to physicians, who use largely ambiguous language that confuses everybody. The parental stress is enormous, and the contact with physicians is rough and distanced. At one point, Romeo says to Juliette, "No outsmarting the doctors, no idiotic theories, no Internet."

DIALOGUE

Declaration of War

Parents	*Are there possible aftereffects?*
Neurosurgeon	*There must not be any.*
Parents	*But if there are?*
Neurosurgeon	*There will be no aftereffects. [Puts hands on mother's shoulder.] Get some rest. Don't count eggs in the hen's ass. Sleep well. See you tomorrow.*

---

[79] See Omuro A, DeAngelis LM. Glioblastoma and Other Malignant Gliomas: A Clinical Review. *JAMA*. 2013;310:1842–1850; and Ma R, Taphoorn MJB, Plaha P. Advances in the Management of Glioblastoma. *J Neurol Neurosurg Psychiatry*. 2021. Online ahead of print.

[80] *AFI's 100 YEARS ... 100 PASSIONS*. American Film Institute (United States). June 11, 2002.

The movie is about how having a very sick child affects parents. It is a must-see film for pediatric neurologists and residents. There are family frictions, strangers who have an opinion, irritations in the hospital, extreme financial burden (even in "free healthcare Europe"), and irreparable strains on their marriage. The narrator says, "They stopped working for two years. They separated, got back together several times, and then separated for good. Each started a new life." The end shows a final visit with their (this time) compassionate neurosurgeon, and when seen five years later, the child is cured. The war has been won.

The film is useful because of several neurologic aspects. First, the presentation that "something might be wrong" and the delay to come to a final diagnosis in a young child are not uncommon. In children less than two years old, behavioral changes, seizures, vomiting, and head tilt are common (and non-specific). Not infrequently, only one-third of the children are diagnosed within one month of onset of presentation due to a doctor's delay but also parental delay. The film does inappropriately show the neurologist vacillating on outcome with a generally pessimistic outlook. Most concerning, however, is the presentation of a tumor diagnosed as "rhabdoid." It will not be apparent to most viewers and even general neurologists, but atypical teratoid rhabdoid tumors are very aggressive, with high mortality in the first year. It would be very unusual to survive disease-free from this diagnosis. (A "10%" survival is mentioned here, and even that may be too optimistic.) Ifosfamide carboplatin and etoposide (ICE) treatment is mentioned (a common approach in Europe, and different in the United States, where methotrexate, high-dose chemotherapy, and stem cell rescue are considered).[81]

Some other lesser-known films deserve mention. In the Dutch movie *Turkish Delight* (1973) ◄◄◄ , one of the most accomplished works of Paul Verhoeven, the protagonist, Olga (Monique van de Ven), is diagnosed with a brain tumor after she loses concentration at her work (bottles fall off the conveyor belt). She is then found unresponsive and, in the next scene, crying in the middle of a pneumoencephalogram procedure. Her response to this cruel procedure is well depicted here and very real. The scene showing (now obsolete) pneumoencephalography is among the most memorable shocking moments in this film.[82] In the rest of the film, she displays infantile, aggressive behavior. A nurse runs in to give her sedative drugs. ("Bad, bad Missus. What are we? Wild and naughty.") In a deeply sad ending, she dies the next morning. Again, there is a misrepresentation here of wild psychotic behavior in a patient with a newly diagnosed brain tumor.

Finally, for an invasive glioblastoma that is responsible for enhanced mental abilities in the outrageously silly *Phenomenon* (1996), see Chapter 9.

Infections of the Brain

Surprisingly, few films deal with meningitis and only with outbreaks. The main difficulty for screenwriters, I suppose, is that meningitis affects just one person, and diseases are more compelling when they affect and kill many (and do so in short order). Such outbreaks (usually a virus of some kind) occasionally appear as Hollywood themes. The ultimate medical disaster movie about a prevalent virus is *Contagion* (2011) ◄◄◄◄ directed by Steven Soderbergh. The fictional virus MEV-1 is a mix of bat and pig virus ("somewhere the wrong bat met up with the wrong pig") and is modeled after the Nipah virus outbreak of April 1999 in Malaysia, when 265 cases of febrile encephalitis were reported. Because the virus is neurotropic, the initial symptoms are headache

---

[81] See Huttner A. Overview of Primary Brain Tumors: Pathologic Classification, Epidemiology, Molecular Biology, and Prognostic Markers. *Hematol Oncol Clin North Am.* 2012;26:715–732; and Crawford J. Childhood Brain Tumors. *Pediatr Rev.* 2013;34:63–78.

[82] Several prominent neurologists and neurosurgeons were alarmed by the "side effects" of the procedure, and it was very uncomfortable at best. See also Lutters B, Koehler PJ. Cerebral Pneumography and the 20th Century Localization of Brain Tumors. *Brain.* 2018;141:927–933.

and dizziness followed by respiratory symptoms, seizures, and rapid-onset coma. *Contagion* does not show specific neurologic manifestations or neurologic involvement except for one terminal seizure. The filmmakers consulted Ian Lipkin, an epidemiologist and Professor of Neurology at Columbia University, before devising the imaginary virus. The film asks the important questions of how the public health organizations respond in such a disaster scenario and how quickly vaccines would be developed.

How could we have known the portending quality of this film? During the height of the SARS-COV-2 pandemic, there was a spike in the streaming of the film.[83] *Contagion* opens with a black screen, and we hear a woman coughing. The fictional virus MEV-1 hits the brain (and not the lungs as in the current pandemic), and we see deadly seizures and exposed brains with surprised pathologists. In *Contagion*, the virus spreads quickly across the globe and kills its victims via a simple chain of germs—from a credit card to a bartender's hand, to the cash register, to the glass on the bar. It is a great depiction of fomite transmission (i.e., the proven concept that some infectious agents remain detectable on plastic and stainless-steel surfaces for days) and how one person can set a pandemic in motion. We even get an explanation of R-naught. *Contagion* has another clear message: it appropriately asks viewers to question how our leaders and public health organizations respond to such situations but also how quickly industries can manufacture a vaccine. Sadly, we now know and must conclude that the COVID pandemic was a global public health disaster and may remain until billions of people worldwide are vaccinated and no more new far more serious variants arise.[84] *Contagion* portrays an infectious disease spreading at an alarming rate, a world with public overreaction, and slow, clueless governmental response, although the WHO and CDC are presented as trustworthy and accountable. While trying to find the source of the virus, a CDC-dispatched researcher dies, and others take considerable risks. The carnage is tremendous, and the Red Cross runs out of body bags—another nod to the current pandemic, in which New York City needed freezer trucks to haul away cadavers when morgues reached capacity. *Contagion* mentions social distancing by name, handwashing, and isolation but does not address the ongoing concern of intensivists that hospitals may suddenly become overwhelmed with severe viral (and bacterial) pneumonia patients, all needing ventilators. However, in this movie, the virus is even more deadly. A vaccine is found very quickly but in a strange way. A CDC research scientist speeds up the process by inoculating herself with the vaccine, and it becomes available for general use in just a few months. *Contagion* is a great movie, not because it now looks so plausible, but because the filmmakers asked epidemiologists Larry Brilliant and Ian Lipkin to participate in the writing of the screenplay and to build a clinical scenario of such an epidemic.[85]

There are two interesting movies on meningitis outbreaks. *The Courageous Dr. Christian* (1940) stars Jean Hersholt, Dorothy Lovett, and Robert Baldwin and was directed by Bernard Vorhaus. It is one of several movies made about the character Dr. Christian in the late 1930s and early 1940s. Dr. Christian is an eminent country doctor played by Danish actor Jean Hersholt. This movie, set at the end of the Depression, has as its major theme a meningitis epidemic, the outbreak of which apparently starts in "Squatter Town," a section of town with poor sanitation. The people—the poor and the

---

[83] For some paradoxical reason, this fictional film was reassuring to some and helped them to cope with quarantine Testoni I, Rossi E, Pompele S, Malaguti I, Orkibi H. Catharsis through Cinema: An Italian Qualitative Study on Watching Tragedies to Mitigate the Fear of COVID-19. *Frontiers in Psychiatry*. 2021;12 :622174.

[84] *The Lancet* editor Richard Horton offers a brilliant and peerless analysis of the current pandemic and explains the public health failure. See Horton R. *The COVID-19 Catastrophe: What's Gone Wrong and How to Stop It Happening Again*. 2nd ed. Cambridge: Polity; 2021. Equally informative are documentaries on the early days of the pandemic in Wuhan by Nanfu Wang (*In the Same Breath* 2021) and Weixi Chen and Hao Wu (*76 Days* 2020).

[85] There are important articles about how the collaboration of scientists can make films more plausible. See Bernstein R. Science on Set. *Cell*. 2013;154:949–950; Shah S. Viral Disaster Movie. *The Lancet*. 2011;378:1211; Lipkin WI. The Real Threat of "Contagion." New York ed. *The New York Times*. 2011.

needy—are a constant concern ("people living around the bend"), and the city board decides to remove them. It finally comes to a major confrontation between Dr. Christian and the police.

DIALOGUE

Dr. Christian	*Chief, there is a child in here with spinal meningitis.*
Chief	*That does not sound serious to me, doctor. …. It is just a stall.*
Dr. Christian	*It is a highly contagious disease with [a] high mortality rate. A single case may rapidly spread over the whole district.*
Mayor	*This meningitis is just a kid disease, isn't it?*
Dr. Christian	*Hardly, it hits all ages and classes.*

The film shows a child sensitive to light and sound who cries easily. (Mother: "Don't be such a cry-baby.") Dr. Christian (stroking his chin while looking serious, see also Chapter 1) thinks the child may have meningitis. He performs a lumbar puncture, and the film shows him finding the characteristic inflammatory polynucleated cells under the microscope. The mayor asks if it is only the "squatters," but Dr. Christian—irritated by the lack of compassion for the poor—tells him the infection may also get to the town administrators.

Dr. Christian orders everybody to be inoculated, and he creates makeshift hospitals. Newspaper headlines are shown: "Crisis Looms. Disease Getting Beyond Control." We see numerous people on gurneys, but there soon is a respite with no new cases, a decline in the number of cases, and improvement in the condition of patients.

Most likely, the outbreak in *The Courageous Dr. Christian* represented meningococcal meningitis, which attacked major American cities in the early 1900s. (The meningococcus bacterium was identified in 1905 by Simon Flexner.[86]) The film accurately mentions treatment with sulfa drugs and the use of serotherapy (administration of meningococcal horse anti-serum). Epidemic meningitis was a major concern in the United States, particularly in a country mobilized for war. The first randomized trial involved nearly 14,000 men at US Army basic training centers, and the polysaccharide vaccine proved to be safe, with a 90% reduction in cases.

Throughout the world, meningococcal meningitis remains a formidable problem (0.5 cases per 100,000 in the United States, but 10–1,000 per 100,000 in Africa). Meningitis epidemics caused by meningococcal disease are seen in one- to two-thirds of infected persons, with sepsis in 30% of the cases resulting in hypotension and intravascular coagulation (causing petechiae and purpura). Survivors face major disability including hearing loss, seizures, and spasticity. These outbreaks may lead to rapid demise of many children, and outbreaks in the Western world still occur.[87] Every outbreak is met with alarm, and therefore, the response is accurately depicted in this film.

Another film with meningitis as a plot driver is *In Enemy Hands* (2004) ◄ , which stars William Macy, Til Schweiger, and Thomas Kretschman and was directed by Tony Giglio. The plot primarily involves a US Navy submarine in the Second World War. The movie names, for the first time, meningococcal meningitis as a diagnosis. One of the crew members starts coughing, then detects a rash, and starts vomiting later. The medic—although not sure—suggests meningococcal meningitis but, due to patient

---

[86] Flexner S, Jobling JW. Serum Treatment of Epidemic Cerebro-Spinal Meningitis. *J Exp Med*. 1908;10:141–203.

[87] See Halperin SA, Bettinger JA, Greenwood B, Harrison LH, Jelfs J, Ladhani SN, et al. The Changing and Dynamic Epidemiology of Meningococcal Disease. *Vaccine*. 2012;30 Suppl 2:B26–B36; and Stephens DS, Greenwood B, Brandtzaeg P. Epidemic Meningitis, Meningococcaemia, and *Neisseria meningitidis*. *Lancet*. 2007;369:2196–2210.

refusal, is unable to quarantine the man, who soon dies. The boat gets torpedoed by the Germans, and they abandon the ship only to be rescued by the German crew. Once aboard, the American captain has the same symptoms but decides not to tell. "Keep it between you and me. I do not want to startle the crew." Soon eight members fall ill. One of the crew members recognizes the rash because his sister had it and died in seven days. Soon the whole boat is coughing, but the outbreak gets little further attention. Nonetheless, the environment where the epidemic emerges is well chosen. Many of these epidemics occurred in military barracks and college dorms, and vaccination is now mandatory.

Two films show a scene with a missed diagnosis of meningitis. In *The Men* (1950) ⫷⫷⫷⫷, one of the traumatic spine injury patients develops fever. It shows testing for neck stiffness, a lumbar puncture, and the surgeon in charge going bonkers after the patient dies. The movie *Barbara* (2012) ⫷⫷ also shows a missed diagnosis of meningitis. Barbara (played by Nina Hoss) is a physician sent to a small sea town in northeast Germany close to the Baltic Sea. A girl is admitted, confused, and belligerent. The physician prepares a sedative because this patient had been admitted many times with fake diseases. (It is later revealed that she is in a hard-labor camp and tries to escape using fake medical illness as an excuse.) Barbara discovers neck stiffness and proceeds with a lumbar puncture. Apparently, the girl had hidden in the woods while attempting to escape and contracted tick-borne meningoencephalitis. It realistically shows meningoencephalitis presenting with behavioral problems. The patient recovers after she is treated with "serum." This is quite timely, particularly because tick-borne encephalitis is prevalent in Eastern Europe and Russia—in the summer. Most cases occur in Germany and the areas formerly known as Czechoslovakia and the USSR. The median incubation time is eight days after a tick bite. The mentioned "serum treatment" is unexplained because there is no specific treatment for tick-borne encephalitis, only prevention by active immunization.[88]

Infections of the central nervous system are only of interest to filmmakers when they occur as panic-inciting epidemics. Rapid death is more often shown than coma or seizures. Sporadically, a case of meningitis is introduced but only to show that the disorder is not recognized or not diagnosed by physicians. Some scenes (*Barbara*, 2012) can be lifted for study because the representation is accurate (for example, showing neurologic examination for neck stiffness) and because the film also suggests that even known malingerers can become seriously ill.

The epidemic of encephalitis lethargica or Von Economo's disease (1917–1927) was the first pandemic to affect the brain tissue directly. Constantin von Economo, to whom identification of the disorder is attributed, described cases seen in a psychiatry ward. The infection became intermittently pandemic through 1918 throughout Europe and the United States. The cause (presumably a virus) has never been identified, and a widespread outbreak has not recurred. This disorder has been mistakenly attributed to the major influenza epidemic, also known as the Spanish flu, during the final year of the First World War (1918). In his paper (Figure 4.10),[89] von Economo suggested that the responsible lesion was in a sleep-promoting area in the hypothalamus, and indeed, lesioning these areas could induce sleep in animals. This encephalitis may have remained an obscure footnote in the history of medicine until Oliver Sacks wrote up his experiences that led to a well-known movie.[90]

Awakenings (1990) ⫷⫷⫷⫷ stars Robert De Niro and Robin Williams and was directed by Penny Marshall. *Awakenings* is centered upon Leonard Lowe (Robert De Niro), who is afflicted with encephalitis lethargica and then has a miraculous improvement on L-dopa—but only temporarily.[91] Robin Williams plays Oliver Sacks as Dr. Sayer with all the mannerisms and aloofness of a befuddled neuroscientist (Figure 4.11). The patients are all in a frozen, immobile (catatonic) state, but Dr. Sayer—much to the surprise of the staff—shows they can catch a ball, catch a dropping pen, and respond to music.

[88] See Lindquist L, Vapalahti O. Tick-Borne Encephalitis. *Lancet.* 2008;371:1861–1871.

[89] von Economo C. Encephalitis lethargica. *Wiener Klinische Wochenschrift.* 1917;30:581–585.

[90] Sacks OW. *Awakenings.* New York: Summit Books; 1987.

[91] I find it interesting that most people regard this movie as a depiction of awakening from a coma, which it most definitely is not.

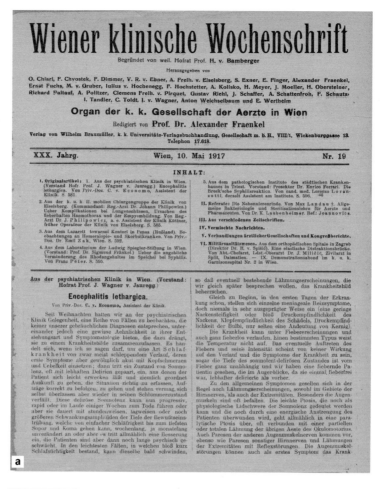

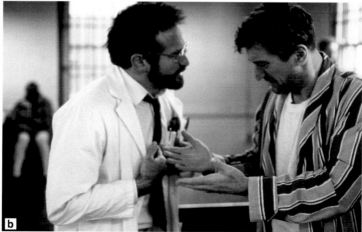

FIGURE 4.11   (a) Title page of the article on encephalitis lethargica by Constantin von Economo. (b) Robin Williams and Robert de Niro as Oliver Sacks and Leonard the patient (Everett Collection, Inc.).

After Leonard improves dramatically, other patients receive L-dopa and show immediate improvement, turning a sedate institution into a lively place. This over-the-top presentation has been criticized, but the portrayal of parkinsonism is quite correct including the later dystonic movements. (The ability to catch a ball is another story and extremely unlikely.)

What is currently known about the disorder is that after a flu-like illness, patients with encephalitis lethargica develop marked sleepiness, ocular movement disturbances, and fever. Abnormal posturing (dystonia) was not initially part of the manifestation, and stupor (hence, the word lethargic) was most prominent and persistent. Some patients could become immediately alert; others had more cyclic responsiveness, with sleep during the day and wakefulness during the night. In earlier descriptions, paralysis of eye muscles was very common, but very often, other cranial nerves were involved. Oropharyngeal dysfunction could lead to early demise. This combination of upper cranial nerve involvement and stupor now, in retrospect, would fit well with an upper brainstem lesion, and indeed, the mesencephalon showed necrosis and perivascular lymphocytic infiltrate. In some patients, the hypothalamus was involved. Many of these patients either developed a catatonic state or recovered with narcolepsy. The parkinsonian manifestations occurred often after a period of years after the infection, but more than 50% of the survivors developed parkinsonian symptoms within 5 years and 80% within 10 years. Oculogyric crisis was a common manifestation.

No treatment was available for these patients. Beth Abraham opened in 1920 as a home for incurable post-encephalitics and victims of permanent war injuries. This created an opportunity to observe patients with "stillness punctuated by sudden explosions of movements."[92]

DIALOGUE

Awakenings

Leonard's mother	*I do not understand it. He was never any trouble before. He was good, quiet and obedient.*
Dr. Sayer	*Because he was catatonic, Mrs. Lowe.*
Dr. Sayer, in conversation with Dr. Ingham	*What must it be like to be them? What are they thinking?* *They are not. The virus didn't spare the higher faculties.* *We know that for a fact?* *Yes, because the alternative would be unthinkable.*

Oliver Sacks remembered that he originally planned a three-month, double-blind clinical trial of L-dopa in institutionalized patients with parkinsonism and stupor from encephalitis lethargica; this was prompted by earlier work on the use of aromatic amino acids in improving parkinsonism. Nine cases improved greatly. That became the basis of the main manuscript, which was initially rejected by several medical and neurologic journals but was ultimately published in 1972 in *The Listener* under the title "The Great Awakening."[93] Oliver Sacks remembers sending a long article to *Brain*, which was returned with the comment "paper so unsuitable that no revision is recommended." Eventually, parts were published as letters."[94] Later, with 11 more case histories, the book *Awakenings* was published, which was the inspiration of this movie. Oliver Sacks described his observations in *Awakenings* as follows: "These 'extinct volcanoes' erupted into life … occurring before us was a cataclysm of almost geological proportions, the explosive 'awakening,' the 'quickening,' of eighty or more patients who had long been regarded, and

---

[92] Weschler L. *And How Are You, Dr. Sacks?* New York: Farrar, Straus and Giroux; 2019:81.

[93] The article in *The Listener*, a now-defunct BBC publication, is referenced in Weschler and includes raving reviews, ibid.

[94] Sacks OW, Kohl M, Schwartz W, Messeloff C. Side-Effects of L-Dopa in Postencephalic Parkinsonism. *Lancet*. 1970;1:1006.

regarded themselves, as effectively dead." Two excellent books[95] have suggested that encephalitis lethargica was significantly overdiagnosed despite distinctly recognizable indications. *Awakenings* focuses on post-encephalitis Parkinson's disease, but the syndrome as described by von Economo could present as meningitis, ophthalmoparesis (oculomotor and abducens), and increasing somnolence to deep stupor. Remarkably, new cases of encephalitis lethargica continue to be diagnosed, and some have described children with basal ganglia encephalitis. N-methyl-D-aspartate antibodies were found in 10 of 20 patients with encephalitis lethargica, which suggest an autoimmune encephalitis that, importantly, may respond to immunotherapy. Many of these patients (young females) have dystonic movements involving face and arms.[96] (Also, see Chapter 8.)

Awakenings is often the first movie that comes to mind in discussions of neurologic portrayal in the movies. However, for many viewers, the "takeaway message" appears to be that "comatose patients" can awaken after 20 years with a simple drug administration. Not everyone was pleased with this film, and the depiction of the seemingly haphazard administration of L-dopa (i.e., secretly doubling the dose despite the serious side effects) has led two bioethicists to use it as an example of an unethical drug trial targeting a disabled, vulnerable population.[97] However, it is unfair to apply current standards for clinical trials to a study done 40 years ago. In any case, Sacks's meticulous notes attest to the rigor of the original study.[98]

The overlap with the Spanish influenza epidemic has been intriguing, and some cases of influenza may have been misdiagnosed as encephalitis lethargica. When post-encephalitic parkinsonism appeared, it presented with a catatonia (being frozen in a certain position). Facial expressions disappeared, and very often upward, involuntary eye movements (oculogyric crises) occurred. Rigidity was common, but tremor—as is typical in Parkinson's disease—was not. The number of patients who developed post-encephalitic Parkinson's disease was small despite hundreds of descriptions. This episode was a significant period in the history of neurology, and sufficient proof of concept has been established.

Epidemics caused by some viral mutant of rabies are part of the horror genre and discussed in Chapter 9. Rabies, one of the oldest communicable diseases known to man and caused by an RNA virus of the rhabdovirus family, was of particular interest to screenwriters because of described drooling, hydrophobia, inspiratory spasm, and wild agitation. This symptomatology was subsequently linked to the behavior of zombies. Rabies encephalitis is rarely seen in the western world.

Spinal Cord Injury

Acute, traumatic spinal cord injury immediately and disastrously changes a person's life. It occurs most commonly in young active males (in their late teens and twenties), mostly as a result of car crashes, hazardous winter sports, after a flash of foolishness such as diving off a rock into shallow water (*The Sea Inside*, Chapter 5), the use of trampolines, and as a result of violence or extreme circumstances such as war. Inability to walk is one of the first neurologic themes in silent film (see Chapter 2). Mary Pickford plays a paraplegic in both *Stella Maris* (1918) ◄ and *Pollyanna* (1920) ◄ . Brilliant surgeons operate (on something) so she can walk again. Acute paraplegia in film often involves coping with varying degrees of success. Most films simply show the rejection by others and the threat of isolation, but a few provide fresh insight into the changed circumstances of the patient with paraplegia. The most important film in

---

[95] See Vilensky JA, ed. *Encephalitis Lethargica: During and after the Epidemic.* New York: Oxford University Press; 2010; and Foley PB. *Encephalitis Lethargica: The Mind and Brain Virus.* Berlin: Springer; 2018.

[96] See Dale RC, Irani SR, Brilot F, Pillai S, Webster R, Gill D, et al. N-Methyl-D-Aspartate Receptor Antibodies in Pediatric Dyskinetic Encephalitis Lethargica. *Ann Neurol.* 2009;66:704–709; Dale RC, Church AJ, Surtees RA, Lees AJ, Adcock JE, Harding B, et al. Encephalitis Lethargica Syndrome: 20 New Cases and Evidence of Basal Ganglia Autoimmunity. *Brain.* 2004;127:21–33.

[97] Wolitz R, Grady C. Use of Experimental Therapies. In: Colt H, Quadrelli S, Friedman L, eds. *The Picture of Health: Medical Ethics and the Movies* 1st ed. New York: Oxford University Press; 2011:560.

[98] Weschler and Vilensky had full access to these notes and commented on the trial design in their respective books.

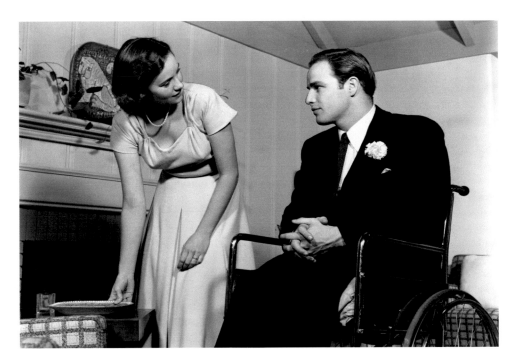

FIGURE 4.12   Marlon Brando and Teresa Wright in *The Men* (Everett Collection, Inc.).

this regard is *The Men* (1950) ◄◄◄◄ , directed by Fred Zinneman and starring Marlon Brando and Teresa Wright[99] (Figure 4.12), which focuses on how couples re-adjust to the "new normal."

DIALOGUE

The Men

Doctor	*In almost every case, the word "walk" must be forgotten. It no longer exists.*
Mother	*My boy is only 19.*
Doctor	*But with proper care he may live to be 90.*
Doctor	*The legs are gone now. The head has to take over.*

Marlon Brando made his film debut playing an introverted, depressed paraplegic. The film was shot in Birmingham Veterans Administration Hospital in Van Nuys, California (close to Hollywood), and included a cast of actual patients. A key scene comes early in the movie when the crass prima donna, Dr. Brock, explains (in the hospital's chapel) to spouses of affected veterans that this is a lasting injury. Living with a paraplegic is an overarching theme in this film. It also daringly (noting the year it was filmed) approaches not only the topic of sexuality ("I am not a man; I cannot make a woman happy") but also fertility ("It is not very probable but in the realm of possibility"). Even Bud's in-laws weigh in ("Is it so wrong for us to want a grandchild?"). Bud marries but returns to the hospital after a spat. Several times, during stressful moments, he jerks his right leg to imitate

---

[99] Teresa Wright was an overlooked Hollywood star who also played Mrs. Lou Gehrig in *Pride of the Yankees.* (See Chapter 7.)

(reasonably correct) spasms. The film highlighted the major injuries of the Second World War and appeared four years after *Let There Be Light,* which dealt with functional disease and PTSD in returning soldiers (see Chapter 8).

The long Vietnam War was next. This time filmmakers used paraplegia in war casualties to point out—in their view—deficiencies in care of the disabled. These movies (inaccurately) suggest deplorable healthcare in VA hospitals. *Born on the Fourth of July* (1989) ◄◄ indicts the Bronx Veterans Hospital—with a horrendous display of medical care provided to T7 paraplegic Ron Kovic (Tom Cruise). The VA hospital is a dirty, unorganized cesspool with rats crawling under the beds. Cynicism is rampant when, in the morning, the nurse calls, "Everybody rise and shine." When Ron asks a doctor if he will be able to have children, he answers resolutely, "No, but we have a very good psychologist here." Massive decubitus is seen, and patients seem to be lined up for "group defecation." When Ron walks unassisted with crutches in a show of "alpha male" behavior, he falls and fractures his leg. The care at home is frustrating, and acceptance is non-existent. Ron Kovic is left alone with poor skin and bladder care and lack of any compassion. This film and so many others supposedly illustrate the national consciousness against the war and against the Department of Veteran Affairs' medical institutions.

Similar scenarios of life after war-related spinal cord injury are found in *Coming Home* (1978) ◄◄◄ . The film also shows a deplorable hospital with paraplegics in the Vietnam War era. Thorazine is used to calm Luke (Jon Voight) when he is aggressively swinging a cane and yelling at the healthcare workers about the poor care he receives. Urine spills from his catheter when he collides with Sally (Jane Fonda), an officer's wife who volunteers at the hospital. They subsequently begin a relationship.

DIALOGUE

Coming Home

Luke to Sally

People look at me, but they see something else; and they do not see who I am. Do you know when I dream, I dream I do not have a chair in my dream?

Another notable film is *The Waterdance* (1992) ◄◄ by the paraplegic director Neal Jimenez. The film is virtually fully set in a VA hospital for spine injury and shows the anger and frustration of going through the rehabilitation process. The title is based on a dream of one of the paraplegics in which he imagines he must dance on water to avoid drowning. The film is largely focused on prolonged rehabilitation but also on the loss of sexuality and the struggles with that adjustment. The screenwriter here is fascinated by sexuality in the paraplegic. The screenplay often strongly leans toward vulgarity.

Another major film, based on the true story of skier Jill Kinmont, is *The Other Side of the Mountain* (1975) ◄◄◄ starring Marilyn Hassett and Beau Bridges, which correctly depicts the challenges of living with a cervical spine injury. The confrontation of the physician with parents is telling. ("All we can do is hope." "Hope that she will walk?" "No, hope that she will live.") She remains wheelchair bound, and the movie focuses on toughness, avoiding self-pity, and a theme of "anything can be overcome." (Parenthetically, the film shows Jill's best friend, crippled by polio, chastising her not to be so self-centered and to try to find a way to live with this handicap.) She becomes a successful teacher but not without encountering prejudice. ("People think that when your toes are numb, your brain is numb." "Paraplegics are unacceptable as teachers in this country.") The film provides less detail but even in this prim and proper tearjerker, making love and having no feeling is discussed. ("You want more than me; you get tired of it.")

Much later, another notable and lauded film—and unprecedented European box-office hit—was *The Intouchables* (2011) ◄◄◄◄ starring François Cluzet, Omar Sy, and Anne Le Ny; written and directed by Olivier Nakache and Éric Toledano; and based on a true story. *The Intouchables* describes in detail the physical care and emotional challenges of a well-to-do aristocrat, Philippe (François Cluzet), with acute high cervical cord injury after a paragliding crash. Paragliding was his favorite form of recreation because he felt grandiose and was on top of the world ("he felt he could pee on the world"). Philippe—a man of means—has a plethora of caregivers. Omar Sy plays the Senegalese Driss, who incidentally has a criminal record and spent six months in jail for robbery. Philippe decides to hire Driss in part because Driss doesn't show him any pity and because the other caregivers are humorless and boring.

The film suggests that the wealthy may have a better deal when it comes to such a major handicap, and it all seems quite droll. Nonetheless, the film provides some unique insights and is very well researched. In showing the burdens of a quadriplegic person, no film before has provided such detail for the audience. Driss is portrayed here as an ignoramus laughing about major pieces of art and music. He is most satisfied when he hears the motor of a Philippe's Maserati roar and when he can dance to his own favorite music. The film is about two fully dependent persons—one on full medical support, the other on government money. In a key conversation, Philippe says, "You don't mind living off others' backs?" and Driss pointedly answers, "No, how about you?"

A bothersome scene occurs when Driss discovers that Philippe does not feel the hot silver teapot. He then pours a little more potentially scalding tea on Philippe's legs until another caregiver intervenes. Other notable scenes involve "hyperventilation" attacks as a result of "phantom pain" and an episode that suggests painful cramping due to spasticity. Driss takes Philippe out in the early morning, where Philippe explains his difficulties controlling these excruciating attacks. During a subsequent attack, Driss offers him a joint, and the film clearly suggests marijuana as a therapeutic option. Driss and Philippe find these sessions an enjoyable, bonding experience. This is problematic territory, particularly as addiction is more common in patients with severe spinal cord injury and chronic pain.

DIALOGUE

The Intouchables

Philippe

> *The medication has its limits .... Doctors call them phantom pains. I feel like a frozen steak tossed onto a red-hot griddle. I feel nothing but suffer anyway.*

The film admirably illustrates the problem of pain management in patients with acute spinal cord injury. Pain after a spinal cord injury is a dull musculoskeletal joint ache or dull abdominal pain, but the most severe pain is generated centrally. Allodynia is common (pain with simple touch), but so is hyperalgesia. Spontaneous sharp, shooting, unrelenting pain, often described by the patient as a feeling of hot stabbing knives, may occur and may be resistant to medication. Surgical approaches (dorsal root entry zone lesioning, or cordomyelotomy) are often insufficient, and there are varying results with transcutaneous electrical nerve stimulation.[100]

The film discusses manual fecal removal and Driss's refusal. ("I don't go for this sick stuff.") The film appropriately discusses bowel dysfunction because most reflex activity below the level of spinal cord injury is lost. Defecation in patients with cervical cord lesions requires diaphragmatic contraction because the abdominal muscles required for straining are lost. Constipation is common, with some

---

[100]Bryce TN, Biering-Sorensen F, Finnerup NB, Cardenas DD, Defrin R, Lundeberg T, et al. International Spinal Cord Injury Pain Classification: Part I. Background and Description. March 6–7, 2009. *Spinal Cord*. 2012;50:413–417.

incontinence. Manual evacuation and digital stimulation are commonly used in combination with mini-enemas, and some patients with chronic obstruction may need a colostomy.[101]

Problems with sexuality are also prominently mentioned in this film, and sex through erogenic zones is discussed. Psychogenic arousal requires thoracolumbar spinal cord function and thus is absent. In spinal cord injury, males may have reflex erections but no orgasms or ejaculation. Patients often discover that nipples, earlobes, or inner thighs evoke genital awareness, and men can experience orgasms despite absent erections.[102]

The film hints at mortality, and the protagonist mentions his shortened life expectancy. It correctly implies that a 50-year-old who suffers a cervical injury will have a mortality of 30% in 20 years (three-fold higher than a healthy person). Complications are directly related to immobilization and associated with infections, such as urosepsis, respiratory failure, pulmonary embolus, and increasing risks of renal stones and pressure sores, but there is also the uncomfortable issue of suicides.

Philippe has a scar from a tracheostomy, which is accurate considering the level of cord injury he has suffered. The phrenic nerve, which innervates the diaphragm, originates from the C4 spinal segment, with some contributions from C3 and C5. Patients with a C3/C4 lesion—such as Philippe—will likely be ventilator dependent; however, patients with a C5 lesion are far more likely to be weaned successfully. The abdominal component to breathing—mostly coughing up—is lost due to absent tone in paralyzed muscles. Many of these patients visibly use their accessory (sternocleidomastoid and scalene) muscles to assist in respiration. Philippe's breathing in the film does not seem to be compromised at all. Often, only short sentences can be spoken with deep inhalations in between and the use of accessory muscles. For the filmmaker, it must have been too much of an additional downer to show all that.

The Intouchables is a complex film on the challenges of being paralyzed from the neck down and an important addition to the collection of *Neurocinema*. The credits of *The Intouchables* say that 5% of the profits from the film were donated to the Association Simon de Cyrène in Paris, whose purpose is to create shared living spaces for disabled adults and friends. Hence, something good came out of this financial blockbuster movie.

The theme of sex after paralysis is seen in Lars von Trier's *Breaking the Waves* (1996) ◄◄◄◄ . In this film, Jan (Stellan Skarsgard) is quadriplegic due to an accident on a rig. The film accurately shows the secondary complications of acute spinal cord injury and has graphic scenes of a craniotomy and cervical stabilization. *Breaking the Waves* also uses a common trope that the tetraplegic is eager to end a relationship or marriage. Following spinal-cord injury, family members often undertake the caregiving role, which can lead to emotional, psychological, and relationship challenges. There is limited research on how individuals with SCI and their family caregivers adapt to their new lives post-injury, but divorce rates may approach 50%.[103] The film, however, focuses less on the injury but explores other complex themes (being good, sacrifice, and faith). The recovery is miraculous, essential to the story, and should not dissuade the viewer.

Paraplegia is a far more common topic in cinema than quadriplegia, and there are numerous actors playing paraplegics. A major distinction should be made between amputees and paraplegics. Amputees are better rehabilitated, and often a transition to better lives is shown in the movies after wearing prostheses (recall Gary Sinise as Lieutenant Dan in *Forrest Gump* [1994] and, more recently, Marion Cotillard as Stephanie in *Rust and Bone* [2012]).

---

[101] Zollman FS, ed. *Mayo Clinic Guide to Living with a Spinal Cord Injury: Moving Ahead with Your Life*. Paperback ed. New York: Demos Health; 2009.

[102] Hess MJ, Hough S. Impact of Spinal Cord Injury on Sexuality: Broad-Based Clinical Practice Intervention and Practical Application. *J Spinal Cord Med*. 2012;35:211–218.

[103] See Jeyathevan G, Cameron JI, Craven BC, Munce SEP, Jaglal SB. Re-Building Relationships after a Spinal Cord Injury: Experiences of Family Caregivers and Care Recipients. *BMC Neurol*. 2019;19:117; and Kreuter M, Sullivan M, Dahllof AG, Siosteen A. Partner Relationships, Functioning, Mood and Global Quality of Life in Persons with Spinal Cord Injury and Traumatic Brain Injury. *Spinal Cord*. 1998;36:252–261.

The films scrutinized here provide a good representation of the emotional duress of paraplegics, but some films use the isolation and major handicap of a paraplegic as a somewhat objectionable device to evoke pity and devastation. Many disabled people are poor, and wars cause increased traumatic paraplegia. Is quality of life after a paralysis all a matter of support and access to care? I cannot tell, but cinema has placed a great emphasis on the major societal issues in patients with acute spinal cord injury. How do the medical professionals at the VA hospitals with their renowned and innovative spinal cord programs feel about the implication it is all a dirty, chaotic mess? I can only imagine.

Poliomyelitis

Although poliomyelitis is very rare today and most neurologists see the sequelae after many decades have passed, this was not the case at the beginning of the 20th century. Here we discuss two key films, separated by half a century. An impressive but overly dramatized biopic is *Sister Kenny* (1946) ◄◄◄ starring Rosalind Russell, Alexander Knox, Philip Merivale, and John Litel and directed by Dudley Nichols. The film shows Kenny taking the nurse's oath: "With loyalty will I endeavor to aid the physician in his work." (At the time, the term "sister" was used to indicate nurse, but Sister Kenny actually had no formal nursing training.[104]) Several confrontational scenes occur in the movie; for example, when Sister Kenny questions the orthopedic surgeon, Dr. Brack (Philip Merivale), regarding his treatment (Figure 4.13). According to Dr. Brack, "The only thing that offers any hope is prompt and complete immobilization" and "Stick to nursing and don't meddle with orthopedic medicine." The movie suggests that all cases treated by Sister Kenny recovered, that the overwhelming majority treated by orthopedic surgeons became crippled, and that most orthopedic surgeons wanted nothing to do with her methods. The film is more about a major nurse–physician conflict than about Kenny's treatment methods and efficacy (or lack thereof). The film clearly suggested that patients would be cured only by her methods and only if physicians were more accepting and less arrogant.

DIALOGUE

Sister Kenny

Kenny to Dr. Brack	*I do not think you are ignorant, only pigheaded. I get improvements even with your failures.*
Kenny to Dr. Brack	*If you need any more braces, steel corsets, or other instruments of medieval torture, I can send them to you. I have taken plenty off your patients.*

The film opens in Australia, but in the second half of the film, Sister Kenny moves to the United States, where she feels she is getting the runaround. In the final scene, she demonstrates her method to orthopedic surgeons, but the film ends with her being informed that a US committee does not support her methods. She sits defeated in a chair but lights up when children (recovered patients) sing happy birthday to her. (Reportedly, Sister Kenny did not like the ending of the film, and it is easy to see why.)

So, what really happened with Sister Kenny? Although poliomyelitis is a neurologic disease, it became orthopedic surgeons' territory during the fin de siècle, when restoration of function and transplantation of tendons was commonplace. Neurologists often would see patients to confirm the diagnosis, but actual care was provided by rehabilitation physicians, and, when severe respiratory failure occurred,

---

[104]See Rogers N. *Polio Wars: Sister Kenny and the Golden Age of American Medicine.* New York: Oxford University Press; 2013. This is the most comprehensive analysis of Kenny's travels and rejection in the United States. Was she a pioneer? In the end, the author feels the answer is complicated. Rogers concludes—correctly avoiding condescension by using the standards of the present—that she does not know whether Sister Kenny's therapy helped.

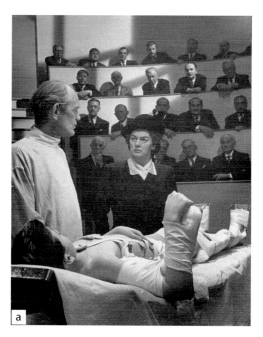

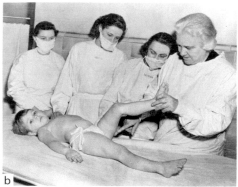

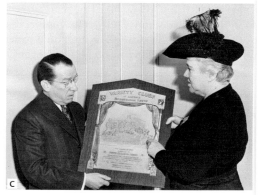

FIGURE 4.13   (a) Scene from *Sister Kenny* showing a confrontational scene with Dr. Brack over a patient's treatment. (Used with permission of Getty Images.) (b) Elisabeth (Sister) Kenny. (Used with permission of Minnesota Historical Society.) (c) Kenny awarded by the Variety Clubs of America Humanitarian Trinity.

by anesthesiologists. However, three neurologists, W. Ritchie Russell, A.B. Baker, and Fred Plum, made major contributions to the respiratory management of poliomyelitis. Each recognized that airway obstruction and respiratory compromise in a neurologic disease shared some similarities with acute neuromuscular disease (myasthenia gravis and Guillain-Barré syndrome), such as pooling secretions and predictive signs of early hypoxemia, but other observations, such as brainstem-associated respiratory failure, were new and original.[105] Care seems to have been established until Sister Kenny appeared.

Elizabeth Kenny (Figure 4.13) has been accused of showing fanciful optimism. She came to the United States in 1940 and wrote a major text, *And They Shall Walk*, in 1943. A Queensland commission

[105]Wijdicks EFM. W. Ritchie Russell, A.B. Baker, and Fred Plum: Pioneers of Ventilatory Management in Poliomyelitis. *Neurology.* 2016;87:1167–1170.

concluded that her management of wrapping stiffened limbs in hot woolen sheets and "re-educating" the underused muscles by exercising and avoidance of orthopedic splints was no more beneficial than orthodox treatment.[106] At the time, the standard of care was based on the hypothesis that stretching paralyzed muscles reduced deformities. Massage was avoided due to extreme tenderness but also the use of splints (steel frames) and plaster casts, even if needed to keep the legs in a good position. Treatment involved warmth and heat lamps. Therapy for poliomyelitis was mostly hydrotherapy, massage, and controlled exercises. Electrotherapy was popular in France, but nothing was proven.

The principles of Kenny's treatment, however, were different and were keeping a bright mental outlook, maintenance of "impulse," hydrotherapy (including alternating hot and cold douches), maintenance of circulation, and avoidance of generally accepted methods of immobilization. She did not believe polio affected the nerves but pointed to the muscles that were in spasm, which could be relieved with hot packs and hot blankets. (What she meant by these "spasms," however, remained unresolved, and when over 3,000 muscle groups were examined by neurologists, none of these "spasms" were found.[107])

The treatment, with all its controversies, became politicized, particularly after the 1952 epidemic a decade later. Kenny established the Sister Kenny Institute in Minneapolis (now Courage Kenny Rehabilitation Institute) after it appeared that her method remarkably improved outcomes in polio patients.[108] When questioned, Kenny said, "Let my record speak." She wrote a book in 1943 with the supportive orthopedic surgeon J.F. Pohl, *The Kenny Concept of Infantile Paralysis and Its Treatment*.

According to personal accounts, Sister Kenny could be abrasive. (Neurologist Donald Mulder recalled, "Sister Kenny was a feisty person who, one observer noted, would continue to fight long after one agreed with her."[109]) In other accounts, she was frequently down in the dumps and found it hard to cope with the large waves of negative publicity. There is no question, however, that Sister Kenny improved care with early mobilization, possibly avoiding unnecessary reconstructive surgeries, and a generally far more optimistic approach. Kenny's emphasis on the alienation of a paralyzed limb is a real phenomenon, and the phenomenon is not only seen in polio but in any long-term immobilized limb. Most of the quibbles about the best treatments in poliomyelitis disappeared with the Salk vaccine. David Oshinsky's Pulitzer Prize-winning book, *Polio: An American Story,* is the place to go to revisit another conflict—the far-from-pleasant development of vaccines.[110]

The Sessions (2012) ◀◀◀ , which stars John Hawkes, Helen Hunt, and William Macy, was directed by Ben Lewin, who is a childhood polio survivor. It is based on a true story. Mark O'Brien died in 1999 after being confined to an iron lung following childhood poliomyelitis. He recalls getting weak and coming out of a coma while encased in an iron lung. (Poliomyelitis often involves the brainstem and respiratory centers and may lead to coma from rising unchecked CO_2.) His parents were told the life expectancy of polio survivors was poor. ("They took me home and gave me a life—gave up theirs.") He was the topic of an Oscar-winning short documentary by Jessica Yu in 1996, *Breathing Lessons: The Life and Work of Mark O'Brien* ◀◀◀◀ . (The documentary is a necessary supplement to this film and demands viewing.) Mark O'Brien attended the UC Berkeley Graduate School of Journalism in Berkeley, California, and became a poet and journalist. In 1997, he co-founded Lemonade Factory, a press that publishes work by people with disabilities. His books include the memoir *How I Became a Human Being: A Disabled Man's Quest for Independence* (2003) and the poetry collections *The Man in the Iron Lung* (1997) and *Breathing* (1998). *Sessions* is structured around an article he wrote, "On Seeing a Sex Surrogate," and handles the topic of sex and disability discreetly.

---

[106] Treatment of Infantile Paralysis by Sister Kenny's Method. *Br Med J.* 1938;1:350.

[107] Pollock LJ, Boshes B, Finkelman I, et al. Absence of Spasm during Onset of Paralysis in Acute Anterior Poliomyelitis. *Arch Neurol Psychiatry.* 1949;61:288–296.

[108] Kendall FP. Sister Elizabeth Kenny Revisited. *Arch Phys Med Rehabil.* 1998;79:361–365.

[109] Mulder DW. Clinical Observations on Acute Poliomyelitis. *Ann N Y Acad Sci.* 1995;753:1–10.

[110] Oshinsky DM. *Polio: An American Story.* 1st ed. New York: Oxford University Press; 2005.

The film shows the devastating effects of living in an iron lung (he was able to get out of the device for 3 or 4 hours per day and slept in it) and living supine for most of the time. A portable respirator allowed him to go outside. Respiratory involvement usually affected 10% of the cases, but in some instances, it involved up to one-third of the afflicted adults. Patients with severe poliomyelitis often develop sleep apnea, with breathing stopping at the onset of sleep; in some, the automatic respiratory control during wakefulness may disappear.

DIALOGUE

The Sessions

Mark O'Brien

This most excellent canopy, the air, look you,
Presses down upon me
At fifteen pounds per square inch,
A dense, heavy, blue-glowing ocean,
Supporting the weight of condors
That swim its churning currents.
All I get is a thin stream of it,
A finger's width of the rope that ties me to life
As I labor like a stevedore to keep the connection.
(Start of the film and excerpted from his poem.)

John Hawkes plays Mark O'Brien and imitates his voice using short sentences but not the staccato speech so typical of neuromuscular respiratory failure (catching a breath in between a few words). His body is appropriately skinny (patients may weigh no more than 60 kilograms), and he appropriately imitates the often-seen severe spinal deformities (such as kyphoscoliosis) that often exacerbate respiratory problems over time. The movie also shows the severe pain with movements of limbs in severe contracture.

Poliomyelitis has appeared in several screenplays in the past but has disappeared with the near disappearance of the disorder. One of the first films to deal with the burdens of poliomyelitis is the cold-blooded noir, *Leave Her to Heaven* (1945) ◀◀◀ about Ellen (Gene Tierney) and Richard Harland (Cornel Wilde). Ellen and Richard are newlyweds, and Richard's brother Danny (Darryl Hickman) is recovering from poliomyelitis in the well-known rehabilitation center, the Warm Springs Foundation in Georgia. Danny is a Hollywood feel-good example of a happy-go-lucky (see what I can do despite crutches!) optimist who can soon leave the rehabilitation center. Ellen is glad to comply with his care, but after his physician suggests to her that he can return home, she gets visibly upset with the idea of having to take him home ("after all, he is a cripple"). His presence puts a wedge in the relationship of the married couple. He seems to recover and can move his legs and do swimming exercises. The film is a thriller, and the femme fatale Ellen watches him drown in an iconic scene, where she fakes a rescue attempt after he has drowned. Interestingly, nowhere in the script is poliomyelitis specifically mentioned; it is only implied.

Poliomyelitis is used to great effect in *The Five Pennies* (1959) ◀◀◀ . Danny Kaye plays a band leader whose daughter is affected by polio. We see her in a few scenes in an iron lung, recovering in a hospital bed through rehabilitation, eventually walking with a cane, and dancing again with her father. The director knew what the audience wanted to see—full recovery of poliomyelitis against all odds and physician prediction. (This clinical course is not very likely.) It also shows Sister Kenny's hot compresses and Danny Kaye goofing off to try to raise his daughter's spirits. He puts blankets on her legs ("the most delicious thing your mother cooked since we're in this house … blanket a la mode"), buys her a puppy, and so forth, but the film is not only about poliomyelitis and a major musical biopic. It was a family blockbuster in 1959.

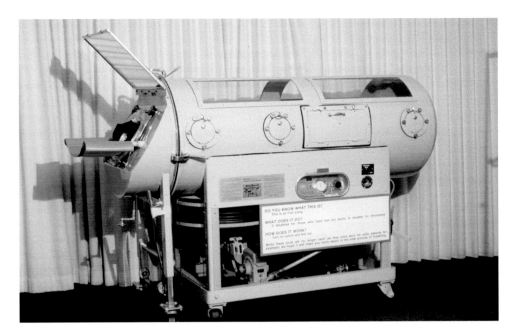

FIGURE 4.14   Iron lung. (Used with permission of Mayo Historical Unit and Archives.)

What can be said about poliomyelitis to understand the portrayal? In the overwhelming proportion of cases, poliomyelitis is a viral infection by an enterovirus that causes a non-distinctive viral illness and, in some, a devastating paralysis from the involvement of the anterior horn of the spinal cord. When the brainstem becomes involved, patients develop oropharyngeal weakness, which causes difficulty in clearing secretions and compromises respiration. Many patients in the past had back stiffness and severe pain from hypertonicity. Many patients developed intercostal paralysis and severe weakness of the diaphragm, an early paralytic stage of anterior poliomyelitis. Other patients were able to create sufficient respiratory movements using the accessory muscles and the diaphragm. Over a few days, the paralyzed intercostal muscles improved, and the patient went on to almost complete recovery.

Respiratory support involved the infamous "iron lung." This machine incorporated electrically driven blowers and created inspiration with negative pressures and expiration with positive pressure (Figure 4.14).[111] Within the chamber—sealing the patient at the neck—a negative pressure caused the abdomen and thorax to expand with air flowing in. A cycle is produced by returning to atmospheric pressure. Patients in the iron lung have their chest expanded every four seconds. Many patients could be liberated from the device or transitioned to a cuirass ventilator. During the major epidemics, the iron lung was perceived as a temporary lifesaving machine, but later it became clear that weaning was not always possible and respiratory support would now have a permanent impact on the quality of the patient's existence.

Film deals with poliomyelitis in different ways—the burden of "a cripple," the arrogant orthopedic surgeons not accepting a nursing approach, a life in an iron lung, and, in general, living with a paralyzed body. The spectrum covered cannot be more all-encompassing and is of more than just historical interest. It acknowledges the importance that poliomyelitis epidemics played in people's lives, in medical history, and in the history of critical care medicine. Poliomyelitis still has not been eradicated. (For further discussion on poliomyelitis in documentary film, see Chapter 6.)

---

[111] Drinker P, Mckhann CF. The Use of a New Apparatus for the Prolonged Administration of Artificial Respiration: I. A Fatal Case of Poliomyelitis. *JAMA*. 1929;92:1658–1660.

Multiple Sclerosis

Multiple sclerosis (MS) leads to disability, but the prognosis is often uncertain. Indeed, it has improved over the last decades due to disease-modifying therapies, but poor communication regarding MS disease progression remains consistent.[112] MS entered the catalog of neurocinema very early and was used in an atrocious way to justify mercy killing. The film *Ich Klage An* (1941) ⫷⫷⫷ describes a terminal condition from MS and the decision to determine one's own fate.[113] The film was directed by Wolfgang Liebeneiner, who took it from a script by George Fraser and Eberhard Frowein, which, in turn, was based on the novel *Sendung und Gewissen* by Hellmuth Unger. During a musical recital, Hanna Heyt suddenly stops playing the piano because of numbness in her left hand. She also complains of dizziness as she stares in the sun. Dr. Lang examines Hanna, using an ophthalmoscope (seeing but not mentioning temporal pallor of the optic nerve) and a nerve conduction test (telling her after he sees a twitch that it is not a muscle disorder). He diagnoses MS but decides not to tell her. The head of the neurology department helpfully adds, "it's like telling a prisoner the date of the execution" and convinces Thomas, Hanna's husband, that telling her may negatively affect her outcome. (He reacts similarly with "My God! This is a death sentence.") Her husband also shows denial and anger and a willingness to find the cause. ("A real doctor never gives up.") The film shows multiple frantic scenes of (ultimately futile) experiments to find a cure. Hanna tells her husband that if she "ceases to be a person anymore, just a lump of flesh," she would become "torture" for him. She anticipates being "deaf, blind, and idiotic" and asks him to promise her that he will do something before it happens. The film shows significant deterioration in her condition. She starts to suffer excruciating pain and dramatic attacks of dyspnea suggesting she is beyond help. Eventually, Thomas provides her a "soothing drink," which results in her death. She says, "Oh, Thomas, if only that was death," to which he replies, "Yes, Hanna, it is death." She seems markedly at peace in the film as she passes. The subsequent courtroom drama seeks to prove that this was a good deed intended to make her end less painful. The courtroom scenes include major arguments supporting euthanasia, and even Paracelsus (Swiss German philosopher and physician) is cited as saying "medicine is love." In a key speech, one of the colleague witnesses says: "the legal system that allows to endure pointless suffering without the benefit of relief is unnatural and inhumane … nature lets things die quickly when life is no longer viable … medical science with pills and drugs insists on artificially delaying the mercy of a quick and natural death."

In the final scene, Professor Heyt challenges the court (*Ich Klage An*) to agree he is guilty of mercy killing only because he loved his wife and could not stand to see more suffering. A final verdict is not shown, and the film ends after his plea.

Ich Klage An was acclaimed at the Venice Biennale and, by January 1945, was seen by 50 million people. The film was favorably received and discussed by critics, and Nazi party leadership agreed that the film made a deep impression. Many years after the war, the controversial director Liebeneiner explained it away as it "a document of humanity in an inhumane time."[114] *Ich Klage An* suggests that MS leads to a devastating illness, which it does not. Liebeneiner did discuss the film with a neurologist to identify an potentially rapid progressive illness that would be appropriate to the film's theme. Moreover, he had to prove that all attempts were made to conclude the disorder was incurable.[115] It was banned by the Allied Governments of Germany in 1945 but later became a

[112] Celius EG, Thompson H, Pontaga M, Langdon D, Laroni A, Potra S, et al. Disease Progression in Multiple Sclerosis: A Literature Review Exploring Patient Perspectives. *Patient Prefer Adher.* 2021;15:15–27.

[113] Wijdicks EF, Karenberg A. Mercy Killing in Neurology: The Beginnings of Neurology on Screen (II). *Neurology.* 2016;87:1289–1292.

[114] Burleigh M. Selling Murder: The Killing Films of the Third Reich. In: Burleigh M, ed. *Death and Deliverance: "Euthanasia" in Germany, 1900–1945.* Cambridge: Cambridge University Press; 1995:183–220.

[115] Rost KL. Sterilisation und Euthanasie im Film des Dritten Reiches. *Nationalsozialistische Propaganda in ihrer Beziehung zu rassenhygienischen Maßnahmen des NS-Staates.* Husum, Germany: Abhandlungen zur Geschichte der Medizin und der Naturwissenschaften; 1987.

"Vorbehaltsfilm" indicating it was available for loan and presentation with restrictions, primarily for educational purposes.

MS returned to the screen 45 years later, although therapies were still few and far between. *Duet for One* (1969) ⚔ was directed by Andrei Konchalovsky and starred Julie Andrews as Stephanie Anderson, a virtuoso concert violinist disabled and wheelchair-bound by MS. Andrews studied for weeks to give the appearance of playing the violin, and she spent time meeting people with MS at a clinic in Bromley, Kent. The film is an emotional roller coaster ride. (She described her role as "the most desperate and emotionally pained woman I've ever played.") There are odd moments of suddenly losing muscle power and falling. A psychiatrist (Max von Sydow) helps her cope with her frustration. ("There are only two things we can do with fear - succumb to it or confront it directly.") The film was inspired by British cellist Jacqueline du Pré and was overshadowed by the only marginally better *Hilary and Jackie* (1998) ⚔⚔ discussed in Chapter 7. Historian Karenberg found that only a few nations have released films with an MS motif and mostly for television (Germany, Great Britain, Poland, the Netherlands, Sweden, Canada, and Greece.) He noted that most of these films come from regions characterized by a high MS prevalence (and a well-developed film industry.) Many films are not easily accessible, and all of them are associated with major disability and the prospect of moving to a nursing home (unfortunately, a reality for some).[116]

Another notable film, *Go Now* (1995) ⚔⚔⚔⚔ , stars Robert Carlyle, Juliet Aubrey, and James Nesbitt and was directed by Michael Winterbottom. It follows Nick (Robert Carlyle) and Karen (Juliet Aubrey) and their struggle with progressive MS. Nick, a working-class Glaswegian, develops a useless hand followed by numbness, ataxic-spastic gait, and, eventually, double vision. The ophthalmologist refuses to tell him the diagnosis, afraid it will lead to more stress. The neurologist procrastinates and adds to the long waiting time. *Go Now* shines light on the frustrations of diagnosing MS and coping with the handicap. The film takes place back when achieving a diagnosis was more difficult due to widely unavailable magnetic resonance (MR) imaging and perhaps also because cautious physicians would not commit to definitive conclusions.

DIALOGUE

Go Now

Karen	*All those questions you are asking him. He has got MS?*
Ophthalmologist	*Not necessarily. It is a possibility.*
Karen	*Why the hell did you not tell him?*
Ophthalmologist	*Do you know anything about MS?*
Karen	*A bit.*
Ophthalmologist	*The symptoms can come and go. Sometimes they disappear altogether.*
Karen	*If he's got it, he has the right to know.*
Ophthalmologist	*It is stress related. Telling him might induce an attack.*
Karen	*What are you going to do?*
Ophthalmologist	*Nothing; but if you want to tell him, you should do so.*

The first sign of Nick's MS is numbness and hand weakness, resulting in a sledgehammer falling down a shaft during work. Soon he has blurred vision, leading to an extensive ophthalmologic evaluation with visual field

---

[116] Karenberg A. Multiple Sclerosis On-Screen: From Disaster to Coping. *Mult Scler.* 2008;14:530–540.

testing. "You won't make the dart team," his girlfriend Karen (Juliet Aubrey) jokingly remarks. The oph-thalmologist calls it a "trapped nerve and overcompensating," resulting in a new eyeglass prescription. These symptoms worry Karen, and she goes to the library and finds out that these signs could mean MS. Another meeting follows, and the film shows a conversation with the ophthalmologist, who suggests withholding the diagnosis. As previously noted, such reluctance has been predicated on the uncertainty of predicting the course of MS. The scene reflects practice in the 1960s but not currently. Neurologists tell patients the diagnosis when there is a reasonable certainty of MS based on actual evidence.

In the ensuing scenes, Nick has great difficulty moving his foot and cannot avoid crashing his car. Next, we see him walking in the hospital with a spastic gait but without any information. ("There is something wrong with me. They are testing for AIDS.") He leaves the hospital, and much to his surprise, discovers that his girlfriend has an MS self-help book. This leads to a confrontation and finally accep-tance. Nick's MS progresses with incontinence and impotence but has a "happy ending," in which they dance at their wedding to the Moody Blues' song, "Go Now." The film has some banalities, but it is a relief to see a more credible representation than the ghastly *Ich Klage An*.

A very different and strange film is *Dreamland* (2006) ⌃ , which shows a young woman with MS and "killer spasms." She uses bee stings and touches electrical wires to improve her condition. The films that use MS in their plots, unfortunately, use it to show a major disabling disease ending in major handicap and ignore the much more common, unpredictable, and often benign nature. Treatments are rarely mentioned, if ever.

The worldwide prevalence of MS is approximately 2 million individuals.[117] Although it remains incurable, progression of MS nowadays is constantly influenced by new therapeutic approaches in the acute and chronic phases. In fact, it has been stated that the emergence of new MS therapies is unequaled in any other area of neurology. Cinematic portrayals of MS commonly show rapidly progressive—likely primary progressive—disease. (For a documentary, see Chapter 6.) They may cer-tainly convince the viewing public to believe that MS rapidly leads to the use of a wheelchair and fatality.

Amyotrophic Lateral Sclerosis

ALS is characterized by the degeneration of motor neurons in the brain and spinal cord. It begins insidi-ously with focal weakness but spreads relentlessly to involve most muscles, including the diaphragm, with death from respiratory paralysis in as little as three years.[118] The clinical course in ALS, however, remains very difficult to judge. The foremost ALS expert, Hiroshi Mitsumoto, said, "When I see patients, I try to find any factors that might be associated with a better prognosis and emphasize these factors"[119] but also admits that "we do not have strong evidence regarding how to discuss diagnosis and prognosis appropriately and effectively."[120] Motor neuron disease is not a topic readily chosen by screenwriters, and when it is used, it seems to fall into the general categories of "severe disability" and "dying from an untreatable disorder."

The key film to see is *You're Not You* (2014) ⌃⌃ , directed by George Wolfe and starring Hilary Swank as Kate. She is an affluent fashion designer and an accomplished pianist. Her symptoms become apparent

[117] In many, after 10 to 20 years, a progressive clinical course develops eventually leading to impaired mobility and cogni-tion, but unfortunately, 15% of patients have a progressive course from onset. See Reich DS, Lucchinetti CF, Calabresi PA. Multiple Sclerosis. *N Engl J Med*. 2018;378:169–180; and Thompson AJ, Baranzini SE, Geurts J, Hemmer B, Ciccarelli O. Multiple Sclerosis. *Lancet*. 2018;391:1622–1636.

[118] Brown RH, Al-Chalabi A. Amyotrophic Lateral Sclerosis. *N Engl J Med*. 2017;377:162–172; and Francis K, Bach JR, DeLisa JA. Evaluation and Rehabilitation of Patients with Adult Motor Neuron Disease. *Arch Phys Med Rehabil*. 1999;80:951–963.

[119] Mitsumoto H. What If You Knew the Prognosis of Your Patients with ALS? *Lancet Neurol*. 2018;17:386–388.

[120] See also Aoun SM, Breen LJ, Howting D, Edis R, Oliver D, Henderson R, et al. Receiving the News of a Diagnosis of Motor Neuron Disease: What Does It Take to Make It Better? *Amyotroph Lateral Scler Frontotemporal Degener*. 2016;17:168–178.

when she strikes the wrong key during a piano recital. The film quickly fast-forwards; 18 months later, Kate is in a wheelchair being tended to by her husband, Evan (Josh Duhamel). Kate is looking for a new nursing aide because the last one "made her feel like a patient" and is mostly wheelchair-bound. Her full dependency on others is well depicted. So, too, is the occasionally nefarious effect of the disease on relationships. Kate experiences the infidelity of her husband, abandonment by close friends, and a tense relationship with toxic parents. When Kate discovers that her husband is having an affair, her anger is quickly replaced by guilt. "I'm the one who got sick, not him," she says. "This isn't the life he built, the life he deserves. He turns me over in my sleep. He feeds me. He bathes me. He does everything but breathe for me. Believe me, he'd do it if he could." And Kate's friends, caricatured as "the ladies who lunch," offer little comfort. One sees her struggling to eat a salad and tells her, "It's going to get a lot easier when you're stronger." She angrily replies, "I'm not getting stronger, so please don't say that." The film captures the emotional ups and downs of the illness. At various points, Kate responds to her daily challenges with dismay, flatness, and desensitization—and what appear to be some elements of a pseudobulbar affect. As the disease progresses, Kate's voice becomes nasal and unintelligible. Kate has major coughing and choking spells, but during a birthday party, she drinks a martini with a straw, which apparently causes no difficulties.

At the end of the film, Kate is hospitalized after her breathing deteriorates. A major family conflict ensues over the decision to intubate her. Kate's parents are visibly upset and try to convince her husband to change the advance directive at the last moment, which he refuses to do. Eventually, she is sent home to die, in keeping with her wishes. Without any respiratory support or the commonly used Trilogy ventilator, Kate dies in the presence of her caregiver and not her husband. One scene is remarkable and very disturbing. In her last moments, Kate's hands clasp at her chest as she tries to catch her breath. She is sobbing. The sound is muted during this scene, ending with Kate's loud, chilling final gasp. It is very unfortunate that the film depicts the end of life as a terrifying struggle. ALS patients and their families often assume that the end will entail a choking death, but neurologists know from the experiences of ALS nurses and palliative care physicians that most patients with ALS die peacefully, either asleep or in a comatose state. Coughing attacks due to mucous airway congestion are very uncommon. So are restlessness and anxiety, as most patients are adequately sedated with morphine or benzodiazepines in the terminal phase. Although *You're Not You* depicts ALS with sensitivity and care, capturing the loneliness and indignity of a fatal neurodegenerative disease, I was hoping for a film with a more measured, less manipulative representation of the final trajectory of ALS. Whether this constitutes irresponsible filmmaking or simply dramatic license is up to the viewer to decide. But Kate's enthusiasm and infectious personality and resilience are what we often see in ALS patients. A small majority of ALS patients rapidly transition to early withdrawal of care, but many feel their life still has a purpose and they make the most of it.[121]

There are very few other fiction films to consider, but the best-known movie is *Tuesdays with Morrie* (1999) ✻ starring Jack Lemmon and Hank Azaria and directed by Mick Jackson. The film is based on Mitch Albom's tremendously popular best-selling novel about Morrie Schwartz, who died of ALS. The film is about one of Morrie's students, Mitch Albom, who travels every week from Detroit to Boston to meet with him. The film's main theme is for Mitch to come to the realization that a fatal illness can be unnecessarily prolonged.

Morrie decides that he will not proceed with a tracheostomy and mechanical ventilation when he reaches the inevitable progression to severe swallowing difficulties. The film is about acceptance. ("Don't treat me. I'm already dead.") It is about what matters in life more than about the disorder of ALS. In Albom's book, Morrie never mentions his illness or his own coping with becoming disabled. The film shows young people witnessing the life experiences of the old and dying. Both the film and the book may be characterized by some as a touchy feely story about the gradual decline of a virtuous man and "love

---

[121] Rabkin JG, Wagner GJ, Del Bene M. Resilience and Distress among Amyotrophic Lateral Sclerosis Patients and Caregivers. *Psychosom Med.* 2000;62:271–279.

conquers all" but does not provide insight into the specific tortuous decline of ALS. Overall, the main criticisms of the book involved its simplicity, which can also be applied to the movie.

Two other films have specifically used motor neuron disease (and ALS), and both actors seem to be modeled after Stephen Hawking (see Chapter 7). His posture, with a lateral head deviation, is used by both actors. *The Theory of Flight* (1998) ◄ stars Helena Bonham Carter, Kenneth Branagh, and Gemma Jones and was directed by Paul Greengrass. Jane (Helena Bonham Carter) is a disabled woman with a "rare form of motor neuron disease." The film is mostly about how she loses her virginity. She communicates with a voice box and seems to closely imitate Stephen Hawking's appearance. She lifts one of her shoulders to her head, creating a similar look, and speaks with poor articulation and lack of mimicry.

Hugo Pool (1997) ◄ was directed by Robert Downey, Sr., and stars Patrick Dempsey as Floyd. He is in a wheelchair and has a voice box. In the film, it becomes clear that he wants everyone to know that ALS is not contagious and that his lovemaking is not fully affected. His role is central in the movie—in a wheelchair, not moving, not speaking (only a whisper), being spoon-fed, and drinking through a straw. His head is constantly tilted to one side, also likely mimicking Stephen Hawking's posture. Predictably, in one of the final scenes, he has sexual intercourse with Hugo (Alyssa Milano) and soon thereafter passes away.

DIALOGUE

Hugo Pool

Minerva	*My daughter says you got this thing, ALS. What does it do to you? It attacks the nerves and then they die. The only part that does not get destroyed is the brain.*
Floyd	*I got a twitch in my right arm. That is what happens before I lose it.*
Hugo	*You are going to beat it.*
Floyd	*I like the way you think.*

Both these films have little to say about motor neuron disease and are about living with a major disability and—how can it not be—about sex in a markedly disabled person. All films represent ALS poorly—in an end stage but with major inconsistencies, unable to speak but still able to safely eat. Serious viewers should turn to the documentaries (discussed in Chapter 6).

Leprosy

Diseases of the peripheral nervous system only show up in films with leprosy, which might be the most interesting for filmmakers (and medical historians). The discovery of the pathogen was ethically compromised. Hansen discovered the Mycobacterium leprae. Hansen inoculated the pathogen of leprosy into the eye of a patient who had been treated for this disease for 17 years and supposedly without the patient's full knowledge. Hansen lost his position as physician of the Bergen leprosy hospitals but functioned as leprosy medical officer for the entire country of Norway and continued conducting research on the discovered leprosy bacillus.[122] Human leprosy has been documented for millennia in ancient cultures. Leprosy is a granulomatous infection of both nerves and skin caused by Mycobacterium leprae. It is still a significant health problem, and the World Health Assembly continues with measures to eliminate leprosy throughout the world. A significant improvement occurred after

---

[122]Grzybowski A, Sak J, Pawlikowski J, Iwanowicz-Palus G. Gerhard Henrik Armauer Hansen (1841–1912)—the 100th Anniversary of the Death of the Discoverer of Mycobacterium leprae. *Clin Dermatol.* 2013;31:653–655.

initiation of multi-drug therapy following many centuries of dapsone treatment. Leprosy is typically diagnosed as hypopigmented or reddish patches with loss of sensation, markedly thickened peripheral nerves, followed by nerve injury and weakness, and documentation of acid-fast bacilli on skin smears or biopsy material. Nerve damage involves the peripheral nerve trunks and, more specifically, on a radial cutaneous nerve, medial nerve, postural tibial nerve, and the lateral popliteal nerve. Enlargement of these nerves may cause pain but eventually also produces hypesthesia and hyperhidrosis, which results in infections and ulceration. Treatment is rifampicin, clofazimine, and dapsone. There is uncertainty about transmission, and it has been known for many years that proximity to leprosy patients increases the risk. However, bacteria do not enter intact skin and do not spread through touch.[123] Leprosy has not been eradicated outside the Western world, with a prevalence of more than 1 per 10,000 in Asia, Africa, and South America. The World Health Organization has found major concentrations of leprosy in India, Brazil, Burma, Madagascar, and Nepal. There has been an increase over the last decade, possibly explained by improved case findings.

The public health issues with leprosy are well depicted in *The Motorcycle Diaries* (2004) ⫷⫷⫷ starring Gael Garcia Bernal and Rodrigo de la Serna and directed by Walter Salles. It is based on a memoir of Argentinian Marxist revolutionary, Ernesto (Che) Guevara's journey from Argentina through Chile, Peru, Colombia, and Venezuela, which included the San Pablo leper colony. The leper colony is a key element in the film. His friend, Alberto Granado, who had already worked in a leprosy hospital in Cordoba, Argentina, proposed the trip. Ernesto Guevara de la Serna (later known as Che Guevara) was an Argentine medical student who dropped out of medical school to join Alberto on this defining trip. The film has little to say about his later political activism. Here, it concentrates on his confrontation with the leprosarium, where approximately 600 patients, mostly Peruvian, were under the care of missionaries.

The island is separated by the Amazon River, and the medical staff lives on the other side of the river. When Ernesto crosses the river, a physician asks him to wear gloves, but he refuses, and when he visits the colony, he shakes hands, to the surprise of a patient. ("Doctor, haven't you explained the rules?") Most of the patients with leprosy live there after having been fired from their jobs, and now they raise farm animals. The film shows real patients affected by leprosy with their major mutilations and nodular skin lesions resulting from granulomatous disease. In the three weeks that Ernesto and Alberto stay in this leprosarium, they attend to wound care and convince Sylvia ("a rebellious patient") to proceed with surgery to save her arm. The visit ends with a historically accurate farewell scene by Ernesto in which he swims across the Amazon River. The film correctly depicts the concentration of leprosy in leprosariums, often on islands. These leprosariums stigmatized patients but provided accurate management of the disease, often under the guidance of missionaries.

DIALOGUE

The Motorcycle Diaries

Doctor	*I suggest you wear these gloves, although leprosy is not contagious under treatment. The nuns are quite insistent on this point.*
Ernesto	*If it's not contagious, then it is just symbolic.*
Doctor	*Yes, but I'm telling you so you don't make any mortal enemies. Don't say I did not warn you.*

---

[123]See Britton WJ, Lockwood DN. Leprosy. *Lancet*. 2004;363:1209–1219; Foss NT, Motta AC. Leprosy, a Neglected Disease That Causes a Wide Variety of Clinical Conditions in Tropical Countries. *Mem Inst Oswaldo Cruz*. 2012;107 Suppl 1: 28–33; and Rodrigues LC, Lockwood D. Leprosy Now: Epidemiology, Progress, Challenges, and Research Gaps. *Lancet Infect Dis*. 2011;11:464–470.

The film clearly identifies the presence of missionaries and their role in treating leprosy. In the early 1900s, thousands of European missionaries served in many parts of the country with their objective not only to serve lepers, but also to engage in evangelization. Often, the Biblical underpinning of their mission was based on New Testament passages that include miracles Jesus performed on lepers who came to request cleansing and casting out of demons. (This is also clearly reflected in *The Motorcycle Diaries*, when Mother Superior refuses food to Ernesto and Alberto because they did not attend Holy Mass.) However, the role of missionaries in treating those affected by leprosy cannot be overstated.[124] Their work is best portrayed in *Molokai: The Story of Father Damian* (1999) about a Belgian priest canonized by Pope Benedict XVI who worked in a leprosy settlement in Hawaii and died from it. This inspirational film is about sacrifice, courage, compassion, and the Gospel message. It is not about neurology unless Father Damian's repeated close contact with dying, untreated patients is intended as a warning of what should have been avoided. (The Kalaupapa settlement, Molokai in Hawaii, was notorious, mostly because many young children were sent there for indefinite confinement. Several memoirs highlighting their anguish have been published.)

City of Joy (1992) ◄◄ with Patrick Swayze, shows slums in Calcutta, India, with actual leprosy patients, and the non-infectious origin is again emphasized. ("I have it, but my daughter does not.") A remarkable line by one of the doctors states that the people are simple and not educated and will never accept lepers in their midst. (City of Joy Aid is an actual humanitarian organization in Calcutta, and the network of clinics, schools, rehabilitation centers, and hospital boats bring relief to the neediest.)

In *The Hawaiians* (1970), there is a very brief scene showing crippled lepers separated on an island who are pushed away by the lead actor (Charlton Heston) in the film but without much further insight into the disorder. The lepers look like zombies, an offensive portrayal, but prejudice and misunderstanding continue to this day.

A more or less identical theme is found in the more recent delightful film *Yomeddine* (2018) ◄◄◄◄ , directed by Egyptian director AB Shawky and expanded from his earlier documentary short entitled *The Colony,* about the Abu Zaabal leper colony in Cairo. Bashay is played by a true leper Rady Gamal and is essentially a film about the unwanted and abandoned grotesques.[125] A flashback shows Bashay moving into the colony with a hopsack cover over his head. (*The Elephant Man* immediately comes to mind.) In this fiction film, he travels to the province where his family lives after the death of his wife. In a bus, he scolds everyone shrinking from him in disgust: "I am a human being!" *Yomeddine* addresses cultural myths in the Arab world that discriminate against people with leprosy and misconceptions about high transmission rates. This film and others highlight the inhumanities of being affected by scarring neurologic disease and thus fully belong in this book.

Cerebral Palsy

Cerebral palsy is a brain injury that occurs before birth and can dramatically affect a person's functioning and activities. Cerebral palsy—the name and the diagnostic frame—emerged in the mid-19th century. The English surgeon William Little is credited with the first description, in a series of lectures to the Obstetrical Society of London between 1843 and 1844. Little wholly inaccurately framed the condition as the result of "asphyxia neonatorum, and mechanical injury to the fetus immediately before or during parturition."[126] In 1946, the US National Society for Crippled Children and Adults

---

[124]Kipp RS. The Evangelical Uses of Leprosy. *Soc Sci Med.* 1994;39:165–178.

[125]See also Wijdicks EFM. Grotesques: Unwanted and Abandoned. In: *Cinema, M.D.* New York: Oxford University Press; 2020:245–268.

[126]Accardo P. William John Little and Cerebral Palsy in the Nineteenth Century. *J Hist Med Allied Sci.* 1989;44:56–71; and Kavcic A, Vodusek DB. A Historical Perspective on Cerebral Palsy as a Concept and a Diagnosis. *Eur J Neurol.* 2005;12:582–587.

established an advisory council on cerebral palsy, which became the American Academy for Cerebral Palsy.

One of the first major feature films to address cerebral palsy was *Gaby: A True Story* (1987) ⫷⫷ starring Rachel Levin, Norma Aleandro, Liv Ullmann, and Robert Loggia and directed by Luis Madoki. It is based on the upbringing and development of the Mexican writer Gabriela Brimmer. The original book features three voices: Gaby, her mother, Sari, and her caregiver, Florencia Morales Sánchez. Gaby became the leading spokesperson in Mexico for people with disabilities; she died at the age of 52 in 2000.

Dialogue

Gaby: A True Story

Gaby

How can I scream when I can't talk? God, if life is so many things that I am not, and never will be, give me the strength to be what I am.
How can I stop loving with the seed of a woman inside me?

Norma Aleandro, who plays Gaby, mostly acts out manifestations of chorea but shows no signs of pseudobulbar palsy. In the beginning of the film, the family is incorrectly told that cerebral palsy is a consequence of Rhesus incompatibility and that she can be mentally retarded or "locked inside her body." Her mother, played by Liv Ullmann, plays a somewhat remote role, but her nanny, Florencia, acts as an interpreter and is the first to discover that Gaby can communicate using her feet. At eight years old, she enters a rehabilitation center's elementary school. There, her language arts teacher persuades her to write. As readers of this book can expect by now, this film predictably includes sexual awakening, when she falls in love with a disabled schoolmate. There is some insight into the disability with cerebral palsy, but the film is easily overshadowed by *My Left Foot*.

My Left Foot (1989) ⫷⫷⫷⫷ stars Daniel Day-Lewis and Brenda Fricker[127] and was directed by Jim Sheridan. The painstakingly crafted film represents cerebral palsy best. Hugh O'Conor plays young Christy Brown with Daniel Day-Lewis in the adult role. The film opens with him at a charity event and then flashes back to his birth. ("Your son has been born. There have been some complications.") The film (inaccurately) suggests a fetal anoxic event during labor, but the onset of this static lesion of the cerebral motor cortex is unknown. Very few cases of cerebral palsy are likely to be caused by severe acute hypoxia during birth. Multiple births, maternal infection antepartum, vaginal bleeding, and fetal infection are all risk factors, but the prevalence is very low. The diagnosis of cerebral palsy is based on a major manifestation of spasticity coexisting with dystonia. The film suggests that psychotherapy and occupational and speech therapy can be applied successfully, but there is little evidence that these are helpful. In some children, motor skills improve. Long-term effects are common including joint dislocation, scoliosis, and deformities.

Christy Brown came from a family of 13 children, and his mother taught him to write and paint. Dublin in the 1930s housed working people and the poor in large sections of town. Children with disabilities would "go to a home," and there were no facilities. The Catholic Church provided shelter and food to the poor but had no practical solution for severe disability. Christy was born under problematic circumstances and apparently was unresponsive after birth and floppy. His mother knew he was different, but she also taught him.

---

[127] Daniel Day-Lewis received a Best Actor award, and Brenda Fricker received Best Actress in a Supporting Role.

DIALOGUE

My Left Foot

Man in bar	*Are you gonna put him in a home, Paddy?*
Paddy Brown	*I'll go in a coffin before any son of mine will go in a home.*
Man in bar	*Now, Paddy, I believe it's the end of the road.*
Woman	*And there he was, lyin' at the bottom of the stairs like a moron.*
Priest	*You can get out of purgatory, but you can never get out of hell. He's a terrible cross to the poor woman.*

According to his biographer, Anthony Jordan, "Every spare moment she had was spent trying to communicate with her son, trying to unlock the brain she knew was within the twisted frame."

The film shows the first discovery of intelligence when Cristy writes the letter "A" on a chalkboard. The film clearly shows many community members assuming the presence of major cognitive deficits, labeling them as instances of major mental retardation.

Daniel Day-Lewis (Figure 4.15) is incomparable in depicting cerebral palsy with its pseudobulbar signs and dystonic postures and avoids overuse of grimacing. The uncontrollable outbursts of screaming and crying may seem a bit unrealistic, but similar outbursts may occur in real life under stressful circumstances. The happy ending (he marries his nurse in the film) should be contrasted to the real Christy Brown (Figure 4.13), who became an alcoholic. (Some of it is shown in the film, which shows him drinking with a straw from a bottle hidden in his pocket.) According to his biographer, he was an "erudite and a philosophical man, who endured a long apprenticeship, but when success did come, he succeeded to 'Vanity Fair.'"[128]

Christy Brown's book *My Left Foot* was followed by *Down All the Days*, an autobiographical work about living in the slums of Dublin in the first part of the 20th century. The book showed drink and violence but also hopelessness and recklessness. ("We are all jarred, Christy, you know. You're not the only one. We all need a bit of help.") His tremendous unchanneled urge, energy, and frustration may have resulted in depression and alcoholism. He married Mary Carr, who neglected him. He apparently died by choking on a lamb chop.

The movie shows Christy's relationship with Dr. Collis, who became the founder of Cerebral Palsy Ireland. Dr. Collis developed a specific program in training and movement and generally getting the athetoid to work in whatever position was easiest. This was usually the sleeping posture. Speech therapy would provide control of the respiratory muscle and swallowing muscle.

Christy also joined the New Association for Disabled Artists and began painting. He gave exhibitions throughout Ireland. A major problem was Christy's alcohol abuse, and this also affected his writing and output.

Two other films on cerebral palsy should be mentioned. *Oasis* (2002) ⏪ portrays an abandoned young woman with cerebral palsy and a complicated courtship. The correct display of dystonia and spastic dysphonia won Moon So-Ri a Best Actress award at the Venice Film Festival. She is constantly grunting, in spasm, with eyes turning, and grimacing. The film is also unique because of several scenes in which she has fantasies of being normal and not spastic. This may occur in patients with cerebral

---

[128]Jordan AJ. *Christy Brown's Women: A Biography Drawing on His Letters, Incorporating the Founding of Cerebral Palsy Ireland by Robert Collis.* Dublin: Westport Books; 1980.

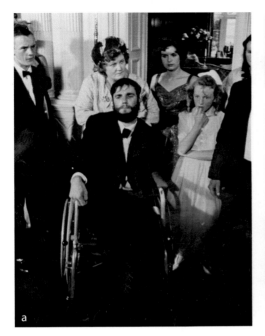
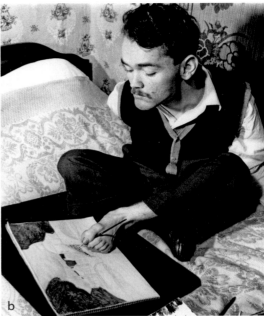
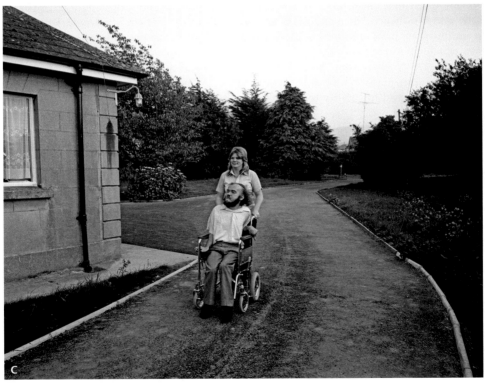

FIGURE 4.15 (a) Daniel Day-Lewis playing Christy Brown. (b) Christy Brown painting with his left foot. (c) Christy Brown in later life. (Used with permission of Irish Photo Archives and Ferndale Films/Hells Kitchen and Getty Images.)

palsy, but the desire to be considered normal is more often seen in patients with much less severe manifestations.

Door to Door (2002) ◄◄ was a TV film in the United States that gained prominence because of its theme of persistence. It is based on the true story of Bill Porter, a door-to-door salesman who could not drive well, speak well, and walked clumsily as a result of a "mild" cerebral palsy. These skills are needed for any door-to-door salesman, but he muscled through. (In real life, he was the top sales-man for the grocery that employed him.) The film stars William H. Macy, who accurately plays his challenge—walking up to 10 miles daily and selling almost anything to everybody. This comparatively mild case of cerebral palsy is acted with unusual distorted faces, unlike Daniel Day-Lewis, and is of some interest.

Several films portray the major physical disability of cerebral palsy. The films celebrate creativity and normal intelligence. Many of those affected by cerebral palsy are wrongly considered mentally handi-capped. It is good to see that this topic has interested directors.[129]

Autism

Autism spectrum disorders are present in nearly 1 in 70 US children. In 1911, Swiss psychiatrist Eugen Bleuler (1857–1939), coined the term autism (from the Greek autos, meaning "self"). The British psychiatrist Lorna Wing (1928–2014) noted that autism is a "spectrum condition" mani-fested in a variety of ways. There are many specialized autism clinics in the United States, and these disorders require a multi-disciplinary evaluation and mostly include neurologists. Films about autism can be divided into films where autism is mentioned in the script and a large part of the narrative and films where the diagnosis of autism is left for the audience to decide. Because autism spectrum disorders have unknown boundaries, interpretation can go wild. Indeed, the number of films in which we might think that autism was clearly intended is very large. Take, for example, *Forest Gump* (1994), where some have recognized Forrest as autistic. His literal interpretation of speech, his superior performance of sequential tasks ("Why did you put that weapon together so quickly, Gump?"), and his ability to maintain a singular focus (ping-pong, running). For many viewers, *Rain Man* (1988) ◄◄ is the key movie portraying autism but not to experts in the field. Most criticize the film for associating autism with savant syndrome (hyper-systemizing, presence of a memory brilliance), with which it is only rarely linked. The wild screaming scene induced by seeing hot water running in a tub and anxiety due to flying on an airline without a perfect crash record are the most memorable scenes, and such tantrums are common in autism. Dustin Hoffman's mannerisms otherwise seem contrived, and sentimentality wins. Pauline Kael—one of the most revered film critics—called it "wet kitsch."

After *Rain Man* (still a very enjoyable film with some good insights), films appeared with a more differentiated depiction of autism. *Fly Away* (2011) ◄◄◄◄ stars Beth Broderick, Ashley Rickards, and Greg Germann; it was written and directed by Janet Grillo and distributed by New Video Group. *Fly Away* is largely about Jeanne's (Beth Broderick) realization that her autistic teenage daughter Mandy needs help and cannot stay in her current social environment. Her attacks are muted by the lullaby "Lady Bug, Lady Bug, Fly Away." The film shows an extreme behavior disorder attributed to autism, with Mandy screaming and attacking other children at school and at play-grounds. The mother, Jeanne, is completely overwhelmed, burned out, and beaten up, living in a messy house. Mandy is a frightening child, and Jeanne is the persevering mother who endures against all odds. The movie has little to say about autism, but Mandy's moments of quiet drawing followed by night terrors are realistic. Jeanne continuously refuses to find a better solution. Because

---

[129]Hambleton GL. *Christy Brown: The Life That Inspired My Left Foot*. Edinburgh: Mainstream Publishing; 2007.

Mandy's flailing around in a car nearly causes an accident, she is transferred to a residential home for autistic children.

DIALOGUE

Fly Away

Schoolteacher	*Realistically, we have to provide her with skills.*
Mother	*Skills? … Like pushing a broom?*
Schoolteacher	*If it makes her feel good?*
Mother	*Mandy is smart. Inside all of that, she is so smart. Just because you cannot handle it, it does not mean my daughter belongs in an institution.*
Schoolteacher	*If you want to play the martyr, that is your choice, not mine.*

Autism spectrum disorders include Asperger's syndrome, and the differences between these disorders are shown in Table 4.3.[130] The films *Adam* (2019) and *Extremely Loud & Incredibly Close* (2011) deal with Asperger's syndrome. Both display repetitive behaviors and fixation on topics.

Adam (2009) stars Hugh Dancy, Rose Byrne, and Frankie Faison and was directed by Max Mayer. It very specifically addresses the social interactions and relationship problems of people with these autism spectrum disorders or, as the character of Beth says in the movie, "not prime relationship material." Adam is preoccupied with the solar system and the universe, and conversations often start with minute numerical details of the Big Bang and later expansion of the universe. He tells his girlfriend Beth (Rose Byrne) that his brain works differently than "neurotypicals." Examples of problematic behavior are many and include applying for nearly 100 jobs after getting laid off and being unable to go to a restaurant and eat something different than macaroni and cheese. Adam is angry with Beth's father, which leads to a major confrontation and the couple finally breaking up. Beth gives him chocolates after this because she feels sorry, and he responds, "I am not Forrest Gump." The disorder is accurately presented as a social interaction problem with outbursts of anger when his world is rocked. He is not able to handle such situations well.

DIALOGUE

Adam

Adam	*Their sensor systems have detected an error in analyzing space.*
Friend	*Adam, I am having lunch. Speak English. No more black holes, black hole radiation, Mars robots. Lunch time is for guys talking about women, the weather, and such.*

Extremely Loud & Incredibly Close (2011) was directed by Stephan Daldry and stars Tom Hanks and Sandra Bullock. Child actor Thomas Horn plays Oskar, the protagonist. Based on the 2005 Jonathan Safran Foer novel, the film makes no explicit connection to autism, and the plot focuses on the loss of a beloved parent in 9/11. In one scene, Oskar reveals he was tested for Asperger's but never actually

---

[130]Volkmar FR, Pauls D. Autism. *Lancet*. 2003;362:1133–1141.

TABLE 4.3   Diagnostic Features of Autism Spectrum Disorders

Features	Autism	Asperger's Syndrome
Age of recognition (diagnosis)	0–3 years (3–5 years)	>3 years (6–8 years)
Regression	About 25% (social or communication)	No
Sex ratio (male:female)	2:1	4:1
Socialization	Poor	Poor
Communication	Delayed, might be non-verbal	No early delay; qualitative and pragmatic difficulties later
Behavior	More impaired than in Asperger's syndrome	Variable (circumscribed interests)
Intellectual disability	>60%	Mild to none
Cause	More likely to establish genetic or other cause than in Asperger's syndrome	Variable
Seizures	Experienced by 25% over life span	Experienced by 10% over life span
Outcome	Poor to fair	Fair to good

diagnosed. He often brings out his therapy tambourine, which he plays to control his anxiety. He is frequently struck by phobias and curious notions, and several examples deserve mention.[131] Oskar covers his ears to block out the noise of screeching subways and loud planes. He has trouble with social interactions. He uses "stimming" (i.e., repetitive behaviors) such as repeatedly opening and closing a door. He retreats under his bed. Then, he finds a key in an envelope with the name "Black" written on it, and he believes it is a clue to his father's death when the Twin Towers fell on 9/11, which sets him on a mission through New York (Figure 4.16). He fixates on numbers including the number of times someone has hugged him.

The thin line between being a nerd and being afflicted by Asperger's syndrome is clear in *Napoleon Dynamite* (2004) ◄◄ directed by Jared Hess. In a film showing features of teen culture and bullying, Napoleon is a social misfit. *Napoleon Dynamite* is very polarizing. It contains a lot of arch, ironic humor including a famously kooky dance. Psychiatrists Levin and Schlozman (2006) have argued he has a socially disconnected character but may have symptoms consistent with Asperger's syndrome. There is impairment of non-verbal behavior (facing the floor when speaking), abruptly stopping conversations, irritability, and dysphonia. However, some people have strongly argued that Napoleon is simply a geek and nothing more.[132]

Autism has become more prevalent over the last ten years (partly as a result of better recognition). It is rarely (<10%) associated with a severe disorder such as tuberous sclerosis, fragile X, or fetal alcohol syndrome. The association of autism and MMR vaccine has been consistently denied by most experts. Volumetric studies and neurotransmitters have been studied, and some abnormalities have been found, but most MRIs in children diagnosed with autism are normal.[133]

Historically, autism spectrum disorders have rarely been considered part of neurology, but recent work has identified the likelihood of an anatomical variant (6–12 months post-natal hyperexpansion of cortical surface areas). A pediatric neurologist may help to ensure a thorough and accurate diagnosis but could also help with seizure management because seizures are more common with autism. The unusual

---

[131] These examples show that director Daldry did thorough research. In fact, he screened the film for experts and children with Asperger's before release, soliciting their input.

[132] Levin HW, Schlozman S. Napoleon Dynamite: Asperger's Disorder or Geek NOS? *Acad Psychiatry*. 2006;30:430–435.

[133] Manning-Courtney P, Murray D, Currans K, Johnson H, Bing N, Kroeger-Geoppinger K, et al. Autism Spectrum Disorders. *Curr Probl Pediatr Adolesc Health Care*. 2013;43:2–11; Pellegrino L, Liptak GS. Consultation with the Specialist: Asperger Syndrome. *Pediatr Rev*. 2011;32:481–488; quiz 489; and Yates K, Le Couteur A. Diagnosing Autism/Autism Spectrum Disorders. *Paediatr Child Health*. 2016;26:513–518.

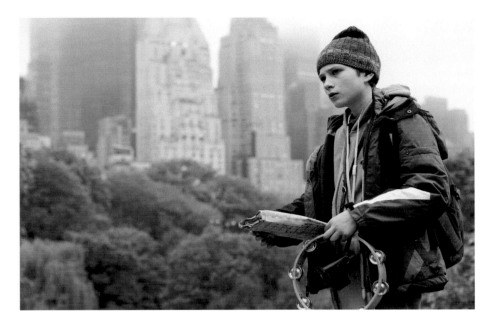

FIGURE 4.16   Oskar on a mission to find the owner of the mysterious key in *Extremely Loud & Incredibly Close* (Everett Collection, Inc.). Note the tambourine, which he plays when in a fearful situation.

behaviors associated with autism spectrum disorders attract filmmakers. The above-mentioned films have used this disability to fill entire screenplays.

Tourette's Syndrome

Tourette's syndrome is autosomal dominant by complex segregation techniques, but no genome linkage has been found. Treatment is a combination of psychological techniques and pharmacologic management, mostly dopamine antagonists or atypical neuroleptics.[134]

George Gilles de la Tourette's first patient with the characteristic behavioral disturbances was Countess Picot de Dampierre, who was known for her involuntary verbal outbursts, coprolalia, in salons frequented by the 19th-century Parisian aristocracy. Within her family, she was perceived to have a comic, caustic personality, not unusual in this society, and she remained socially integrated despite additional extraordinary contortions and grimaces.[135] Not long ago, Tourette's was seen as a psychiatric disorder ("acute nervous and convulsive disease") and treated with psychotherapy. It is now a reasonably treatable medical disorder.[136] Gilles de la Tourette's syndrome is rare (worldwide prevalence of 1%), and one would expect that the strange vocalizations such as sniffing, throat clearing, snorting, and tics with twitching and head nodding would interest filmmakers writing comedies. Several fiction films have used this syndrome and other tics and are successful. Obscenities in cinema are shown as coprolalia or copropraxia but, in reality, these manifestations are uncommon (25 % and 5%).

[134]See Cavanna AE, Seri S. Tourette's Syndrome. *BMJ*. 2013;347:f4964; Robertson MM. The Gilles de la Tourette Syndrome: The Current Status. *Arch Dis Child Educ Pract Ed*. 2012;97:166–175; Plessen KJ. Tic Disorders and Tourette's Syndrome. *Eur Child Adolesc Psychiatry*. 2013;22 Suppl 1:S55–S60; 4. Robertson MM. Tourette Syndrome, Associated Conditions and the Complexities of Treatment. *Brain*. 2000;123 Pt 3:425–462.

[135]Walusinski O, Feray JC. The Marquise de Dampierre Identified at Last, the First Described Clinical Case of Gilles de la Tourette Syndrome. *Rev Neurol (Paris)*. 2020;176:754–762.

[136]Walusinki has written an extensive biography on the life and the works of Gilles de la Tourette. See Walusinski O. *Georges Gilles de la Tourette: Beyond the Eponym*. Illus. ed. New York: Oxford University Press; 2018.

Niagara, Niagara (1997) ⚔ stars Henry Thomas, Robin Tunney, Michael Parks, and Stephen Lang and was directed by Bob Gosse. *Niagara, Niagara* is a love story between two misfits with an unclear plotline. Tourette's plays predominantly in this film and is the basis of violent eruptions and, eventually, a fatal outcome. Marcy (Robin Tunney) and Seth (Henry Thomas) meet while shoplifting, and their relationship progresses to drugstore holdups. The film implies that Tourette's syndrome leads to violent behavior. Tourette's is shown with phonic tics, and the representation is remarkable. The fact that they occur during times of personal stress is accurate. The symptoms of echolalia (imitation of sentences or sounds of others), coprolalia (expression of socially unacceptable words) and copropraxia (obscence gestures) are all shown to excess. Marcy explains that all the girls in her grammar school called her nick-names: "Mental Marcy," "Spazzy," and "Twitchy." She explains that drinking helps her and "for some reason, sex helps." She even discusses incorporating tics into a voluntary movement. At one point, she goes to a drugstore and asks for Haldol and Cogentin (appropriate medication for Tourette's). Symptoms of obsessive-compulsive behavior are shown and explained (repeatedly tapping on her boyfriend and organizing pencils and nail-polish bottles). A major fight breaks out at the end of the film, likely to show the social difficulties implicit in the condition. ("They are calling it explosive-aggressive behavior.")

The Tic Code (1997) ⚔⚔ was directed by Gary Winick and stars Christopher Marquette, Gregory Hines, and Polly Draper. *The Tic Code* shows uncontrollable facial tics under stress in a film with a major melodramatic tone. The protagonist, Miles (Christopher Marquette), is a jazz piano prodigy. The movie shows Miles's father's denial of this syndrome as a neurologic disorder. The film becomes a buddy movie when Miles finds a saxophonist with Tourette's syndrome. (The film's screenwriter, Polly Draper, modeled him after her husband, who has Tourette's.) *The Tic Code* is quite impressive in its portrayal of involuntary (and mostly muted) mimicry. Miles makes guttural repetitive sounds/ vocalizations and tries to hold his breath. "I am not holding my breath, just holding my feelings." He also displays compulsory touching of objects. He is unable to play when stressed. His father left the family because of his tics, and his mother, Laura (Polly Draper), explains Tourette's as, "He's got a few less inhibitors in his brain." His father wants a genetic test because his new girlfriend is "creeped out by that Tourette's thing," but he is told angrily by Laura that genetic testing does not exist. Miles is nervous about seeing his father again after many years and puts on a patch (the type not mentioned, but likely a clonidine patch).

DIALOGUE

The Tic Code

Laura	*I think it means a lot to him to see someone with a similar neurologic problem.*
Tyrone	*Neurologic problem? I heard it called many things but never a neurologic problem.*
Laura	*What do you call it?*
Tyrone	*I call it something I don't like to talk about.*

Several other films briefly use Tourette's syndrome. An absurdly funny and massively exaggerated portrayal is in *Deuce Bigalow: Male Gigolo* (1999) ⚔, where one of the protagonist's female clients has long-lasting major tics and persistent echolalia and coprolalia to humorous effect. Her normal speech is constantly interrupted by sexual verbiage, but Deuce offers her a solution. He takes her to a baseball game, where others in the stadium interpret her outbursts as a critique of the game, and the crowd begins to shout out using her same language.

Tics and "hemifacial spasms" are common in Nicolas Cage in *Matchstick Men* (2003) ⚔⚔ and are associated with a considerable obsessive-compulsive disorder with compulsions and ritualistic behavior (closing the door three times). Inappropriate vocalizations are also apparent, suggesting Tourette's syndrome, but the full "syndrome" depicted in this film is not easily classifiable and seems a deliberate patchwork of overheard or read symptoms. Most recently, Tourette's has been used purely for comedic effect in *The Square* (2017). During a press conference, a Tourette's patient in the audience suddenly starts yelling obscenities, and others in the audience do not know where to look. One person steps up and tells the audience to accept this man's disorder. The film is about the absurdities of the art world and not specifically about Tourette's. The purpose of using it is unclear. The director Östlund responded: "I'm making fun of everyone. I'm very thorough in that way. No one escapes from this satiric approach."[137]

Hollywood's use of Tourette's syndrome allows the screenwriter to have the character curse and fight whenever it comes in handy. Whether anti-social behavior is related to Tourette's syndrome is a topic of discussion among experts. Severe Tourette's syndrome is rare, and anti-social behavior is uncommon. I hope, at some point, that there will be some appreciation of the seriousness of the disorder, its complex presentation, and associated compulsive behavior.

Neurogenetics

Genetics will likely appear more often in film now that the field of neurogenetics dominates major discoveries and new treatments. In film, neurogenetics started in 1992 with *Lorenzo's Oil*, which created controversy as a result of its therapeutic claims. Without precedent, it prompted editorial comments in the *New England Journal of Medicine* and *The Lancet*.[138]

Lorenzo's Oil (1992) ⚔ , starring Nick Nolte, Susan Sarandon, Peter Ustinov, and Zack O'Malley Greenburg, was directed by George Miller. The film is based on Lorenzo Odone (Figure 4.17). Lorenzo (played, as he ages, by several actors) is a six-year-old child who becomes irritated easily, develops tantrums, and is diagnosed with adrenoleukodystrophy (ALD). The film starts with teachers pointing out to the parents (Augusto and Michaela Odone, played by Nick Nolte and Susan Sarandon) that Lorenzo has a disturbed behavior and suggests he needs a special-ed class, to which his mother replies, "The special aid our son needs will be provided at home." In fact, Lorenzo was an unusually gifted five year old who started demonstrating bizarre behavior in 1983. He received the mixture of two cooking oils three years later. The visit with the pediatric neurologist, Professor Nikolais (see also Chapter 3) after the diagnosis is established is realistic, and the disorder (with "abnormal very long-chain saturated fat" and "they have no enzyme to break it up," and "all we can hope for is to slow the cascade of symptoms") is explained reasonably well including the genetics. "ALD is passed only through the mother. It goes from mother to son." Myelin is explained as a plastic coating around electrical wires. The parents seek a treatment, and there seems to be an initial improvement, but the rest of the film shows the boy's decline (with spastic ataxic gait, likely acted by a double) to a minimally conscious state. At the end of the film, during the credits, several perfectly healthy-looking running children (with their names listed) tell the audience they have been on Lorenzo's oil for years.

DIALOGUE

Lorenzo's Oil

Pediatric neurologist	*It is the cruelest kind of genetic lottery. … No one is to blame.*
Lorenzo's mother	*All these experts working in isolation, each one on its own piece of the jigsaw.*

---

[137] Phillips-Carr C. Little More Than a Temper Tantrum: On Ruben Östlund's "The Square." *Another Gaze.* 2018; January 5.

[138] See Moser HW. Lorenzo's Oil. *Lancet.* 1993;341:544; and Rizzo WB. Lorenzo's Oil–Hope And Disappointment. *N Engl J Med.* 1993;329:801–802.

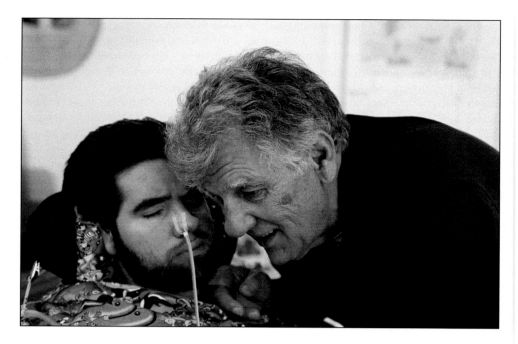

FIGURE 4.17   Lorenzo Odone and his father. (Used with permission of the Myelin Project.)

ALD is a rare X-linked disorder affecting 1 in 20,000 males. At the time of his diagnosis, Lorenzo's parents were told he could live a few years at the most, but he lived until age 30. The parents desperately tried to find a therapy to halt the relentless progression. The disorder results in dementia, loss of senses (sight, hearing), and ataxia due to storage of the so-called very-long-chain saturated fatty acids, resulting in demyelination. The accumulation of these lipid chains is a result of impaired degradation through peroxisomal β-oxidation.

In the film, clinical efficacy is suggested using oleic acid (unsaturated short chain) and erucic acid, which are potent competitive inhibitors.[139] This drama of a miracle cure prompted a strong critique by one of the leading experts, Dr. Hugo Moser. Lorenzo's oil may prevent progression in some patients but mostly when they are asymptomatic. Once the disease has advanced, there is no benefit. Still, it prevented the onset of ALD in two-thirds of susceptible boys who otherwise would have progressed and died.[140] The film also dramatizes the parent–physician conflict and inaccurately introduces a scene where the United Leukodystrophy Foundation objects to use of the oil. Rosen summarized the film as portraying "nurses as heartless, physicians as pompous fools, and parent support groups as mindless as a herd of sheep."[141]

Current opinion is divided. For Lorenzo, the oil did very little, resulting in the eventual progression of the disease and his ultimate demise at the age of 30 in 2008. Therefore, ALD continues to be a devastating disease without a cure or even effective treatment if not detected early. Consequently, the search for novel treatments is still active, and hematopoietic stem cell transplant and gene therapy are viable therapies for boys with early progressive cerebral disease.[142]

[139] Aubourg P, Adamsbaum C, Lavallard-Rousseau MC, Rocchiccioli F, Cartier N, Jambaque I, et al. A Two-Year Trial of Oleic and Erucic Acids ("Lorenzo's oil") as Treatment for Adrenomyeloneuropathy. *N Engl J Med*. 1993;329:745–752.

[140] Moser HW, Raymond GV, Lu SE, Muenz LR, Moser AB, Xu J, et al. Follow-Up of 89 Asymptomatic Patients with Adrenoleukodystrophy Treated with Lorenzo's Oil. *Arch Neurol*. 2005;62:1073–1080.

[141] Rosen FS. Pernicious Treatment. *Nature*. 1993;361:695.

[142] Moser AB, Liu Y, Shi X, Schrifl U, Hiebler S, Fatemi A, et al. Drug Discovery for X-Linked Adrenoleukodystrophy: An Unbiased Screen for Compounds That Lower Very Long-Chain Fatty Acids. *J Cell Biochem*. 2021. 2021 ;122(10):1337–1349.

Finding a cure for another devastating neurologic illness is the theme of *Extraordinary Measures* (2010) ◄◄ , starring Brendan Fraser, Harrison Ford, and Keri Russell and directed by Tom Vaughan. Brendan Fraser is John Crowley, a biotechnology executive with three children affected by Pompe disease (first described by a female Dutch pathologist in 1932). Pompe disease is a result of a deficiency of the lysosomal enzyme acid alpha-glucosidase, which breaks glycogen links.[143] The film immediately confronts the viewer with a child in a motorized wheelchair and another severely paralyzed. Both are tracheostomized and fed through a gastrostomy. Megan's eighth birthday party is the setup of the story. An underlying respiratory infection brings Megan to the ICU, and in an accurately portrayed physician–parent interaction, the physician tells the family that nothing more can be done and she is already past the normal life expectancy (classic Pompe rarely survives the first infantile year). After a successful resuscitation, the parents feel something needs to be done. Contact with an expert, Dr. Stonehill (Harrison Ford)—representing a fictional composite of scientists—leads to the discovery of an enzyme that halts progression.

DIALOGUE

Extraordinary Measures

Mother to Megan	*I mean, do we just accept our fate and do what we are told by all well-meaning doctors and wait for the worst to happen … or do we fight it?*
John to Dr. Stonehill	*The man is a genius. He is on the verge of a scientific breakthrough.*
Dr. Stonehill	*I am not on the verge of anything. … It is just a theory. … I am just an academic.*

The film is generally neurologically and scientifically accurate, but it remains difficult to have a child actor portray a major scoliosis, marked difficulty with breathing, and an absent smile due to facial muscle involvement. (In the movie, Megan smiles all the time.) Since 2006, enzyme-replacement therapy for this devastating glycogen-storage disease has resulted in some success in less-affected patients (predominantly in those with normal muscle architecture). *Extraordinary Measures* fortunately shows excellent representation of physician–parent interaction, the complex science behind the disease, and the funding of research by universities versus the industry. The film is based on the book *The Cure* by Geeta Anand.[144]

The Cake Eaters (2009) ◄ was directed by Mary Stuart Masterson and stars Kristen Stewart, Aaron Stanford, Jayce Bartok, Bruce Dern, and Elizabeth Ashley. The film introduces Friedreich's ataxia—a neurologic disorder for which there is no treatment. It results in progressive ataxia, dysarthria, spasticity, and cardiomyopathy.[145] The disorder was clearly chosen to add pathos to the life of a teenager afflicted with a neurodegenerative disease. The director contacted several persons with Friedreich's disease and sought input from the Friedreich's Ataxia Research Alliance (FARA). Kristen Stewart plays Georgia, a 15-year-old who falls easily and locks herself up in her home. She displays marked ataxia and slurred speech. She walks holding on to a wall in school or is assisted by friends. She refuses a wheelchair when one is offered. None of the common difficulty with fine dexterity is shown. She feels a sense of urgency now that she has been diagnosed, which leads to poor decisions. However, the progression and potential fatality of the cardiac disease is discussed. There is no further

[143] van der Ploeg AT, Reuser AJ. Pompe's Disease. *Lancet.* 2008;372:1342–1353.

[144] Akst JA. A review of *Extraordinary Measures*. The Scientist. Wilmington, DE: LabX Media Group; 2010.

[145] Parkinson MH, Boesch S, Nachbauer W, Mariotti C, Giunti P. Clinical Features of Friedreich's Ataxia: Classical and Atypical Phenotypes. *J Neurochem.* 2013;126 Suppl 1:103–117.

neurologic insight or discussion of the consequences of the disease, and therefore, the film is of little interest to physicians.

The Cake Eaters

Georgia	*I have Friedreich's ataxia.*
Boyfriend	*Is that why you talk drunk?... Are you going to get better?*
Georgia	*This is pretty much as good as it gets until my heart goes out. I wonder when that is going to be.*

The Madness of King George (1994) ✄ , which stars Nigel Hawthorne, Helen Mirren, Ian Holm, Amanda Donohoe, Rupert Graves, and Rupert Everett and was directed by Nicholas Hytner, focuses on the agitation and eccentric behavior associated with acute porphyria. In the opening footage, King George III develops excruciating abdominal pain and then suddenly recovers from what he says was one of his "smart bilious attacks." Attention focuses on his urine color, which is, at one point, dark and, at another point, blue. In 1966, Macalpine and Hunter[146] proposed that the King's illnesses were due to recurrent attacks of acute porphyria, an inherited metabolic disorder with paroxysms of physical and mental disturbance, which could be identified in succeeding generations and traced as far back in the King's ancestry as Mary Queen of Scots. Simultaneously, signs and symptoms of encephalopathy appeared: talking "with uncommon rapidity and vehemence," sensitivity to light and sound, emotional lability, uninhibited behavior, and nocturnal confusion. Total insomnia supervened; at one point, he had no sleep for 72 hours ... and to his death his physicians reported his sleep in quarters of an hour." "Great irritability of frame and temper" was accompanied by "turbulence" and frank delirium: "he baffled all attempts to fix his attention," and showed "gross errors of judgment."[147]

Acute porphyria may include neuropsychiatric symptoms, although its true spectrum is often misunderstood and exaggerated.[148] Neuropsychiatric manifestations of porphyria—significant confusion, hallucinations, and psychotic breaks—have been reported repeatedly in the literature, but there is very little to support such a connection. However, it is well known that acute porphyria can cause posterior reversible encephalopathy syndrome, which can present as acute confusion, seizures, and a decreased level of consciousness. These symptoms are all reversible after an attack has subsided. Another clear neurologic manifestation is peripheral motor neuropathy.

Apparently, King George III had four bouts of mental derangement in October 1788, February 1801, January 1804, and October 1810. This incapacity could last up to six months, resulting in "dementia" and the king's replacement by the Prince of Wales. There has been significant speculation about whether these events can be explained by acute porphyria. Attending physicians to King George III recorded the unusual colors in his urine including a blue pigment and blue ring on glass.[149]

The historical arguments against acute porphyria for King George III's spells and attacks are the rarity of the disease, lack of clinical features in his descendants in a disorder with a high penetrance, the atypical presentation, and the (often inaccurate) association of psychiatric disorders with acute porphyria. Attacks of acute porphyria are associated with increased urinary excretion of porphobilinogen as well

---

[146]Macalpine I, Hunter R. The "Insanity" of King George 3d: A Classic Case of Porphyria. *Br Med J*. 1966;1:65–71.

[147]Macalpine and Hunter, ibid.

[148]Crimlisk HL. The Little Imitator–Porphyria: A Neuropsychiatric Disorder. *J Neurol Neurosurg Psychiatry*. 1997;62: 319–328.

[149]Arnold WN. King George III's Urine and Indigo Blue. *Lancet*. 1996;347:1811–1813.

as increased excretion of aminolevulinate. Many patients have significant abdominal pain and vomiting. Pain may also affect muscles, back, buttocks, and thighs, and the abdominal pain may suggest peritonitis. A significant dysautonomia includes tachycardia and hypertension. These racing-heart symptoms are also mentioned in the film. The King's behavior (agitation, rambling incoherent speech, and episodes of violence and sexual impropriety) was treated by restraint. A recent linguistic analysis of King George's letters showed that during periods of mental illness, he wrote with a reduced vocabulary, fewer distinct word types, and a tendency to greater redundancy compared to the letters written prior to the onset or after recovery.[150] Others remain wholly unconvinced and attribute his illness to bipolar disease but also acknowledge such an assertion of porphyria fits well with a number of very questionable retrospective diagnoses in other historical figures (e.g., Mary Darwin, Vincent Van Gogh, and Admiral Beaufort; see also Chapter 9). [151]

Genetic aberrations may lead to rapid disability and, in some, a major neurodegenerative disease. The promotion of drug development in rare diseases is at the heart of a worldwide collaboration, and many countries have introduced a combination of regulations and policies for orphan drugs in the last two decades. Over 500 rare conditions have been designated.[152]

End Credits

This review of the signs and symptoms of neurologic disease and neurologic syndromes indicates that very few neurologic disorders have failed to merit a screenplay. We can show respect and admiration for the filmmakers and screenwriters who have brought these topics to the screen; it encapsulates an outright achievement. When a presentation is frankly wrong, we need to ask ourselves why; the nature of the inaccuracy may eventually highlight differences of perception between physicians and laypeople. When it is right, we should call it out and recommend it to colleagues and trainees. Soothing sentimentality is expected, as is grandstanding, but we will take it. We recognize that filmmakers or screenwriters do not necessarily share the obligations of the historian or scientist to present facts. Complete veracity is often be an unachievable (and unnecessary) standard. The study of neuroethics is another matter. Some films may be misguided or sensational while others correctly call out actual transgressions; that is the focus of the next chapter.

[150] Rentoumi V, Peters T, Conlin J, Garrard P. The Acute Mania of King George III: A Computational Linguistic Analysis. *PLoS One*. 2017;12:e0171626.

[151] Hift RJ, Peters TJ, Meissner PN. A Review of the Clinical Presentation, Natural History and Inheritance of Variegate Porphyria: Its Implausibility as the Source of the "Royal Malady." *J Clin Pathol*. 2012;65:200–205.

[152] Mariz S, Reese JH, Westermark K, Greene L, Goto T, Hoshino T, et al. Worldwide Collaboration for Orphan Drug Designation. *Nat Rev Drug Discov*. 2016;15:440–441.

5

Neuroethics in Film

The only thing worse than your kid dying on you is him wanting to.

The Sea Inside (2004)

Main Themes

Virtue and morality extends to the practice of neurology. Hospital practices are full of complex decisions and must incorporate neuroethics—the voice of our conscience. Neurointensivists and neurohospitalists have it no easier than intensivists, who must often decide to discontinue dialysis or to stop reintubating critical patients when the situation calls for it. Neurologic injury is often more calamitous, and the comatose or minimally aware patient cannot communicate. The burden of decision falls more frequently on families, and we must guide them in multiple conversations. Withdrawal of support or "comfort measures" are often quickly accepted by families because they fully and quickly grasp the scale of the injury. Serious illness conversations about severely affected neurologic patients should (and frankly must) include decisions on whether to go permanently on a ventilator and be fed through feeding tube, and to stay home or go to a hospice. All too often, unfortunately, these conversations do not take place preemptively, and they are nearly impossible to convene during a crisis. You cannot "just do nothing" for a patient with severe amyotrophic lateral sclerosis in acute distress. The ethics of acute neurology are vexing, but clear solutions to problems can be argued either way. Moreover, in limiting support, what is ethical and what is legal are often at odds.

For serious screenwriters, these situations offer some very interesting themes, particularly for those who have personally experienced these situations with a family member. Progressive or devastatingly disabling neurologic disease with its complex decision-making may certainly invite cinematic treatment. These decisions are commonly encountered bioethical concerns and involve multiple specialties with diverse skillsets. At the outset, we should be concerned about accurate portrayals of comprehensive palliative measures, specifically because most screenwriters are not qualified ethicists. (The venerable filmmaker Terrence Malick, who taught philosophy at the Massachusetts Institute of Technology, is perhaps a notable exception, but he has not yet ventured into neurology.[1]) We should not be surprised by the use of major topics such as euthanasia in devastating neurologic disease because the effect on the audience will be chilling, and it may produce exasperated sighs in medical professionals. But medicine has its own set of "skeletons in the closet" such as unethical experimentation and lack of informed consent. These are bound to provoke the audience with screenwriters willing to go an extra mile.

---

[1] Malick's streams of consciousness and landscapes were very suitable for cinema, but recently he ventured into a major ethical quandary with *A Hidden Life* (2019). See Rossouw MP. There's Something about Malick: Film-Philosophy, Contemplative Style, and Ethics of Transformation. *New Rev Film Telev Stud.* 2017;15:279–298.

DOI: 10.1201/9781003270874-5

Early in the history of US neurocinema, we encounter *An Act of Murder* (1948) ◄◄◄ , which involves a "mercy killing" when a brain tumor causes unbearable pain.[2] In this film, the patient's husband causes a car crash in an attempt to end it all. She is killed, but he survives. He successfully stands trial to argue his motivation and avoids a conviction for at least second degree homicide. It is not much better decades later, when Frankie (Clint Eastwood) in *Million Dollar Baby* (2004) ◄ sneaks into the hospital ward to disconnect a paralyzed ex-boxer from the ventilator. The film offered only one answer to her physical and emotional pain. Such scenes get media attention, but we do not know if filmmakers (or Hollywood, for that matter) care about this misrepresentation. Their whys are often untraceable, and they need not worry about accountability. We, as physicians, care deeply about intractable pain but are not always consistent in our practices. However, not all pain is intractable, and much can be effectively treated without resorting to the final extreme of ending the patient's life. But it is a major issue. Marcia Angell, a former editor of the *New England Journal of Medicine*, could not say it any better: "Pain is soul destroying. No patient should have to endure intense pain unnecessarily. The quality of mercy is essential to the practice of medicine; here, of all places, it should not be strained."[3]

Nevertheless, there are major challenges to face, and some aspects of decision-making are desperately sad. For example, there are decisions to withdraw care in patients when treatment is considered futile, patients deciding not to proceed with long-term care, and conflicting situations within families.

There are also sociologic concerns. The decision to move a family member with advanced dementia to a nursing home has been addressed in feature films.

Only recently have we seen these major bioethical situations addressed in film. Earlier ideas may have been rejected as too controversial or unable to pass Hays code restrictions. We had to wait for cinema to become more rebellious.[4] The bioethical topics portrayed in many films touch all specialties and, thus, are a potentially rich source of teaching and discussion. I have selected films where neurology is front and center. Sporadically filmed and presented neuroscience topics such as brain death and organ donation, psychosurgery and lobotomy, and psychologic experiments are covered elsewhere.[5] For cinematic accounts of ethics in the whole of medicine, I refer to other works.[6]

Physician-Assisted Suicide

Rising numbers of the public may support physician-assisted suicide (PAS). Surveys of physicians have low response rates and are limited by the same biases and heuristics as public surveys. Surveys in the United States, Europe, and Australia demonstrate lower support for euthanasia and PAS among physicians than the public.[7] PAS is currently available for Americans living in states where it is legally authorized. (Currently, "death with dignity" laws are present in 9 states.) In most cases, patients are prescribed lethal medications to be ingested at home. But in hospitals in states where assisted death is allowed, most physicians elect not to participate. In 2017, the American College of Physicians (ACP) concluded that "On the basis of substantive ethics, clinical practice, policy, and other concerns

---

[2] Angell M. The Quality of Mercy. *N Engl J Med.* 1982;306:98–99.

[3] Angell, 1982, Ibid.

[4] Post-war creativity in the arts developed into a "freedom from everything" movement that started in the late 1950s and continued through the 1970s. Filmmakers became more daring and created "new waves" in several European countries but also the US. See Menand L. *The Free World: Art and Thought in the Cold War.* New York: Farrar, Straus and Giroux; 2021.

[5] Wijdicks EFM. *Cinema, MD.* New York: Oxford University Press; 2020.

[6] Colt H, Quadrelli S, Friedman L, eds. *The Picture of Health: Medical Ethics and the Movies.* New York: Oxford University Press; 2011 and Shapshay S, ed. *Bioethics at the Movies.* Baltimore: Johns Hopkins University Press; 2009.

[7] Emanuel EJ, Onwuteaka-Philipsen BD, Urwin JW, Cohen J. Attitudes and Practices of Euthanasia and Physician Assisted Suicide in the United States, Canada, and Europe. *JAMA.* 2016;316:79–90.

articulated in this position paper, the ACP does not support the legalization of physician-assisted suicide. It is problematic given the nature of the patient-physician relationship, affects trust in the relationship and in the profession, and fundamentally alters the medical profession's role in society."[8] The answer to a question of a possible change in policy has remained a resounding "no" for the American Medical Association, although they fully embrace and support patient autonomy. PAS remains illegal in most countries, including Canada, Australia, all of Asia, and most European countries, including Germany and France. Occasionally, a controversial verdict surfaces.[9]

An important general observation is that over the last century we have reached a point where medicine can help most patients avoid severe symptomatic suffering, and this is a direct result of major advances in palliative care. Most physicians still would support a basic Hippocrates tenet: "I will give no deadly medicine to anyone if asked nor suggest such counsel." There are very few physicians in the world who play a central role in euthanasia or who would like to be identified as playing a central role.

And then there was Jack Kevorkian; characterized as a hero, sinner, and murderer. Dr. Jack Kevorkian, arguably one of the most controversial physicians in the United States, has been portrayed by Al Pacino. Because progressive neurologic disease, including non-terminal disabilities such as multiple sclerosis, is a commonly used justification for PAS—at least in Kevorkian's view—this film is highly relevant for neurologists. *You Don't Know Jack* (2010) ◄◄◄◄ stars Al Pacino, Danny Huston, Susan Sarandon, and John Goodman and is directed by Barry Levinson. *You Don't Know Jack* is an important, nearly documentary-style film because it unknots the real story from the myth. The movie does not glorify Kevorkian—far from it. It is more about the man than the cause. Alternative options for end-of-life care (i.e., comprehensive palliative care) are unfortunately not provided. Had the movie been a documentary, we might have been shown such options. Pacino received a well-deserved Emmy and a Golden Globe Award for his depiction of Kevorkian, whom he portrays as a bullheaded, obstinate, and principled person. In the Special Features section of the DVD, Kevorkian himself appears and seems pleased with the portrayal[10] (Figure 5.1).

The euthanasia movement did not start with Jack Kevorkian. The Euthanasia Society of America was founded in 1938. The initial successes in swaying public opinion were rapidly nullified after the Second World War, when euthanasia became associated with the Nazi euthanasia program. The right-to-die movement gained some momentum after the Karen Ann Quinlan and Nancy Cruzan cases of persistent vegetative state, but Jack Kevorkian is a different story. Medical organizations have always felt a great unease with Kevorkian's ideas, which is clearly stated early in the movie: "I love you, Jack, but most colleagues think you are nuts." Kevorkian's zeal became controversial when the *British Medical Journal* in 1996 published an editorial entitled "Jack Kevorkian: A Medical Hero," claiming that he had the "rare heroism to make us all feel uncomfortable."[11] The journal published a more nuanced paper in 1999, in which the US bioethicist physician Howard Brody stated, "Kevorkian, who by his own count, has assisted over 100 deaths, has always been a master at manipulating the American media. Early on, some defenders of assisted suicide complained that Kevorkian's personality and methods had been allowed to obscure the pros and cons of the issue itself." His obituary in the *British Medical Journal* in 2011 was far from laudatory and cited the palliative care physician and proponent Timothy Quill, who said "clearly his approach was the wrong one. It was always as much about Kevorkian as it was about the patients."[12]

---

[8] Snyder Sulmasy L, Mueller PS, Ethics P, Human Rights Committee of the American College of Physicians. Ethics and the Legalization of Physician-Assisted Suicide: An American College of Physicians Position Paper. *Ann Intern Med.* 2017;167:576–578.

[9] A pharmacist in the United Kingdom gave his father a morphine-laced fruit smoothie and later additionally injected him with insulin as he slept and died and then pleaded guilty. He was a free man after the judge imposed a sentence of suspended nine months. See Dyer C. Seven Days in Medicine: 15–21 November 2017. *BMJ.* 2017;359:j5382.

[10] Levinson B. *You Don't Know Jack.* HBO Films April 24, 2010.

[11] Roberts J, Kjellstrand C. Jack Kevorkian: A Medical Hero. *BMJ.* 1996;312:1434.

[12] Brody H. Kevorkian and assisted death in the United States. *BMJ.* 1999;318:953–954 and Stafford N. Jack Kevorkian. BMJ. 2011;342:d4100.

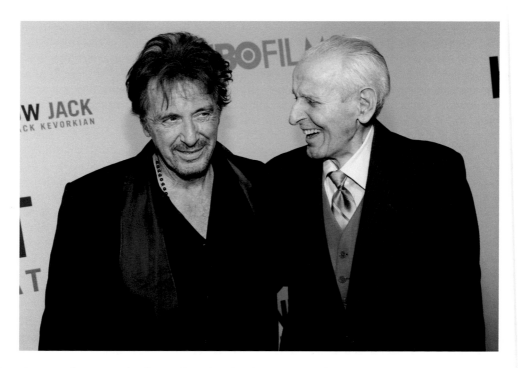

FIGURE 5.1 Al Pacino and Jack Kevorkian. (Used with permission of AP.)

(It should be noted that two years earlier, Brody co-authored a paper with Dr. Quill in the *New England Journal of Medicine* supporting the idea that physician-assisted suicides should be legal with a strictly regulated policy, each case being thoroughly examined by an independent committee.[13]) The debate[14] has continued and will certainly become interesting with the recent appointment to the US Supreme Court of strong opponent Neil Gorsuch.[15]

Jack Kevorkian has been admired, ignored, and caricatured. He was a celebrity who was greeted with applause on many talk shows. His infamous Volkswagen minivan—where he assisted patients in their suicide after driving to meet them in remote places—has been for sale on eBay. His macabre artwork shows Nazi symbols and decapitations. One of his paintings has been used as an album cover by the sludge metal band Acid Bath.

The medical side of Jack Kevorkian's story has been well documented. Dr. Kevorkian, a pathologist, claimed to have assisted in multiple deaths. He was tried in court multiple times and was acquitted multiple times. He built two devices. The first, called the Thanatron (*thanos* = death), was a machine built from scraps that provided barbiturates, a neuromuscular blocker, and potassium chloride. Later, when his medical license was revoked (and possibly because the necessary drugs could not be easily obtained anymore), he switched to the Mercitron (connoting mercy), consisting simply of a carbon monoxide canister and a mask. However, after he administered a lethal injection to a patient (Thomas Youk, a patient with amyotrophic lateral sclerosis) and used the television show *60 Minutes* to broadcast the video of Youk's euthanasia in 1998, he was charged with first-degree murder

[13] Miller FG, Quill TE, Brody H, Fletcher JC, Gostin LO, Meier DE. Regulating Physician-Assisted Death. *N Engl J Med.* 1994;331:119–123.

[14] See Quill TE, Battin MP, eds. *Physician-Assisted Dying: The Case for Palliative Care and Patient Choice.* Hardcover ed. Baltimore, MD: The Johns Hopkins University Press; 2004; and Foley K, Hendin H, eds. *The Case against Assisted Suicide for the Right to End-of-Life Care.* Baltimore: The Johns Hopkins University Press; 2004.

[15] Gorsuch NM. *The Future of Assisted Suicide and Euthanasia.* Princeton, NJ: Princeton University Press; 2006.

and delivery of a controlled substance. Kevorkian spent 8 years in prison. Think of him that way and then look at the film.

The film portrays the evolution of assisted suicide, according to Jack Kevorkian, very well, but the viewer should be warned that some clips from the original Kevorkian files show actual patients, intermingled with clips of actors. The film shows patients with Alzheimer's disease, amyotrophic lateral sclerosis, multiple sclerosis, and spinal cord injury. (The inclusion of neurologic disease in the film is an overrepresentation based on a review of his cases of euthanasia in Oakland County, Michigan, 1990–1998, which showed that 38% had neurologic disease.[16])

The movie also shows two patients rejected by Kevorkian, suggesting that he had personal criteria for selecting patients. To one patient with Parkinson's disease, he says it is not the right time. In another scene, a paraplegic patient with severe facial scarring—shown after a botched suicide attempt—is diagnosed by Kevorkian as depressed and is told with little compassion, "We cannot help you." Here the screenwriter suggests that Kevorkian is not available for anyone in despair. Kevorkian's criteria for assisting a patient in dying are not addressed. Most disturbing is a scene in which a patient is shown struggling with the mask, after which a plastic hood is placed over his head, eventually requiring two attempts to end his life.

The movie implies that Kevorkian meticulously documented these cases on index cards and used videotaping to show a non-coerced discussion with the patient. In all depicted scenes, the patient flips a switch to set off an infusion or pulls a paper clip from a section of compressed tubing, allowing the drug or gas to flow. The film clearly shows a parsimonious operation, and one of his assistants, played by John Goodman, says, "Jack Kevorkian is cheap."

In the movie, Jack Kevorkian proclaims that self-determination is a basic human right and emphasizes his desire to "cause a national debate." He comes up with an unusual and irrelevant comparison: why is it that mentally competent patients cannot decide whether they want to live or die while physicians are "starving" comatose patients? Susan Sarandon plays Janet Good of the Michigan Hemlock Society, who emphasizes that indignity alone can be a reason for wanting to die. The movie is grim, cold, and sad, and these feelings are further amplified throughout the movie as it counts the number of patients, names them, and then shows the dead in black and white.

DIALOGUE

You Don't Know Jack

Jack Kevorkian	*You know they started to do this in Europe already … Holland … never here, we are too puritanical.*
Reporter	*There are those who would say about Dr. Jack Kevorkian: 'Right message, wrong messenger.'*
Attorney	*And who is the right messenger?*

In the Netherlands since 2002, PAS and euthanasia are not punishable if provided by a physician meeting the requirements of due care. The Netherlands is the only country that also allows assisted dying for minors (0–12 years). Dutch physicians must report all cases. The Dutch Supreme Court has also decided in 2020 to allow euthanasia in dementia with prior written statements and without a rule to

---

[16] Roscoe LA, Malphurs JE, Dragovic LJ, Cohen D. Dr. Jack Kevorkian and Cases of Euthanasia in Oakland County, Michigan, 1990–1998. *N Engl J Med.* 2000;343:1735–1736.

confirm their request. Although the comparison may be contrived, during the Second World War, The Netherlands was the only occupied country whose doctors refused to participate in the German euthanasia program. How this paradigm shift happened (and other EU countries have followed) is not fully clear, but one potential factor was the lack of any organized palliative and hospice care, coupled with a lack of knowledge about complex pain control on the part of Dutch physicians.

What do viewers need to know to interpret this film accurately? Medical societies have already stated that physicians should not actively end life; instead, they should provide comfort and solace. This is a clear distinction from actively ending life. Justification for PAS is thus problematic in many domains (trust, social implications, reputation, and integrity), but adequate pain relief remains necessary, even when it leads to very high doses of medication. For sure, palliative care has rapidly become sophisticated, such that "a good death" is often a reachable goal, and we are much better situated now.

The terms "physician-assisted dying," "death with dignity," or "aiding dying" sugarcoat a bigger problem. In states and countries where PAS is allowed, no physician is required to honor the request of a patient and can transfer the care to others if there is personal reluctance or ambivalence. There is a general understanding that only a fraction of all deaths result from assisted suicide in European countries and the US states where it is allowed. There is an increase in the number of assisted suicides, partly explained by better reporting. Advanced cancer remains the most considered disease, with amyotrophic lateral sclerosis and multiple sclerosis much less common, along with spinal cord injury.

The film unfortunately perpetuates the idea that there is a general lack of end-of-life care in hospitals and that doctors are "cowards." The film suggests that once afflicted, patients lack alternatives to assisted suicide. After the film—if the portrayal of Jack Kevorkian is accurate—a perversity to the entire story appears. Kervorkian died a free man in 2011 at the age of 83 years.[17] The epitaph on Kevorkian's tombstone reads, "He sacrificed himself for everyone's rights." Physicians need to know about Jack Kevorkian and his ways, but then we should consign him to the obscurity he would have hated.

Another film critical to the discussion of assisted suicide is *The Sea Inside* (*Mar Adentro*) (2004) starring Javier Bardem, Belén Rueda, Lola Dueñas, and Mabel Rivera and directed by Alejandro Amenábar. *The Sea Inside* has similar themes but is about assisting the dying process (not by physician but by family) and is based on the true story of Ramón Sampedro, who died in 1998 at the age of 55 (Figure 5.2). Ramón was left quadriplegic after a diving accident and wrangled for 30 years with the Spanish government to obtain the right to end his life. The decision was made after many years of living with his father, brother, sister-in-law, and nephew, who all participated in his complex care. A daily routine had emerged with the required care, but Ramón, despite all the care, had decided that his life had no dignity. He hired an activist lawyer who specialized in end-of-life care. Because she had an inherited neurologic vascular illness, this lawyer "understood" his suffering. His relationship with another woman, Rosa, was different; she supported continuation of his current existence and the general concept that life is worth living. The film also shows a quadriplegic priest arguing the Catholic position, and their meeting results in a shouting match re-emphasizing the position of each. These contradictions—as expected—are the main theme of this film. The ending is memorable and shows what happened in real life—a videotape of Ramón drinking a potassium-cyanide solution and dying on camera. This tape was sent to the media and prompted a special commission in the Spanish Senate. Nothing came of it, and PAS or any active withdrawal of support has remained illegal in Spain. The providers of the solution were never found. This event marked the first time that the media played a role in end-of-life discussions, a topic previously confined to academia. Currently, in Spain, the Constitutional Court has endorsed

---

[17] Murphy TF. A philosophical Obituary: Dr. Jack Kevorkian Dead at 83 Leaving End of Life Debate in the US Forever Changed. *Am J Bioeth*. 2011;11:3–6.

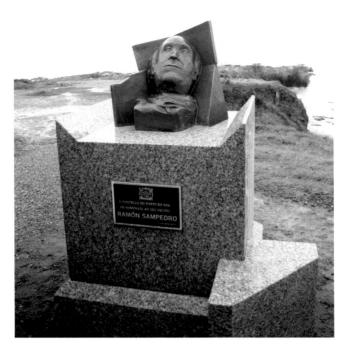

FIGURE 5.2   Sculpture of Ramón Sampedro. The bust was inaugurated in January 2011 and is located at the beach (Playa as Furnas) where Ramón had his accident. (Kindly provided by Manuel G. Teigell.)

the right of the individual to deny medical intervention including lifesaving intervention. This would have been unthinkable in Spain during most of the twentieth century, still under the dictatorship of Franco (1939–1975).[18]

A recent film is *Everything Went Fine* (2021) ◄◄◄ based on a biographic novel by Emmanuelle Bernheim about her elderly father and directed by Francois Ozon. The father, a stroke victim, demands that his daughter move him to Switzerland for his costly euthanasia ("10,000 euros! How do poor people manage?") It attempts to show true love but also coercion by an impossible man ("We can't refuse our father anything") and the potential for later pent-up pain and guilt. Switzerland is the only country that allows assisted suicide for foreigners as well as residents. Assisting in suicide is only punishable when performed with "motives of self-interest." It stars Sophie Marceau as the daughter and André Dussollier as her father, the stroke victim. Adding to the complications, Emmanuèle's mother (Charlotte Rampling) suffers from Parkinson's disease, which impacts her dignity. Andre wishes to avoid such a future and, therefore, seeks an end.

Few practicing US neurologists report significant volumes of assisted-suicide requests, although it depends on the scope of practice. With terminal illness, it is rarely more than 1% or 2%. Our current approach is to hold a series of discussions with the patient and next of kin. Preferably, discussions will also involve a palliative care physician, who will start by exploring alternatives to this request such as anxiolytics and anti depressants as appropriate. If necessary and reasonable, the patient can voluntarily stop eating and drinking, but next-of-kin often objects. Palliative sedation, which relieves pain and

[18] Simon-Lorda P, Barrio-Cantalejo IM. End-of-Life Healthcare Decisions, Ethics and Law: The Debate in Spain. *Eur J Health Law.* 2012;19:355–365.

dyspnea (or fear of dyspnea), is recommended.[19] This stepwise approach is not shown in film because it shows care, consensus, and calm, not necessarily very appealing to filmmakers. Some prefer to glorify individuals as uncelebrated heroes fighting heartless, bureaucratic medical systems.

Self-Determination

Self-determination (creating a sense of relief on your own terms) and assisted suicide obviously overlap. Also, self-determination and withdrawal of support may seem the same, but there are obvious differences. Withdrawal of support is often made after a shared decision of family members and the responsible care team. Here, we review the decision of a patient with all mental faculties intact to call it quits—no matter what, "no ifs, ands, or buts." These rash decisions abound in classic literature, theater, and opera. Cinema saw an opportunity too.

Whose Life Is It Anyway? (1981) ◄◄◄◄ stars Richard Dreyfuss, John Cassavetes, and Christine Lahti and was directed by John Badham. It was adapted from a play by Brian Clark. (It premiered at the Mermaid Theatre in London and won the Laurence Olivier Award for best new play.) The film accurately depicts the ethical discussion taking place in the early 1980s and considers the competency of sick or injured patients to refuse medical treatment. Ken Harrison (played by Richard Dreyfuss) is paralyzed as the result of a severe motor vehicle accident. He also has multiple fractures. To further add to the drama, as a result of trauma to the kidney, he has bilateral nephrectomies requiring permanent dialysis—a strange and unknown surgical indication. He enters the hospital, where Dr. Emerson (chief of medical services, played by the renowned director and actor John Cassavetes) runs into the emergency department, yells at everyone, and slaps Ken in his face, telling him to fight. Ken's condition is discussed with the orthopedic surgeon, who suggests fixing the cervical fracture. Dr. Emerson tells the orthopedic surgeon to keep him alive. After surgery, Emerson tells him he will never walk again or use his arms. Ken, a famous sculptor, decides that this is the end. He does not want to stay in the hospital; he wants to go home and die there. Dr. Emerson is unwilling to discuss such an option and orders Valium. When Ken refuses to take the pill, Emerson simply injects it intravenously without Ken's consent. Moreover, he coerces a psychiatrist to find someone ("a staunch Catholic") who would support declaring Ken incompetent. When challenged by one of his colleagues (Christine Lahti, playing Dr. Scott), he says, "Hey, do not give

---

DIALOGUE

Whose Life Is It Anyway?

Ken	*I decided I do not want to stay alive.*
Dr. Emerson	*You can't decide that.*
Ken	*Why not?*
Dr. Emerson	*Because you are depressed.*
Ken	*Does that surprise you?*
Dr. Emerson	*No, in time, you will learn to accept to let us help you.*
Judge	*Do you think you are suffering from depression?*
Ken	*I am completely paralyzed. I think I would be insane if I wasn't depressed.*
Judge	*Yes, but wanting to die must be strong evidence that your mental state has gone far beyond simple depression.*

---

[19] In states that permit physician-assisted suicide, a barbiturate and antiemetic is prescribed. Time to death is variable, sometimes lasting hours.

me that right-to-die routine. We're doctors. We are committed to life." The film eventually works its way into court, where Ken passionately argues for self-determination. Ken calls this refusal by physicians an "act of deliberate cruelty" and is outraged that "you have no knowledge of me whatsoever, and you have the power to condemn me to a life of torment." Psychiatrists take the stand but are divided on whether this represents a "reactive" depression. The judge deliberates and returns, quoting the Karen Ann Quinlan case that decided the preservation of personal right to privacy and right to protest against bodily intrusions, and he even quotes the Saikewicz case, which holds that incompetent patients should be afforded the right to refuse life-sustaining treatment. (That case, however, dealt with *terminally ill* incompetent patients.[20]) The judge's final verdict is to allow Ken to leave the hospital if he wishes to do so. Dr. Emerson accepts the court's decision but asks Ken to stay in the hospital to provide better comfort. "Why?" he asks. "Because you may change your mind!" Ken dies peacefully in the hospital.

This film is useful because of the good back-and-forth arguments about what constitutes patient autonomy. It may even represent the stance of physicians in the 1970s and 1980s, who were unwilling to commit to withdrawal of support. The film is well researched legally and medically. Due to these acute observations, it is a landmark in the cinematic depiction of the neuroethics of self-determination.

As mentioned in the introduction, another assisted withdrawal of care is shown in the provocative film *Million Dollar Baby* (2004) ◄ . The most shocking scene, which has troubled much of the audience, is where Clint Eastwood disconnects the mechanical ventilator of his trainee boxer. Her urge to end her life included forceful biting and injury of her tongue as an act of auto-mutilation. Her loneliness is further emphasized by her family, who ask her to sign her property away to them. She is left alone and cannot fight (literally and emotionally). This final climactic scene created some uproar when the film premiered, but it did not initiate a discussion and did not prevent the film from receiving the Academy Award for Best Picture. However, most viewers understood that for a visitor to effectively inject a sedative and disconnect the ventilator is highly improbable (even if your name is Clint Eastwood). Disability rights advocates were understandably appalled by the prejudice and inaccuracies about spinal cord injury, medical care, rehabilitation, and reintegration into society.

The problem addressed in both these movies is sudden, devastating, traumatic quadriplegia. Complete cervical transection with apnea usually precludes recovery, but a third of the patients with injuries at the C3 level or lower may recover somewhat. Mortality is around 10% in the first year and doubles in the following decade. The ethical questions in patients with traumatic quadriplegia and ventilator dependency are very difficult to answer. It is highly unusual for a patient with full knowledge of the consequences to ask emphatically to have the ventilator removed. In follow-up interviews at rehabilitation centers, assessments were predominantly positive, with over three-fourths of the patients "glad to be alive."[21] Patients may require five years to find a lasting quality of life after a spinal cord injury. Although many patients express hopelessness and despondency, many also change their mind with the passage of time. Suicide rates are much higher than in a comparable population but are rare overall (less than 5%). Many of us may think we would rather be dead than end up fully paralyzed and ventilator dependent. But prolonged suicide ideation is not common in young patients with a traumatic spinal cord injury. A highly supportive family, marital status, and the availability of resources are important. A productive life is feasible.[22] (See *Intouchables* discussed in Chapter 4.)

Honoring the request to turn off the ventilator requires a comprehensive analysis by an ethics committee. It is difficult to judge whether the patient's request is a rational choice and whether the patient is capable of autonomous choice.[23] The patient should be presented with all relevant facts and rehabilitation

---

[20] For a provocative but balanced discussion, see Annas GJ. Reconciling Quinlan and Saikewicz: Decision Making for the Terminally Ill Incompetent. *Am J Law Med.* 1979;4:367–396.

[21] Charlifue S, Apple D, Burns SP, Chen D, Cuthbert JP, Donovan WH, et al. Mechanical Ventilation, Health, and Quality of Life Following Spinal Cord Injury. *Arch Phys Med Rehabil.* 2011;92:457–463.

[22] Middleton JW, Dayton A, Walsh J, Rutkowski SB, Leong G, Duong S. Life Expectancy after Spinal Cord Injury: A 50-Year Study. *Spinal Cord.* 2012;50:803–811.

[23] Swartz M. The Patient Who Refuses Medical Treatment: A Dilemma for Hospitals and Physicians. *Am J Law Med.* 1985;11:147–194.

options. Postponing the decision is wise, but some patients with a complete transection may forcefully continue to reject any such suggestion. The ventilator can be withdrawn if the patient refuses to reconsider, because any patient may exercise the right to refuse life-sustaining treatment. These decisions are very stressful to caregivers, who may disagree with the decision, and they should seek support. It is well established that physicians—in their own personal judgment—are too pessimistic about "quality of life" for these patients, particularly when there is ventilator dependency. When surviving patients are asked, they rate their quality of life as good and even excellent, and they express a gratitude for being alive.[24]

Withdrawal of Support

Another medical decision in tailoring care is withdrawal of support. Virtually all major ethical and social issues are depicted in *The Descendants*. The stress of families waiting for closure, trying to reach consensus among family members, and the futility of critical care under certain circumstances can all be seen in this film.[25] For the viewer, it provides an opportunity to discuss one's own values and perceptions.

The issue of advance directives is recent, and therefore, this major neuroethical issue is seldom found in film. "Doctor knows best," the "fighting doctor," and the doctor who "never gives up" is what screenwriters were accustomed to presenting. In the real world, there has been a major change in the structure of end-of-life care, and *The Descendants* is a good way to start to examine this. Starring George Clooney, Shailene Woodley, Beau Bridges, Judy Greer, Matthew Lillard, and Robert Forster and directed by Alexander Payne, *The Descendants* (2011) ◀◀◀◀ has many plot elements and is multi-layered. In essence, however, the premise is quite simple: this is a film about withdrawal of care in a futile situation. The film concentrates on all aspects of withdrawal of support in a patient with a major catastrophic head injury. Matt King (George Clooney) is an attorney in Honolulu whose wife, Elizabeth (Patricia Hastie), is hospitalized in a coma as a result of a boating accident. Throughout the film, she tragically is shown comatose; this is one of the best cinematic representations of prolonged coma (for others that are not so good, see Chapter 4). In one of the opening scenes, we see Matt walking into the Queen's Medical Center in Honolulu, thinking that she will wake up, they will talk about their marriage, and he will buy her everything she wants. He is certain that they will rediscover their lost love and can be close again like in their early days. However, after his discussion with Dr. Johnson, it becomes rapidly apparent that she has no chance of waking up and her condition is permanent. Matt ignores this conversation with the neurologist, and when his family inquires about her state, he simply says, "Hope for the best and keep the vital organs working." He has a serious, much different conversation with his daughter. In a heartbreaking moment, he tells her he must let Elizabeth

---

DIALOGUE

The Descendants

Dr. Johnson

I wish I had better news, Matthew, but Dr. Chun and Dr. Mueller agree that her condition is deteriorating. She has no eye movement, no pupillary responses. She has no brainstem reflexes whatsoever. I mean, the machine can keep her alive; but her quality of life would be so poor, basically the way she is now.

---

[24] Whalley Hammell K. Quality of Life after Spinal Cord Injury: A Meta-Synthesis of Qualitative Findings. *Spinal Cord*. 2007;45:124–139.

[25] See Mehta S. The Intensive Care Unit Continuum of Care: Easing Death. *Crit Care Med*. 2012;40:700–701; Gerstel E, Engelberg RA, Koepsell T, Curtis JR. Duration of Withdrawal of Life Support in the Intensive Care Unit and Association with Family Satisfaction. *Am J Respir Crit Care Med*. 2008;178:798–804.

go as stipulated in her living will. He tells her both he and Elizabeth were very clear about that, should anything happen to either of them. Then, out of the blue, his daughter tells him that his wife had an affair. This is followed by a remarkable scene showing a tremendous unloading of stress. Matt—growing more upset upon hearing that his other family members were also aware of Elizabeth's extramarital relationship—projects his anger. He tells them that what they are doing to Elizabeth—trying to care for her in the hospital—makes no sense. ("You are putting lipstick on a corpse.") The film perhaps also implies that the discovery of the affair pushes him over the edge to withdrawal of care.

Matt also discusses the advance directive with his father-in-law, who looks at it and says, "It's like reading Korean ... jibber jabber." Matt suggests walking through it with him, but his father-in-law tells him he knows exactly what the situation is, and he wants to honor his daughter's wishes. Although there is a resolution within the family and appreciation of Elizabeth's wishes to not be kept in such a state, the film captures the family stressors and fragility during such circumstances very well. It quickly becomes a quietly devastating film.

Elizabeth is now in a persistent vegetative state (although the dialogue suggests brain death), and great effort has been made to make her look exactly as these patients are. Her sunken facial expression, lack of any mimicry, and no resemblance to the glamourous photos displayed next to her bed is a stark reminder of what such a condition entails. There is great attention to detail in this film. Observant physicians will note that with every new scene, the writing board in her room changes from "weaning" to "DNR" to "no plan for the day" as she transitions to palliative care. The film is extraordinarily sensitive in showing the family coming to terms with this catastrophe. There is a poignant break in tension and a tender scene in which Matt says goodbye to his wife, followed by scattering her ashes in the ocean off Waikiki. There are very few films that are as frank about withdrawal of care in a futile situation as this one.

Another film on coma is *Dormant Beauty* (2012) ⚔, loosely based on the famous PVS case in Italy (Eluana Englaro) ⚔. The film unfortunately does not provide any insights into this cause célèbre. Englaro's family had to wait 17 years to follow her wishes over objections by the Catholic Church and Italian Prime Minister Silvio Berlusconi, who flat out stated that Eluana looked healthy and could even have given birth to a child. Later, he said that Eluana did not die a natural death but was killed.

Another film that very briefly touches on withdrawal of support is *Steel Magnolias* (1998) ⚔. Shelby (Julia Roberts), who has type I diabetes, successfully delivers a baby, but several months later, she develops kidney failure and starts dialysis. Shelby is found unconscious, and through a window, we overhear that her coma might be irreversible. There is no explanation of the cause of coma, and when she does not awaken, the ventilator is removed. The scene shows the immediate presence of a bradycardia and arrest without showing the patient. The husband is seen signing a form before withdrawal, another highly unusual procedure (and, often in film, confused with signing a consent form).

How do these films reflect real-life situations? Advance directives, used in many countries, are legal documents in which the patient has determined what actions should be taken if they are no longer able to make decisions due to illness or incapacity. The documents can come in many forms. Some specify that an individual with power of attorney may make decisions about the patient; others, such as a living will, leave instructions for treatment. Surrogate decision-makers may be legally established as a durable power of attorney and are usually members of the patient's family. These advance directives typically specify when there is care in a terminal condition, and living wills clearly specify not to prolong care in the setting of futility. Physicians will review advance directives, and they need to be addressed with the patient and family members.[26]

In a persistently comatose patient who is unable to make decisions and never will, a surrogate has a major role. The decision to be made is based on the patient's best interests and, as expected, is dependent on the benefits of treatment versus the burdens of treatment. A family that continues aggressive care in a severely brain-injured patient with additional significant other medical concerns should understand there will be a long road of complications. Treatment required with each of these complications may be reassessed each time they occur.

---

[26] Truog RD, Cist AF, Brackett SE, Burns JP, Curley MA, Danis M, et al. Recommendations for End-of-Life Care in the Intensive Care Unit: The Ethics Committee of the Society of Critical Care Medicine. *Crit Care Med*. 2001;29:2332–2348.

A do-not-resuscitate (DNR) order is part of a decision that can be put forward in a living will. Many hospitals require that resuscitation orders be addressed upon admission. Families typically request full resuscitative measures upon admission but often ask for a DNR status after seeing no progress in care. DNR status may also come into play when physicians see no improvement despite aggressive measures to reverse the condition, or when there is simply an overwhelmingly bad clinical situation. There is a long history of deescalating the level of care in intensive care units (ICUs).[27]

Family-Physician Conflicts

Physicians and other medical staff can be accosted by angry family members; we must remain gracious, and many of us have tried to find ways to accomplish this.[28] One film stands out as a centerpiece, and it is *Critical Care* (1997) ◄◄◄◄ starring James Spader, Kyra Sedgwick, Helen Mirren, Anne Bancroft, and Albert Brooks and directed by Sidney Lumet. The conflicts between family members are very well depicted in this comedy. Although there are exaggerations, the film clearly highlights a common occurrence in ICUs with families who disagree with each other on what the best level of care might be.

Critical Care starts by introducing a new ICU (with futuristic blue lights and anti-decubitus mattresses that look like pool floats) and one of the doctors, Dr. Ernst (James Spader), taking care of several patients. One elderly patient is in a persistent vegetative state after a cardiac arrest. The patient, on a respirator, has been recently moved to the critical care unit. "Why was daddy moved to this floor?" Dr. Ernst explains, "He was getting excellent care on the eighth floor, but this is the newest ICU facility.") The patient's daughters are divided on what should be done. Connie (played by Margo Martindale) wants his life prolonged as long as possible, but Felicia (Kyra Sedgwick) cannot stand it any longer. The movie is a satire on prolonging care and its financial consequences but even more so on family conflicts. Connie is convinced that he responds ("One squeeze is yes; two squeezes is no. You tell me that is some kind of a seizure?"). She knows because she visits him in the hospital every single day. She gets angry at the physician ("My father is not terminally ill; he is convalescing"), accusatory ("For the rest of you, it is all sneers and laughter"), and paranoid ("I heard nurses and technicians laughing and telling jokes … as if he wasn't a living person in the room"). Connie also worries that Felicia might be doing something to him in her absence ("I'd watch myself around her"). The film eventually turns into a conflict about inheritance after the patient dies, and it introduces a commonly perceived myth—withdrawal from care to get the inheritance.

DIALOGUE

Critical Care

Dr. Ernst	*You wanted to see me?*
Connie	*Oh, yes, I know… if you and my sister were discussing my father's care?*
Dr. Ernst	*Her only concern is that your father's suffering is not prolonged.*
Connie	*I'd watch myself around her. My sister is Delilah, Dr. Ernst. My sister is Salome and Jezebel.*
Dr. Ernst	*Really?*
Connie	*Since my sister does not believe my father should be receiving life support, I don't think it's appropriate to allow her to be alone with him.*

---

[27] For a succinct but thorough history of the growing complexity of care over the years, see Luce JM. A History of Resolving Conflicts over End-of-Life Care in Intensive Care Units in the United States. *Crit Care Med.* 2010;38:1623–1629.

[28] See Bloche MG. Managing Conflict at the End of Life. *N Engl J Med.* 2005;352:2371–2373; Fassier T, Azoulay E. Conflicts and Communication Gaps in the Intensive Care Unit. *Curr Opin Crit Care.* 2010;16:654–665; and Studdert DM, Mello MM, Burns JP, Puopolo AL, Galper BZ, Truog RD, et al. Conflict in the Care of Patients with Prolonged Stay in the ICU: Types, Sources, and Predictors. *Intensive Care Med.* 2003;29:1489–1497.

How does this film translate to real-life ICU practices? Some families of comatose patients want to pursue any possible option, do not recognize the seriousness of the situation, and often believe that withholding intensive care is a poor decision no matter what. In their minds, every individual should be given a maximum chance, and they cannot comprehend why the physician does not agree. This film clearly shows a realistic example of such a conflict and is worthwhile as a teachable clip in lectures. Connie continuously cites the Bible and biblical figures to make her point. The extreme puzzlement of the physician inundated with biblical citations is equally well portrayed here. Religious influence—the "our faith lets us continue on" argument—is prevalent in these situations, emphasizing that life always has value, even if there is suffering. On balance, physicians respect all faiths, and their task in this respect is to say words of comfort and express understanding. Family conflicts are a significant threat, not only to quality of care but also to what should be a normal, cordial relationship between the treating physicians and concerned family members. Conflicts may also be present within the family structure, as *Critical Care* so clearly demonstrates. Different opinions may result in the inability to make important decisions for the patient, and additional irritations, such as conflicts with nurses or residents, may further obscure the wishes of the patient. From the family's point of view, conflicts often arise due to ineffective communication, disrespectful behaviors or dismissive attitudes on the part of staff, and the perception that there is a time pressure about the decision to stop critical care. Some families do not accept the limits of medicine. Some spouses simply cannot make the decision to stop, even when physicians suggest curtailing care. This may cause a powerful defensive stance of the family that can lead to continuous requests for treatment.

Dispute resolution should start with a reappraisal of what caused the conflict. First, a physician with significant communication skills must moderate a family conference that includes all health-care workers. There should be clear reassurance to the family that the patient's cultural attitudes and values are appreciated. Barriers to communication should be identified and improvements suggested. Resolution of conflicts can only come by spending an appropriate, necessary amount of time with the family explaining the plan and expectations. The consequences of a conflict do not only jeopardize the patient's safety and quality of care but can also lead to progressive mistrust, dissatisfaction, burnout, misunderstanding with staff, and increased healthcare expenditures due to the increased length of stay.

Decisions about care in critically ill patients have rarely been used as a plot. *Critical Care* should be contrasted with *The Descendants*, where decisions are clear and there is resolution and closure. When seen in its totality, *Critical Care* has many absurdities. It addresses the costs of health care, makes fun of hospital administrators (in a brilliant role of Albert Brooks as Dr. Butz), and suggests that continuation of care in a young, well-insured patient is financially beneficial. One dialyzed patient with vivid hallucinations is fully cared for because the hospital can profit from transplanting kidneys (they don't). Dr. Butz also posits that discussions of feeding tubes in the terminally ill are non-existent. ("You think just because someone's going to die soon, we don't need to feed them? I've news for you! We're all gonna die! So why should any of us eat?") When care of the comatose patient is questioned, he counters, "Where have you been all your life? … It is called revenue." Although it is humorous, it presents a complex topic—family conflict on de-escalation of care when care seems futile and certainly when the courts are involved.[29] There is much dark cynicism and many misperceptions of health care, but that makes the film a topic for discussion and gives us a chance to rebut or agree. Many (neuro)intensivists are very familiar with the conflicts presented, and many would be able to provide a perspective. It is a film that fully deserves scrutiny and perhaps even debate.[30]

---

[29] White DB, Pope TM. The Courts, Futility, and the Ends of Medicine. *JAMA*. 2012;307:151–152.

[30] Another "must-see" film on this topic is *Near Death*, an extensive documentary on decision-making in the intensive care unit and conversations with patients and families about their wishes. It includes neurology (e.g., discussion by staff on brain death and care in a comatose patient) and is a bioethics masterclass (Fred Wiseman. *Near Death*. Zipporah Films 1989). The full 6 hours is worthy of your time.

Institutionalization in Dementia

Cinema (and certainly the American New Wave) likes mistreatment—or the perception of it—and putting someone away is at the pinnacle of many movies in the history of medicine in film. Therefore, we should not be surprised that cinema has looked at this major event for the elderly and has created drama in which the individual enters a featureless care facility and "goes postal."

The traditional thinking has always been that the elderly cope best when they can stay in their homes. However, Alzheimer's disease rapidly increases nursing home placement, from 20% after 1 year, 50% after 5 years, and over 90% after 8 years. This is substantially higher than in elderly patients without dementia (by comparison, 5%–10%).[31] Caregivers' burden is a major factor. In the United States, over 9 million people are caring for relatives with dementia.

The Savages (2007) ◄◄◄◄ , starring Laura Linney, Philip Seymour Hoffman, and Philip Bosco; and written and directed by Tamara Jenkins, is one of the more profound films dealing with children facing decisions to place a parent with dementia in a nursing home, often labeled with the deplorable term *institutionalization*. Jon and Wendy (Philip Seymour Hoffman and Laura Linney) live their own lives, and their father (who has been abusive to them in the past) resides in a well-known senior living community in Arizona (Sun City). Lenny (Philip Bosco) is in a non-marital arrangement, but then his girlfriend dies. He must leave because he has no right to use or inherit any of her property. His dementia is rapidly increasing, requiring assistance. The children have been estranged, and they realize it when they visit his home. ("Did you see there were no pictures of us?")

Jon and Wendy see no way other than to move their father to a nursing home, a move that becomes a certainty after Lenny smears feces on the wall and is admitted to the hospital for agitation. Now in the hospital, they find him in restraints and confused ("They have me hogtied for 2 days."), and he accuses his children of not being there when all this happened. ("I know who you are...the late ones.") Now faced with a difficult situation, both children are frankly overwhelmed by choice of how to handle this situation properly. The neurologist—who thinks Lenny has Parkinson's disease and not dementia because he does not see any strokes on MRI—does not help either with clarifying the situation.

We see Jon and Wendy struggling to find a good nursing home, and Lenny is admitted to a drab place. (When Wendy asks Jon, "Do they smell?," Jon answers, "They all smell.") Wendy cleans out Lenny's house, finding cluttered closets, old-man clothes, useless memorabilia, and even an eight-track cartridge—but more importantly, unseen photos of their youth. These photos remind Wendy of a better time, but Jon remains sarcastic and wants nothing to do with it.

In the nursing home, we see Lenny with a shuffling walk, and he is mostly agitated and disoriented. The tactless nursing home staff want to know what to do when he dies—burial or cremation. The children are now suddenly forced to discuss these sensitive matters. In a key comic-dramatic scene, the children ask Lenny what he would want to do in case "something happens." When Lenny looks non-plussed, Jon adds, "If you would be in a coma, would you want to be on a ventilator?" Lenny is flabbergasted ("What kind of question is that?") but ultimately agrees to let them "unplug" him. When Jon asks him, "Then what?" he yells, "You bury me!" Indeed, the reality of entering such a facility is overwhelming for family members, who are rushed through the admission process and stacks of paperwork. Wendy tries to find a better nursing home, but Jon is not interested, knowing that nothing matters if Lenny does not know where he is. This effort is actually an attempt to make themselves feel better rather than addressing Lenny's needs. As a result of this experience, both Jon and Wendy relive some old painful memories, although we do not learn what really happened.

---

[31] Smith GE, O'Brien PC, Ivnik RJ, Kokmen E, Tangalos EG. Prospective Analysis of Risk Factors for Nursing Home Placement of Dementia Patients. *Neurology.* 2001;57:1467–1473.

In the end Lenny dies, but not much changes, and they go on with their lives, perhaps changed, perhaps not.

DIALOGUE

The Savages

Jon
> *Do not make me out to be the evil brother putting away our father against your will. We are doing this together, right?*
>
> *It is not about Dad; it is about your guilt...that is what these places prey upon; and all this wellness propaganda and landscaping is just to obscure the miserable fact that people are dying.*

Fred Won't Move Out (2012) ◄◄◄ is a film is based on a personal memoir and shot in the house of the director's parents. It is as close as a scripted film can get to a documentary about the troubles with parents and cognitive problems. Starring Elliott Gould, Fred Melamed, Stephanie Roth Haberle, and Judith Roberts and written and directed by Richard Ledes, *Fred Won't Move Out* eloquently shows the socioeconomic effects of dementia on an elderly couple. The film starts with children visiting their parents. In the car, it becomes rapidly clear where the problems are: "The thing is, when he is up there by himself, we have no idea what medication he is taking or how much. We don't know if he is taking her medication … I agree it is totally nuts." Victoria (Mfoniso Udofia) is a caretaker from Ghana and is called "Queen Victoria" by Fred. The morning scene shows both physically in need. Fred can barely come down the stairs, and Susan is afraid to even sit down. "Good morning, Susan," Fred says. "Whoop-de-doo" is Susan's answer. Susan is more affected than Fred. Music therapy is performed with a piano player, and all are singing Susan's favorite tunes. Susan, who has been nearly catatonic, changes dramatically, smiles, and enthusiastically sings and laughs. Fred says, "It makes her happy, and when she's happy, it makes it much better for all of us."

Their children—Bob (Fred Melamed) and Carol (Stephanie Roth Haberle)—are trying to find a solution after an unclear medical event that suggests something serious could happen with their parents. Both soon also find out that the caretaker is overwhelmed and that this situation cannot go on. Victoria tries to do the main errands but also wants to keep Fred as active and participatory as possible. When the children find out he has not done his taxes and confront him, he says, "I do not owe anything." In a civil discussion, the children try to get Fred to agree to move out of his wonderful lake house, and Bob suggests that they are going to live "like in a dorm." That seems agreeable to Susan but not to Fred, and he responds grumpily, not seeing the point of going elsewhere. ("I am not going.")

A tranquil scene shows both children walking through the lot and reminiscing about the past. The film's cutaway scenes show Fred and Susan's house with its fantastic foliage, flowerbeds, and a majestic lake view. We see a seasoned house in all its glory but with the addition of stacks of medication lined up on the cabinets, a visual reminder of the inevitability of growing old. Well timed in the narrative, Bob tells a wonderful myth of the gods. He tells his children that the gods Zeus and Hermes were looking for disappearing hospitality among the Greeks and found nobody to welcome them except for an older couple. As a reward, Zeus and Hermes let them make one wish. Their wish was to die together, so Zeus and Hermes turned them into two oak trees. They could now live together for a long time.

Susan leaves for a nursing home, and Fred stays with a caretaker. When he is told that his children will pick him up, he does not want to go. ("Who will be here when Susan comes back?") It seems that the children remain at an impasse and are unable to resolve it with the best of intentions. Bob decides

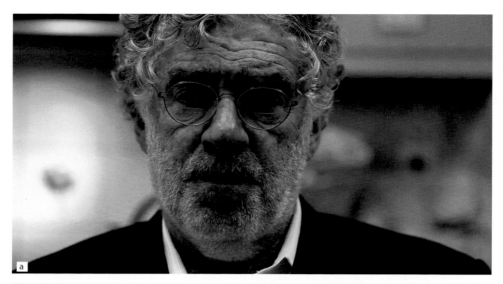

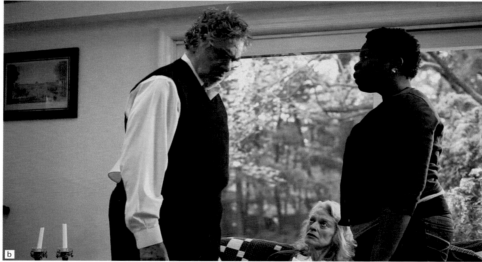

FIGURE 5.3 Scenes in *Fred Won't Move Out*. (a) Fred, played by Elliot Gould; (b) Fred confronted by Victoria, played by Mfoniso Udofia. Susan, played by Judith Roberts, is sitting on the couch. (Used with permission of Richard Ledes.)

in a flash to get Fred a new cinnamon-colored cat ("Ginger"), pretending that he has found her behind a tree. (In reality, Ginger, a beloved family pet, died long ago, but Fred has been asking for her.) Fred is elated that "Ginger" has been found, and this scene suddenly indicates a far more profound dementia than what had been apparent initially. The cat escapes, and the film ends abruptly. In the end, we do not know whether Fred moves out. As the credits came on, I reflected that maybe we should all turn into oak trees when the time comes.

These films show difficult behaviors in dementia (Figure 5.3). Delaying placement with good in-home care could save billions of dollars annually, and efforts to keep patients at home do improve their quality of life. These two remarkable films show how children cope with their debilitated parents—debilitated from a dementing illness, left on their own with nowhere to go. But these are also parents unwilling to accept help, unable to cope, and spiraling into rapid self-neglect. These are the major themes, and these issues are where the strength of these films lies.[32]

Experimentation

Mad scientists and physicians—recognized by a wide-eyed and flyaway-hairdo appearance—have been known since the era of silent film.[33] Characters introduced as "Doctor" or "Professor" are supposed to have their predictions taken as authoritative. Later, when scientists spoke in the movies, they often had a German accent, which recalls Dr. Strangelove (Peter Sellers) in Stanley Kubrick's masterpiece. Mad physicians are mostly found in horror films, most of which have to do with creating humanoid monsters. Both Dr. Frankenstein (from Mary Shelley's classic novel) and Dr. Moreau (from *The Island of Dr. Moreau* by H. G. Wells) have been personified in film and seen experimenting with and surgically reshaping or creating monstrous figures.

But one bothersome film specifically focuses on neurologists. *Extreme Measures* (1996) ⚔ stars Hugh Grant, Gene Hackman, Sarah Jessica Parker, and David Morse and was directed by Michael Apted. *Extreme Measures* is iconic because, for the first time, a film suggests that there are neurologists conducting wild, uncontrolled experiments. The film opens with Dr. Guy Luthan (Hugh Grant) noticing "strange symptoms" in a homeless patient admitted to the emergency department. It becomes rapidly clear that the neurologist, Lawrence Myrick (Gene Hackman), performs experiments on homeless patients in order to find a cure for spinal cord injury. The film addresses several unethical behaviors beyond the obvious lack of informed consent. The film's premise is up-front when Myrick tells Luthan that the homeless (with no benefit to society) can be "heroes" by providing possible cures to millions, even if it leads to their own deaths. This key conversation explains the title of the film. Myrick declares that he has no time to conduct trials for a promising new drug in rats or chimpanzees.

DIALOGUE

Extreme Measures
Dr. Lawrence Myrick

People die every day, and for what? For nothing. What do we do? What do you do? You take care of the ones you think you can save. Good doctors do the correct thing, but great doctors have the guts to do the right thing.

Introducing new therapies to healthy human controls is unusual outside the setting of a randomized controlled trial, and the scenario in *Extreme Measures* is not only highly improbable but criminal. Without giving away too much of the plot, this eventually leads to a major confrontation. After Dr. Myrick is accidentally shot and killed, his widow gives his data to Dr. Luthan, who decides to apply for neurology residency. Here, the film supports the premise that the therapy might work but for the fact that the wrong method was used. It just needs another try.

---

[32] For further reading, see Caron CD, Ducharme F, Griffith J. Deciding on Institutionalization for a Relative with Dementia: The Most Difficult Decision for Caregivers. *Can J Aging.* 2006;25:193–205; Klug MG, Volkov B, Muus K, Halaas GW. Deciding When to Put Grandma in the Nursing Home: Measuring Inclinations to Place Persons with Dementia. *Am J Alzheimers Dis Other Demen.* 2012;27:223–227; and Yaffe K, Fox P, Newcomer R, Sands L, Lindquist K, Dane K, et al. Patient and Caregiver Characteristics and Nursing Home Placement in Patients with Dementia. *JAMA.* 2002;287:2090–2097.

[33] They also wear white coats and are stereotypes; smart, dedicated, and enjoy tinkering in the laboratory. See Frayling C. *Mad, Bad and Dangerous?: The Scientist and the Cinema.* London: Reaktion Books; 2005.

TABLE 5.1   Principles of Medical Professionalism

1.	Commitment to professional competence
2.	Commitment to honesty with patients
3.	Commitment to patient confidentiality
4.	Commitment to maintaining appropriate relations with patients
5.	Commitment to improving quality of care
6.	Commitment to improving access to care
7.	Commitment to a just distribution of finite resources
8.	Commitment to scientific knowledge
9.	Commitment to maintaining trust by managing conflicts of interest
10.	Commitment to professional responsibilities

Extreme Measures exemplifies everything that can go wrong in the professionalism and ethics of neurology research. For dramatic purposes, of course, it avoids the major tenets of ethical medical research, which are to do no harm, practice full disclosure, and offer patients the right to refuse participation without consequences for future care. In fact, the film ignores all major ethical principles.

The ACP has summarized its enumerated principles of medical professionalism (Table 5.1).[34]

Financial conflicts of interest continue to be a major concern in medicine, and medical decisions may still be influenced by monetary considerations. Patient self-determination or autonomy—although a major principle—has been taken to another level in *Extreme Measures*. However, the film also implies another disturbing suggestion—that data derived from unethical research can be used and analyzed.

Unfortunately, the history of medicine is blemished by unethical research. Most notorious are the Nazi human neurologic experiments that included head-injury experiments in children, hypothermia experiments on captured Russian troops, and brain studies at high altitudes. In the US, the Tuskegee syphilis experiments, which studied the natural history of untreated syphilis, are among the most scandalous. The participants were not aware that they had syphilis, and they were not treated with penicillin. A prevailing misunderstanding was that the government infected the men with syphilis. However, this was actually a separate study in which US government researchers infected hundreds of Guatemalan prisoners, psychiatric patients, and sex workers with syphilis and gonorrhea during the 1940s to study the effects of penicillin. For Blacks, the Tuskegee study is a strong symbol of their mistreatment by physicians and was well depicted in *Miss Evers' Boys* (1997). President Clinton apologized on behalf of the government, and there was financial compensation for the survivors. Currently, clinical research is strongly regulated, and academic centers train clinical researchers through close mentorship. All research protocols are overseen by institutional review boards that demand close record keeping. There are also standards for neurology, and teaching has entered simulation centers.[35]

Respect for the individual person is a major moral principle guiding the ethics of research. This means that persons are never asked to be research subjects against their will or coerced into participation. Vulnerable populations must be protected by proxy (a surrogate decision-maker). The concept of *informed consent* relies on several prerequisites: (a) the person has been given all information needed; (b) the person has a good understanding of the pros and cons; and (c) the person is not being deceived. Vulnerable populations include patients with Alzheimer's disease, critically ill patients, sedated and agitated patients, and, of course, any comatose patient.[36] Participation in research should always be

---

[34] ACP-ASIM Foundation. American College of Physicians-American Society of Internal Medicine; European Federation of Internal Medicine. Medical Professionalism in the New Millennium: A Physician Charter. *Ann Intern Med.* 2002;136:243–246.

[35] Kurzweil AM, Lewis A, Pleninger P, Rostanski SK, Nelson A, Zhang C, et al. Education Research: Teaching and Assessing Communication and Professionalism in Neurology Residency with Simulation. *Neurology.* 2020;94:229–232.

[36] Smithline HA, Gerstle ML. Waiver of Informed Consent: A Survey of Emergency Medicine Patients. *Am J Emerg Med.* 1998;16:90–91.

voluntary. Waivers are not allowed if the researcher does not have the time to reach the relatives of the person subjected to research, although waivers are allowed in emergency treatments that potentially could benefit the patient.[37]

Cinema (ideally, through documentary film) is a potential medium to educate and prevent potential ethical malfeasance and to inform of historical violations. However, we must recognize that in many countries these major violations are in the past, and currently we have much better oversight and understanding of the basic principles.[38]

But criminal behavior never goes away, and TV docuseries pick up on it. *Dr. Death* (2021) ◄◄◄◄ , starring Joshua Jackson and Alec Baldwin and directed by Patrick MacManus, explores the crimes of neurosurgeon Christopher Duntsch, a sociopath who was sentenced to life in prison after maiming and even "killing" almost all of the nearly 40 patients he operated on between 2011 and 2013.[39] Drug abuse was a major factor. His colleague surgeons labeled him as the most careless, clueless, and dangerous spine surgeon ever seen. The trial was a criminal conviction against a doctor for his actions in the course of his work—a first. The burden of the prosecution was to show that proven intent to maim or kill those who relied on his skills differed from malpractice, where a mistake leads to a poor outcome for a patient. This horror film will have the audience think twice about spine surgery (which they should do in any case) but also affirms ineptitude protected by his medical center and vagueness in reporting malpractice and wrongdoing. It has a substantial portion of swagger and wisecracking and plays to the god complex (see Chapter 1) used in so many other cinematic portrayals of surgeons.[40]

Compassion Fatigue

Ideally, physicians care for their patients' well-being and do not discriminate; they treat everyone the same and contribute to the healing of the patient. That is true in most circumstances, but such a constant commitment is difficult and must be taught. Physician burnout may occur due to an overwhelmingly high workload, lack of restorative rest, and considerable emotional burden. One major film that addresses all these problems and is recommended, without hesitation, as required viewing for all neurologists, neurosurgeons, and perhaps even all physicians. The film shows a lack of humanity in a hospital system where the staff has been overcome by gruff and sarcastic behavior. *The Death of Mr. Lazarescu* (2005) ◄◄◄◄ , written and directed by Cristi Puiu, threads several themes throughout the story, but in the end, the viewer is confronted by the lack of appropriate neurologic and neurosurgical care. Dante Remus Lazarescu (played by the renowned theater actor Ioan Fiscuteanu) is a widowed, retired engineer in his senior years. His daughter has left for the United States, and he lives with his cats. His pension is handled by his sister, who takes most of it. He has been a heavy drinker, predominantly of mastropol (homemade alcohol). He lives in a run-down apartment in Bucharest, Romania, and the film opens with him calling for an ambulance late on Saturday night because of headache and vomiting. Nobody seems alarmed, and no ambulance shows up. He goes to a neighbor (after no response and no ambulance), who tells him it is his ulcer. When Mr. Lazarescu vomits blood in the neighbor's apartment, the neighbor tells him it is Mallory–Weiss syndrome. Yes, Lazarescu has been drinking, but he knows too well this is different—and nobody seems to believe him. Eventually, the ambulance arrives, and the medic Mioara (played by the equally renowned actor Luminita Gheorghiu) becomes his "guardian angel" throughout

[37] Harnett JD. Research Ethics for Clinical Researchers. *Methods Mol Biol.* 2021;2249:53–64.

[38] Harnett 2021, Ibid.

[39] There are many Dr Deaths, and the nick name is loosely applied, for example, to James Grigson, a US psychiatrist later exposed as a charlatan, who testified in over 100 trials that resulted in death sentences. The most notorious Dr. Death was, of course, Josef Mengele who was also called" the angel of death." Dr. Harold Shipman a British general practitioner and serial killer, also received the moniker.

[40] Wijdicks EFM. *Cinema, MD, A History of Medicine on Screen.* New York: Oxford University Press; 2020.

the long night that follows. Lazarescu keeps on mentioning headache, but, again, all is attributed to his drinking. Mioara tries to find an emergency department that can help him.

Upon arrival at the first hospital, the emergency physician tells him again, when he complains of a headache, that he should stop drinking. The emergency physician gets irritated, pokes in his right upper quadrant, notices an enlarged liver, and concludes that there is little he can do. Lazarescu is told to go elsewhere when an acute multi-trauma comes in.

In another hospital, a young physician detects a subtle arm drift and calls for a neurologist, who orders an emergent CT, but he is told he still has to wait for 3 hours. (The neurologic examination is "interesting," and it is described in detail in Chapter 3.) Gradually, Lazarescu becomes more and more sleepy. The neurosurgeon arrives after the CT scan shows a subdural hematoma and a presumably cancerous mass in the liver. At this point, the film picks up speed and becomes far more dramatic in showing appalling physician behavior. The neurosurgeon seems uninterested in proceeding but asks him to sign a consent form. ("If I operate without his signature, I go to jail.") A conflict arises between the neurosurgeon and the medic, when she suggests the need for a rapid operation. He tells her to take him to a different hospital. (He also sarcastically suggests driving around for an hour, because when the patient becomes comatose, a doctor does not need a signature.) Finally, in the last hospital, the need for surgery is recognized, and we see him naked on a stretcher being washed and head shaven. By now, he is deeply stuporous. The title of the film implies his death, but we do not see it.

There is little compassionate care for Mr. Lazarescu. His first name, Dante, is allegorical, and his surname is a merge of the biblical person Lazarus with resuscitation. Lazarescu's dignity and autonomy are neglected—all because he is an alcoholic and smelly. He is an extremely vulnerable patient in an over-stretched medical system where egotism is rampant. Informed consent is the worst of its kind. There is an attempt to help him sign while someone supports his hand and even attempts to do it for him before he throws out the sheets of paper. He is also told that neurosurgery is nothing more than surgery for an appendectomy. The medic, who follows him through all the niches of all the hospitals, seems the last hope in this Orwellian-Kafkaesque world.

DIALOGUE

The Death of Mr. Lazarescu

Neurosurgeon	*You are not in a coma. You are not lethargic. You feel a bit sleepy. Me too. It is 3:05 a.m.*
Emergency physician	*Hospitals are full of people like you that soak their brains in alcohol and batter their wives and kids.*
Lazarescu	*My head hurts, Doctor.*
Emergency physician	*Good, that means you have one.*

What can we learn from this remarkable film? Poor working conditions—such as those depicted in the film—will lead to dissatisfaction and dwindling of compassion, often first recognized by sarcasm. This impact on the quality of care may result in quick, poorly thought-out decisions (e.g., all alcoholics with headache must have a hangover) and conflicts with coworkers (e.g., "How do you dare to question me?"), and *The Death of Mr. Lazarescu* demonstrates that phenomenally.

The *Oxford English Dictionary* defines the term *compassion fatigue* as "apathy or indifference towards the suffering of others or to charitable causes acting on their behalf, typically attributed to seemingly frequent appeals for assistance, esp. donations; hence, a diminishing public response to frequent appeals." It involves all healthcare workers, and failure to remedy an unworkable situation (such as Ceausescu's damaged Romania) only perpetuates this miserable situation.

The film shows the worst of medicine. Dante Lazarescu is funneled through a hellish medical system devoid of compassion and inadequate in its resources. With every passing hour, Lazarescu gradually deteriorates from a subdural hematoma and develops hemiparesis, dysarthria, and, finally, aphasia and drowsiness—all unrecognized by caregivers. The medic's persistence results in Lazarescu receiving care, but by then it is too late.

The message of the film is that overburdened healthcare workers may overlook major health issues, especially when the person needing care is outside the boundaries of what is expected as normal care. In this case, the reluctance to deal with an unkempt, vomiting patient—instead, handing the patient off to another facility—proved to be a fatal mistake. Most hospitals in Romania are not this way, and most hospitals in many other countries are not this way, but this scenario definitely could occur anywhere. Does this self-important physician behavior have a familiar ring? I am afraid that, sometimes, it does.

Compassion fatigue is common and has been recognized in emergency departments, and those who initially demonstrate high levels of empathy are, ironically, most at risk.[41] Great solutions are not easy to find (certainly not the psychobabble such as "Set boundaries between home and work," "We all need to refuel ourselves," "Take time away from work," and "Practice self-care").[42] This film should be required viewing for all neurologists and neurosurgeons. It is my personal favorite. The director's intention was to depict the fear of dying alone and to "undress" doctors. He was admittedly avenging himself against the medical profession after some personal experiences. The film was based on a true story of an ambulance in Romania that tried to admit a patient to various hospitals, all of which refused to admit him; the patient was ultimately left to die on the street.[43] This morality tale also reminds us of the need for education in bedside manners. For many decades, there has been a concern about the loss (or erosion) of the art of medicine; while that might be partly true, medical schools recognize that their students need to understand that the onset of disease is usually unexpected. The other end of this equation is a deeply suffering human being (and family) confronted with an urgent need to deal with the disease. I always cringe when I hear a resident tell me he or she has a "great case" to present.

End Credits

The examination of neuroethics in film can be thought-provoking, and the reason for including it in this book will become abundantly clear when we watch the discussed films—there are very real questions about compassionate care and palliation. There is very little allegory, and the films with ethical questions are obviously contextual. The appeal is in the subject matter and human cost and the unmistakable follow-up questions: what would you do in a similar situation? Are we capable of moral decision-making and accepting responsibility for our actions? Some of these fiction films are "mandatory" watching, not necessarily because their portrayals are accurate but more often because they are wrong or highly debatable.

---

[41] Cavanagh N, Cockett G, Heinrich C, Doig L, Fiest K, Guichon JR, et al. Compassion Fatigue in Healthcare Providers: A Systematic Review and Meta-Analysis. *Nurs Ethics*. 2020;27:639–665; and Schmidt M, Haglund K. Debrief in Emergency Departments to Improve Compassion Fatigue and Promote Resiliency. *J Trauma Nurs*. 2017;24:317–322.

[42] Rimmer A. How Can I Manage Compassion Fatigue? *BMJ*. 2021;373:n1495.

[43] Puiu remembers: "When I said I was ill, they said, 'Please go home …' When I really was ill, having blood pumped from my stomach, a doctor came to me chewing gum. 'Is this serious?' I asked.; 'Yes, you're going to die,' he said – and left. He could not have been serious, but there was no sign of irony." The director's experiences are cited in Riding A. 'Death of Mr. Lazarescu' Comes after a Bout of Hypochondria. *The New York Times*. National ed. New York: The New York Times Company; 2006:15.

6

Neurology in Documentaries

It kind of grounds you, it brings you back to reality.

But You Still Look so Well (2012)

Documentaries are amalgams of footage and the state of things as they exist in real time — no different with medical or neurologic topics, but they are in a separate class. Some feel the documentary is just a dressed-up fiction genre. I explore here full-length documentaries on major brain injury and progressive neurologic disease. Major topics include dementia, amyotrophic lateral sclerosis, multiple sclerosis, stroke, and rehabilitation of traumatic brain injury but also very common disorders such as migraine. We will encounter filmmakers with neurologic disease, filmmakers with parents with neurologic disease, and filming in nursing homes or in a patient's home environment. We will see experts as "talking heads" and patients taking antagonistic positions. Many documentaries on neurologic disease are immersive, instructive, and educational, but some are deeply disturbing. The evocation of affliction and suffering might be a good summarizing description.

Main Themes

Fictional film gives a dramatized portrayal of neurologic disease, while documentary film is supposed to portray reality. But does it? Film scholars acknowledge, paradoxically, that documentaries have a higher "deception factor."[1] Nick Fraser wrote, "we can agree that documentaries must be truthful but truthful to what?"[2] Viewers may not recognize that the reality behind these documentaries is far more complicated than what is shown. Documentary filmmakers may start with agenda or seek a revelation. They may pose difficult questions or showcase a difficult situation, but much is done simply to shock the viewer. Images can appear out of context. From many hours of footage, the filmmaker may select only the images supporting his or her agenda. Another filmmaker could easily create a completely different film from the same material. Some documentaries intentionally blend fiction and nonfiction. Some realistic, "live-action" scenes may be (unidentified) reenacts. For valid reasons, these works must be viewed with healthy suspicion. They may be what film critic Geoffrey O'Brien called "movies with documents." As another film critic, Gilbert Adair, expressed most eloquently: "The cinema of effect and illusion has always solicited the suspension of collective disbelief."[3] Newer technology has entered this genre, and material can be easily changed or blended in with other material. Most recently, one filmmaker resorted to the unethical practice of placing words in a subject's mouth through artificial intelligence.[4]

---

[1] Barnouw E. *Documentary: A History of the Non-Fiction Film*. 2nd revised ed. New York: Oxford University Press; 1993.

[2] Fraser N. *Say What Happened: A Story of Documentaries*. London: Faber & Faber; 2019.

[3] Adair G. *Flickers: An Illustrated Celebration of 100 Years of Cinema*. Paperback ed. London: Fraser & Fraser; 1995.

[4] Rosner H. The Ethics of a Deep-Fake Anthony Bourdain Voice. *The New Yorker*. 2021; July 17.

DOI: 10.1201/9781003270874-6

Several recent notable medical documentaries may involve healthcare systems (*Sicko* [2007]) or lack thereof (*The Waiting Room* [2012], *The English Surgeon* [2007]); the food we eat and the food that makes us sick (*Food, Inc.* [2008]); and attacks on the pharmaceutical industry (*Big Buck, Big Pharma* [2006]). Some have admirably addressed the loneliness of dying of cancer (*Dying at Grace* [2003]) and AIDS (*How to Survive a Plague* [2012]). Each of these documentaries has unearthed potential problems in the practice of medicine or prevention of disease. Many have a specific agenda. At the end of the day, however, the ability of documentaries to influence public opinion or create awareness is limited.

Patient-advocacy organizations have released short documentaries on neurologic disease, some of which are screened during disability film festivals—most notably, the New York ReelAbilities Film Festival (www.reelabilities.org). This festival primarily features films by and about people with disabilities and exists to "explore, discuss, and celebrate the diversity of our shared human experience." In many films, the difference between developmental intellectual disability and autism is not sufficiently clear. Some short TV documentaries are of interest, such as the film *A Sense of Self* (2017) on the investigative reporter Liz Jackson, who produced documentaries for Australian TV and self-directed her film on coping with (supposed) Parkinson's disease.

Some serious full-length neurologic documentaries have also emerged thanks to readily available footage obtained from user-friendly cameras. Documentaries are problematic if they involve filming of persons who are unaware of their disease, and therefore documentaries of patients with severe cognitive impairment obviously raise ethical concerns. How do we know that the patient wants to be filmed even if the family agrees? Questions of perceived exploitation for film and the ethics of consent should always be addressed. Subjects may agree to participate while still in full possession of their cognitive abilities, but consent becomes problematic when they are no longer able to approve or reject scenes generated during filmmaking. Nonetheless, documentary filmmakers are, for the most part, careful about these ethical concerns. Documentary filmmakers do not make light of people's disabilities. But many medical documentaries are just the "same old, same old" and highly forgettable.[5]

Neurologic documentaries may involve partially eradicated diseases such as poliomyelitis or exceedingly rare disorders such as the mystery of lytico-bodig disease on the island of Guam in the 1950s with its features of amyotrophic lateral sclerosis, Parkinson disease, and dementia in *The Illness and Odyssey* (2013).

Sentimentalization of neurologic illness is also a potential concern. Some documentaries show the full devastation of a life-threatening neurologic disease. These may be very difficult to watch, and some viewers may want to look away or wonder why we even would want to see these films. Despite these concerns and caveats, there are some very significant documentaries the reader should note.

Alzheimer's Disease

Alzheimer's disease is widespread, and thus we can hope for a penetrating film that shows its clinical course and its consequences. We are experiencing a steep increase in elderly patients with dementia, with healthcare costs three times higher than for patients without dementia. There is no cure or even a solid understanding of Alzheimer's disease. Research has focused on a beta-amyloid problem (the "Baptists") and a tau problem (the "Tauists").[6] Others maintain there is an environmental (toxic) cause.

---

5 "Do we need yet another film on autism awareness?" asked one reviewer recently of the documentary *The Reason I Jump* (2021). Harris J. Enough "Autism Awareness." The Necessity Now Is Action. *The Guardian*. US Edition ed. Manchester, UK: Guardian News & Media Limited; 2021.

6 Mudher A, Lovestone S. Alzheimer's Disease-Do Tauists and Baptists Finally Shake Hands? *Trends Neurosci.* 2002; 25:22–26.

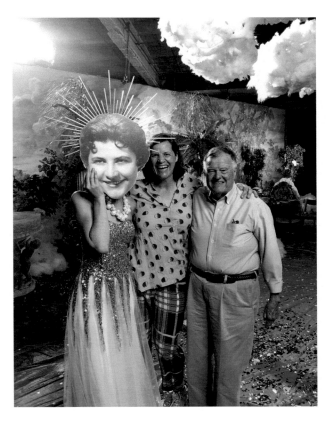

FIGURE 6.1 Dick Johnson and his daughter, film director Kristen Johnson. The other person acts out Dick's wife who died from the consequences of dementia. (Kindly provided by the director.)

Most documentary films concentrate on caregivers facing the burden of managing the behavioral problems of patients still living at home with Alzheimer's disease. Millions of Americans provide unpaid care for their loved ones, and many have stopped working or reduced their working hours as a result. These documentaries elucidate the toll on these caregivers. The caretaker is often the narrator.[7] Some TV documentaries have involved artists or the benefits of creative arts, as seen in *I Remember When I Paint* (2009). The filmmaker may choose, for dramatic purposes, the loss of creativity and, thus, the loss of what could have been. Documentaries on Alzheimer's disease often show spouses and significant others caring for a person who has lost the personality traits that created their bond. It has been called ambiguous loss—missing but not dead, similar to a soldier being missing in action. These films can also show the reality of nursing homes, with all their benefits and drawbacks.

Dick Johnson Is Dead (2020) ◄◄◄◄ is directed by Kirsten Johnson. Both of her parents were diagnosed with Alzheimer's disease (Figure 6.1). She chronicles her father's early decline from Alzheimer's disease. Dick is a psychiatrist, and when we see him at the age of 86, he is resigned to what remains to him and what has been taken away. As a compassionate psychiatrist, he was delightful company and very interested in hearing stories, but now things are different. He speeds through a construction site and completes the 5-mile return trip on four flat tires. His secretary notices mistakes in his prescriptions. Every phone call about him becomes an alarm bell. So, he must retire from practice and leave his

[7] Bullock R. The Needs of the Caregiver in the Long-Term Treatment of Alzheimer Disease. *Alzheimer Dis Assoc Disord.* 2004;18 Suppl 1:S17–S23.

wonderful home in a wooded lot in Beaux Arts Village, Washington, to live with his daughter Kristen, in a high-rise apartment in New York. His daughter now sees his cognitive decline first-hand. He gets dressed at 3 AM "to see a patient" but, after being put back to bed, reappears three more times. Kirsten knows what is coming and so, in a way, does Dick. New York looks overwhelming. When he is nearly fatally hit by a passing truck just to get in a car, the film almost seems to suggest that trading suburbia for downtown New York, albeit necessary, is a bad choice for patients with dementia. Kristen Johnson enlists Dick to play himself in a documentary and uses slapstick to bring levity to the tragedy. The fake deaths are not purely cartoonish but mimic actual freak accidents that plague the elderly with cognitive impairment. Dick not only plays along but seems to enjoy it all. ("She kills me multiple times and I come back to life; it is *Groundhog Day* again.") Stuntmen fill in for him when he is crushed by a falling air conditioner, stumbles and falls flat on the pavement, or falls from the stairs despite holding on to the rail. She also sets up a "living funeral" and has Dick enter the nave in tears to greet his friends and family. Dick is all in, but so are his acting friends and family.

Two scenes are worrisome. In one he is supposed to be accidentally hit by a beam, which then causes profuse bleeding from his carotid artery, drenching his shirt in blood. He looks confused and visibly uncomfortable, not fully recognizing fake blood and the boundary between reality and play ("this is worse than my heart attack"). The other, even more poignant scene happens on Halloween, when he is left alone to watch TV in an unfamiliar apartment. He worries that he has been abandoned and wonders what to do if nobody returns for him. He is emotionally affected ("Oh, man, sweetie, your father is a wreck") and thinks of his late wife, who died in a nursing home.

Dick Johnson Is Dead handles a great number of topics such as imposing on loved ones ("I like living with you so I am not terribly worried about it"), euthanasia ("I give you permission to euthanize me; pass it by me before you do it"), the care of a spouse with Alzheimer and her ultimate demise escalating after a hip fracture ("the brutality"), and the almost certain futility of prolonged cardiopulmonary resuscitation in the old-old (stacked shocks for ventricular fibrillation). The fantasy scene depicting Dick's and his wife's younger selves in heaven with unlimited fudge, popcorn, and new feet (he has congenital toe aplasia) is a pleasant respite.

The director clearly struggles with potentially objectionable scenes and recognizes that she occasionally pushes the envelope a bit too far.[8] A close friend in the living funeral is visibly uncomfortable with the whole idea and must remind himself it is only a movie. However, Dick apparently had creative input despite his fleeting lucidity. (When his neurologist tells him his Mini-Mental Status Exam was less than 20, he jokes that his memory is getting better.) But humor is a coping and healing mechanism often used by relatives of Alzheimer patients (and the patients themselves).[9] It is an effective clinical tool to relieve discomfort, stress, and anxiety, particularly if we know what makes the patient laugh—a quick-witted, sarcastic remark (not necessarily impaired by early cognitive decline) or pure silliness. For some viewers, these scenes initially appear odd; for me and I suspect others, they are endearing and transform the anticipatory prolonged pain and grief into laughter. It worked for the director/daughter (who knows she is at increased risk for Alzheimer's disease) to share a project with her father despite changes in the quality of their relationship. Kirsten Johnson has given us "the beginning of his disappearance" and also "when it gets messy, we hold each other close." It is a riveting, sublime, and transcendent film and an essential tale of regret for what is going to be lost through "the long goodbye"—not suddenly, like her staged accidents. Its uniqueness—a psychiatrist supremely cognizant of his disease course and his filmmaker daughter offering him the opportunity to defy his dementia through a shared film project—sets it apart from other documentary films on dementia. In addition, it clearly shows how changes in environment greatly unveils the neurological deficit. Neurologists know this all too well with patients admitted to

---

[8] My conversation with Kirsten Johnson about Death. San Francisco: Reimagine; 2020.

[9] Hickman H, Clarke C, Wolverson E. A Qualitative Study of the Shared Experience of Humor between People Living with Dementia and Their Partners. *Dementia (London).* 2020;19:1794–1810.

hospitals who are "doing just fine at home, no problems whatsoever,"[10] who become wildly delirious and confused at sundown and can be hardly contained at night.

The documentary *You're Looking at Me Like I Live Here and I Don't* (2012) takes a different approach; we are now confronted with end-stage dementia in need of nursing-home placement. Written and directed by Scott Kirschenbaum, it was filmed inside the Traditions Alzheimer's Unit in Danville, California, and focuses on one nursing-home resident, Lee Gorewitz, who is in her 70s (Figure 6.2). The documentary opens with photos of Lee before her diagnosis, but no backstory is given. The filmmaker then simply shows her going from one activity to another. She is different from the other, more sedate residents. Acting as a tour guide of the nursing home, she hops around from place to place, talking spontaneously. She seems very comfortable, non-agitated, and nonsedated, but she has no insight. Somewhat ironically, early in the documentary, the filmmaker asks her if she knows what Alzheimer's disease is. Her answer is complete gibberish. When asked to read her nametag, she can only read her last name but is able to spell it aloud. Walking through the nursing home, Lee is pleasant, spry, and chuckling. When she meets a caregiver or nursing assistant, she asks, "Are you doing a simple thing that you do not have to do anymore?" When the caregiver responds, "What do you need?" Lee answers, "It all depends on how it goes along." She solo dances, snapping her fingers like a lounge singer, in front of the camera with music playing Frank Sinatra's *Somewhere Beyond the Sea*. The other residents are in varied stages of dementia, some participating in activities, some barely engaging, some just hunched over. When Lee comes across an older woman slumped over in a chair, she comments, "That one looks like it's dead."

DIALOGUE

You're Looking at Me Like I Live Here and I Don't

Filmmaker	*What is Alzheimer's disease?*
Lee Gorewitz	*Alzheimer is the family of ... uh ... God, I have lost it. Alzheimer is the person that goes down and helps to help the person who does and gets to feel what is it once again. Alzheimer? That is kinda funny for me ... weird ... I guess I do not understand how you can have two together.*

A touching moment comes when she looks at family photos and comments, seemingly lucid, "Here is my family who are really doing nothing to help me (chuckles) ... you always did it that way." When her deceased husband is mentioned, she comments, "How do I even say it? The air—was very good."

Her language deficit can be understood as speech devoid of specific words (nouns and verbs), using only pronouns (his, it, they), and often she does not know what she is referring to. Speech is also convoluted, meandering, and disjointed. This loss of vocabulary is characteristic of dementia, with patients answering in short sentences and showing nothing of the verbal sophistication known before to family members.[11] Lee frequently loses her train of thought. Her language is best characterized as an aphasic dementia and not a primary progressive aphasia. She is unaware of her speech deficit.

Poignantly, the filmmaker shows how a protected, closed environment can contribute to patients' contentment. Lee tries to work the code of the exit door (Figure 6.1) but is not frustrated when it fails to open after she randomly punches in numbers. This remarkable minimalistic documentary shows that dementia may not always lead to a distressing situation, and a happier disposition may exist (at least for some time). Lee Gorewitz died in 2012.

---

[10] Or, alternatively, "he is very active," and "no, we have not noticed anything."

[11] Ahmed S, Haigh AM, de Jager CA, Garrard P. Connected Speech as a Marker of Disease Progression in Autopsy-Proven Alzheimer's Disease. *Brain*. 2013;136:3727–3737.

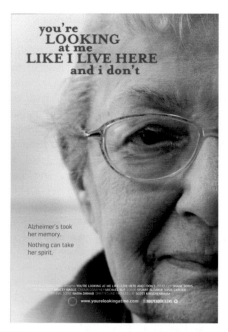

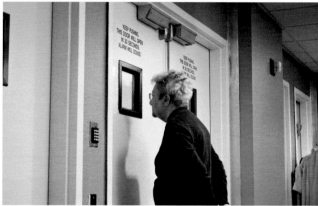

FIGURE 6.2 Film poster of *You're Looking at Me Like I Live Here and I Don't*. Lee Gorewitz before the exit door. (Used with permission from Scott Kirschenbaum.)

The Genius of Marian ◄◄◄◄ is a documentary directed by Banker White, who films his mother Pam White (Figure 6.3) in the early stages of Alzheimer's disease. The title, *The Genius of Marian*, refers to a book Pam was writing about her mother (Marian), who was a painter. Marian developed Alzheimer's disease and stopped painting. Most of Marian's watercolor paintings are featured prominently in this documentary. Pam was a year into the project, but at age 61, she was also diagnosed with Alzheimer's disease. The film shows the considerable burden of care faced by Pam's husband and, thus, provides some new insights into the early stages of Alzheimer's disease. The viewer clearly sees that the early stages of Alzheimer's can be hard to define; however, advancement to other stages may become apparent with the passage of time. Little context is given to the viewer; however, the film does introduce the viewer to the gradual onset of deficits. In Pam's case, one of the most "shocking developments" for her family was revealed when she could not figure out the tip on a restaurant check. Her son, a physician, adds that as he visited his parents, he gradually noted more deficits, and Pam began to behave out of

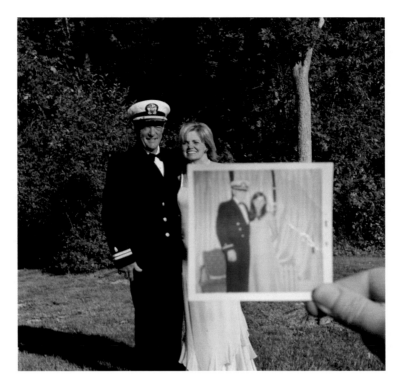

FIGURE 6.3   Pam White and her husband in the years preceding her illness. (Used with permission from Banker White.)

character, verbally attacking her husband. He prescribed medication to keep her "calm and happy." Pam's husband is constantly by her side. ("I like to be with her. I don't mind doing it.") Nevertheless, her care is challenging; he struggles to get her out of bed and to dress her. Most touching is Pam's remark that "I was quite distressed and upset about it, but it does not really matter. It does not really change anything, and I don't feel sad and I don't feel regret. …" This disconnect and lack of insight is well represented. The documentary is notable for its portrayal of a family trying to cope with the not-so-subtle dementia of a wife and mother. The disintegration of her mind is contrasted with beautiful, colorful, and warm watercolors, and these paintings provide some solace from what we are seeing so clearly here— early Alzheimer's disease in a genetically affected family.

Several other documentaries deserve mention. *The Forgetting: A Portrait of Alzheimer's* (2010) is an Emmy Award-winning documentary showing the disease in its different stages, gradually progressing to its nadir. The film provides some useful medical background and shows the 1906 discovery of the disease by Alois Alzheimer—as head of his neuroanatomical laboratory—and his observation of "peculiar changes of the neurofibrils" in his key patient Auguste D. The documentary is narrated by family members, researchers, and clinicians. This film is difficult to watch, showing belligerent behavior as part of the relentless decline, until nothing more than an immobile, dazed body remains.

A similar approach is seen in *Extreme Love: Dementia* (2012) , where we visit Beatitudes, a special "memory unit" in a senior housing complex. It is part of the *BBC Extreme Love* series directed by Louis Theroux, a British journalist with a resumé of shocking documentaries. It shows some interesting aspects of care, such as "going along with an hallucination" and not telling a patient they will be a permanent resident, in order to avoid major upset. This documentary suggests that the husband of one of the couples considers divorcing his wife to have the state pay her medical bills.

Other documentaries on dementia but with no new insight include *Vergiss mein Nicht* (2012) and *Mam* (2009). A major recent project is the series *Living with Alzheimer's* (LivingwithAlz.org), which includes several short documentaries.

A documentary that stands out from all others because of its unique topic—the positive effect of music in Alzheimer's disease. *Alive Inside* (2014) ⫷⫷⫷⫷ directed by Michael Rossato-Bennett follows Dan Cohen, a social worker in a nursing home, who discovered that some Alzheimer's disease patients responded extraordinarily to their favorite music using an iPod. The emotional link to music is very convincing when you see patients becoming markedly animated with music. Music may be soothing and therapeutic for many patients who otherwise would need psychotropic medication.[12]

Music is deeply personal and can elicit strong emotions. Joy and chills predictably return each time we revisit a favorite melody, hook, or rhythm—it seems as if this response is hardwired in the brain. Some of us have also experienced the loss of joy in music during a life-changing event, when we find no comfort in music. What happens to music appreciation after an injury to the brain is tremendously interesting but not fully understood. The "music circuitry"—if there is one—is unknown, but some neuroscientists consider musical memory a separate cognitive domain.

Musical recognition remains relatively spared in Alzheimer's disease and other dementias. In advanced Alzheimer's disease, the delight that comes with familiar music can be fully preserved, even when language is markedly impaired and the emotional state depressed. More tellingly in exceptional cases, patients with frontotemporal dementias develop a preference for a different genre of music (e.g., polka, rap). Music appreciation in advanced dementia seems the last thing to go. The patients seen here seem noncommunicative, bedridden, compacted, and sad until the music starts. Retrieving old memories remains possible in dementia, and so why not through the medium of music rather than photo albums.[13]

Alive Inside is filled with fragments of nursing home residents "awakening" after hearing nostalgic tunes, but there is also an interesting focus on the history of nursing homes in the United States, bureaucracy in nursing home care, and the place of elderhood. The overall theme, however, is the power of music, which Cohen calls connecting to the person's self. The documentary cleverly links patients' childhood-period footage with the experience of revisiting music and speculatively suggests that music, through emotion, is a portal to other hidden, previously untapped memories. However, the emotional link to music is very convincing when you see Johnny (who "kind of exists") and Marylou (crying about her failing daily functioning and aphasia) suddenly become markedly animated.

But some skepticism remains. The director eschews failures or frustrating attempts and, in keeping with the joyful theme, we see only examples of success. Finding the right music may be difficult and time consuming. Does music really bring back sufficiently detailed memories? Does music improve behavior or socialization, and does music reduce the need for antipsychotics to control agitation? Could music do harm when it causes patients to start moving wildly or, as a result of serious comorbidities, become short of breath or develop chest pain? Might they fall while dancing to the music? The documentary also raises "massively overused" antipsychotics and by mentioning that patients have "no control over the medication flowing through them"—an unsubstantiated claim.

These recent documentaries comprise a large contribution to the catalog of medically themed films. Given their focus on one of the most disturbing concerns in neuro geriatric practice, they are a major component of what Sally Chivers cleverly called "The Silvering Screen."[14]

---

[12] A large body of literature shows that engagement with music improves the quality of life, but studies are very hard to do. See Baker FA, Pool J, Johansson K, Wosch T, Bukowska AA, Kulis A, et al. Strategies for Recruiting People with Dementia to Music Therapy Studies: Systematic Review. *J Music Ther*. 2021; 58:373–407..

[13] We already saw the link between music and neurology in Chapter 4. *The Music Never Stopped* (2011) is about profound abulia and antegrade amnesia after removal of a large brain tumor but with full remembrance of songs prior to surgery. Music therapy is used to great effect in *Fred Won't Move Out* (2012), showing exuberance in the main character with advanced dementia during a sing-along.

[14] Chivers S. *The Silvering Screen: Old Age and Disability in Cinema*. Toronto: University of Toronto Press; 2011.

Huntington's Disease

Neurogenetics has found its way into the movies (Chapter 4) but rarely into documentary film. Most familial neurodegenerative diseases have no cure, and there are no medications to delay the manifestations of the disorder. For filmmakers, there may not be much to show other than the relentless decline of the patient. However, further characterization of the genetic code of these disorders, and eventually prediction of its later appearance through laboratory testing, has become a reality. Some scientists have stated that precision (individualized) medicine is just around the corner, and if so, this could create immediate ethical problems with late-onset neurologic disorders. Accurate prediction (i.e., knowing whether you will get it) varies for each neurologic disorder, and actual testing may involve insufficiently validated biomarkers.

One disease in this category is Huntington's disease. The documentary *Do You Really Want to Know?* (2012) ✓✓✓✓ , written and directed by John Zaritsky, accurately addresses these problems. Genetic testing for Huntington's disease has been available since discovery of the gene in 1993 and now is able to prediagnose family members with a high probability, although nothing can be done to prevent disease onset. Genetic testing has outrun understanding of the pathogenesis and treatment of the disease (Figure 6.4). Huntington's disease is a prime example of this medical quandary.[15]

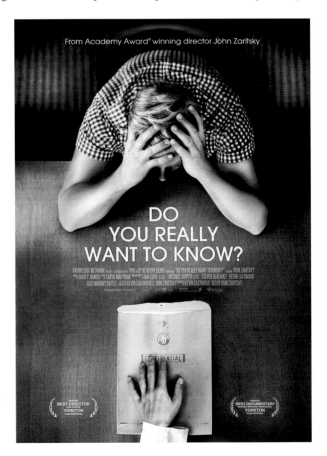

FIGURE 6.4   Film poster of *Do You Really Want to Know?* (Used with permission from Kevin Eastwood, producer.)

---

[15] Roberts JS, Patterson AK, Uhlmann WR. Genetic Testing for Neurodegenerative Diseases: Ethical and Health Communication Challenges. *Neurobiol Dis.* 2020;141:104871.

Huntington's disease is caused by the expansion of a trinucleotide cytosine-adenine-guanine (CAG) sequence on chromosome 4. This expansion within the Huntington gene results in an abnormally damaging protein. However, a positive test does not predict with 100% certainty that the disease will develop, because some patients with certain CAG lengths may be spared. Huntington's disease is a neurodegenerative disease that progresses over many years and includes the development of myoclonus, chorea, dystonia, and rigidity as well as irritability and psychosis. Eventually, it may also lead to obsessive-compulsive behavior and depression. Hypomania is well recognized in patients with Huntington's disease. There are many medications that successfully mute the responses of these symptoms.

The motor symptoms of chorea (when awake) are constantly present and may involve head movements and tongue protrusion. Movements may be difficult to initiate, and dystonia may occur (abnormal positioning and tics). Walking is unsteady with ataxic features and may also include dystonic posturing. Psychiatric symptoms include a combination of irritability and apathy followed by cognitive decline. Hypersexuality and paraphilias have been noted. The last clinical stage is marked by devastating motor symptoms, full dependence on others for care, and marked dementia. Nursing home placement is typical.[16]

Do You Really Want to Know? is the first comprehensive documentary that addresses the symptoms of Huntington's disease and its penetration into families. The documentary goes through the difficult decisions faced by three different families. The three key persons followed throughout the film are John Roder, Jeff Carroll, and Theresa Monahan. John calls it a "genetic sentence." John is a scientist with periods of severe chorea. He knew it ran in his family, but he and his wife decided to have two children, hoping that they would not pass on the gene. In 1993, when he was asymptomatic, he got tested, expecting a negative result, but the result was positive. In this documentary, it is 10 years since his diagnosis, and he is impaired by chorea, dystonia, and spasticity.

A second key person in the documentary is Jeff Carroll, who decides to have the test and also tests positive. When his wife becomes pregnant (twice), they decide to test prenatally, and fortunately, both children are negative. Jeff became a researcher in Dr. Michael Hayden's laboratory, an internationally known Huntington's research facility in Canada.

DIALOGUE

Do You Really Want to Know?

Jeff

You're never going to not know your status again. You can never turn back the clock and go to "maybe" again. You are always going to know one way or the other for sure.

The third person is Theresa Monahan, a woman with a strong family history of Huntington's disease, who decides not to get tested despite her husband's urging. Later, she proceeds with testing without informing her husband for several months. Despite testing negative, this situation caused a period of self-inflicted anguish. She felt she deceived her husband by not telling him she was getting tested and, therefore, is unable to share her good news.

The documentary provides statistical data and a good overview of what Huntington's disease entails. Huntington's chorea, or Huntington's disease, is an autosomal-dominant disease. The prevalence of Huntington's disease has remained about 4–10/100,000. The disorder usually presents between

---

[16] Ross CA, Tabrizi SJ. Huntington's Disease: From Molecular Pathogenesis to Clinical Treatment. *Lancet Neurol.* 2011; 10:83–98.

the ages of 30 and 50, but most family members are aware of the disorder as a result of its considerable penetrance, with half the children of an affected family testing positive. Theresa's family provides a good example. Her grandfather was one of ten children, five of whom died from Huntington's disease, and her mother was one of seven children, four of whom died from Huntington's disease. Theresa calls herself "lucky."

Only 5% to 10% of individuals at risk test themselves for Huntington's disease despite the availability of predictive testing for nearly two decades. Women are more likely to undergo testing, possibly before deciding to pursue pregnancy. However, surprisingly, the decision of whether to conceive offspring differs only slightly between those who carry the gene and those who do not.[17]

The film suggests the risk of suicide, but in general, there has been a decrease in suicides in patients who have tested positive. This is relevant because depression is common in this population and often requires treatment (psychopharmacy and psychological help). The risk of suicide is highest around the testing period. Depression may even occur in the preclinical stage when the uncertainty is the greatest.[18] A related diagnostic problem is that Huntington's disease may present with psychiatric symptomatology before hyperkinesia or chorea starts. Coping with the disease is not easy at all, according to published accounts.[19]

Testing is available, but young individuals (<18 years) or those with severe psychiatric illnesses are excluded. In practice, very few proceed with testing for the disease.[20] Most family members should undergo a multidisciplinary approach before testing (geneticist, psychologist/psychiatrist, and neurologist), which usually is set up in specialty clinics. The mean duration of Huntington's disease is about 15 years; thus, close care is needed.

This remarkable film about a rare neurologic disease admirably shows the major aspects of the disease and the dilemmas families face. Many decisions—wanting to know, not wanting to know, or wanting to know and not telling anyone—is how vulnerable humans respond to these tremendous uncertainties. The benefit of testing for Huntington's disease remains unclear, but now that a test is available, family members have the right to know. Individuals may improve their well-being, and there is a lower prevalence of depression in the group that decided to go ahead with genetic testing. With genetic testing becoming commonplace, these decisions will apply to any late-onset neurodegenerative disease.

Multiple Sclerosis

When I Walk (2013) ◄◄◄◄ , directed by Jason DaSilva, is a diarist's documentary of 7 years living with primary progressive multiple sclerosis (MS) (Figure 6.5). Progressive MS is a universally progressive spinal disease. Clear criteria have been developed, and there is considerable interest in MS therapies that include neuroprotection and myelin repair. The disease is rapidly progressive—the time of onset to using a cane for walking is a median of 7 to 8 years. More recent studies report 14 years, with no clear explanation for the further delay.[21]

[17] Hayden MR. Predictive Testing for Huntington's Disease: The Calm after the Storm. *Lancet*. 2000;356:1944–1945.

[18] Almqvist EW, Bloch M, Brinkman R, Craufurd D, Hayden MR. A Worldwide Assessment of the Frequency of Suicide, Suicide Attempts, or Psychiatric Hospitalization after Predictive Testing for Huntington Disease. *Am J Hum Genet*. 1999;64:1293–1304.

[19] See Mahmood S, Law S, Bombard Y. "I Have to Start Learning How to Live with Becoming Sick": A Scoping Review of the Lived Experiences of People with Huntington's Disease. *Clin Genet*. 2021; Hans MB, Koeppen AH. Huntington's Chorea. Its Impact on the Spouse. *J Nerv Ment Dis*. 1980;168:209–214; and Kessler S, Bloch M. Social System Responses to Huntington Disease. *Fam Process*. 1989;28:59–68.

[20] Krukenberg RC, Koller DL, Weaver DD, Dickerson JN, Quaid KA. Two Decades of Huntington Disease Testing: Patient's Demographics and Reproductive Choices. *J Genet Couns*. 2013;22:643–653.

[21] See Confavreux C, Vukusic S. Natural History of Multiple Sclerosis: A Unifying Concept. *Brain*. 2006;129:606–616; and Wolinsky JS, Group PRS. The Diagnosis of Primary Progressive Multiple Sclerosis. *J Neurol Sci*. 2003;206:145–152.

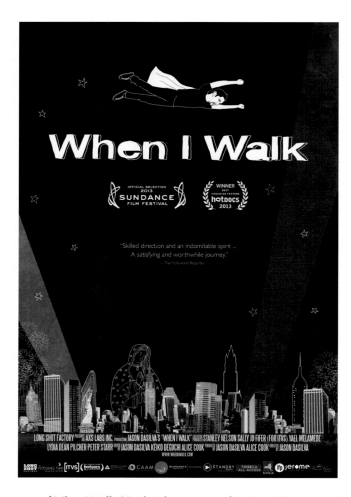

FIGURE 6.5   Film poster of *When I Walk*. (Used with permission from Long Shot Factory.)

Director Jason DaSilva has several short films and feature-length documentary films to his credit. This personal documentary is a major accomplishment by a skilled filmmaker who lets us experience with him his progressive MS, the rapid changes over time, and all the major practical consequences of the disease for a young, vibrant person. Interwoven throughout the documentary is animation that calls attention to the burden of MS.

We are first introduced to DaSilva after his diagnosis, when his legs give way during a vacation in the Caribbean. The film shows the initial stages of primary progressive MS. A brief interlude shows how primary progressive MS is defined and how it is considered an immunological disorder. Coping with an MS diagnosis is presented in a straightforward, unsentimental way. His mother explains that it could be worse and compares it—as many people do when newly diagnosed—with other, more severe, disorders. She tells him he could be in a worse place—"the places where people are stuck."

Next, DaSilva is seen exercising in the gym, hoping that his case and progression will be different. But he soon is confronted with reality. He is shown undergoing a Shriner's gait assessment of his spastic gait. To his surprise, one of the healthcare workers broaches the topic of a wheelchair. He is shown brochures from wheelchair suppliers but wants little to do with it.

The documentary shows, step by step, the relentless progression of this type of MS. Soon we see DaSilva having difficulty climbing stairs and needing a cane for stability. His marked spastic, ataxic walk is prominently shown (hence, the title *When I Walk*). This walking handicap limits his social life. In a moving moment, he tells the viewer that he has had his "share of beautiful women," but as his MS gets worse, the girls seem to have disappeared into thin air (illustrated by photos of his former girl-friends with the faces faded out). It is powerful to see a young person so visibly disabled. His mother plays an important role, often bringing him back to reality, although she can at times be harsh. ("We are really alone in this world.") He visits India, a place he had visited previously, but this time, with his walker, DaSilva notices people staring at him when he walks—a much different experience from his prior, pre-diagnosis visit. For him, the biggest question is whether he will be able to make all the films he had planned. Soon his vision becomes affected, and he develops difficulty focusing and has to stop a project that he had intended to complete while in India. At this point, DaSilva tries alternative medicine including yoga, transcendental meditation, and ayurvedic medicine. Nothing changes.

Dialogue

When I Walk

| Jason | *I just start using a cane, and they are already talking about wheelchairs.* |
| Mother | *Things are tough in life. Get real, you mollycoddled North American kid.* |

DaSilva visits his 87-year-old grand-uncle and asks him if there is a family history of MS. (There is none.) His grandmother, a devout Catholic, suggests he go to Lourdes, which he does.[22] After he bathes in the waters at Lourdes, he dreams of running. ("Maybe a century of my family's prayers will get me out of this.") Nothing changes. The film also follows DaSilva in his search for extremely controversial surgi-cal procedures, and he proceeds with the opening of his apparently obstructed cerebral veins. Again, nothing changes.

He visits an MS support group, where he meets his future wife (and co-writer of this documentary). Alice is much less affected by her MS and is able to assist him. The film shows them having fun riding a scooter around the Guggenheim Museum, going to Hawaii, and eventually marrying. Finally, DaSilva's life changes.

DaSilva's relationship with Alice makes his "depressing" (in his mother's words) situation far more endurable, and they often discuss living with the disease and making a life of their own, maintaining their desires and ambitions. Despite the progressive MS, difficulty getting pregnant, and miscarriage, the film ends on a positive note when Alice again becomes pregnant and an ultrasound shows a fully developed fetus.

When I Walk is one of the first comprehensive films on MS, but there have been other TV documen-taries, notably *"But You Still Look So Well ..." Living with Multiple Sclerosis* (2005 and its sequel in 2012), which emphasize that many patients have no visible signs of disease, and their diagnosis does not seem to impact their daily life in a major way. MS may not always visibly affect patients, and thus the topic

---

[22] MS is also a theme of *Lourdes*, a 2009 film directed by Jessica Hausner. It stars Sylvie Testud as a patient with severe MS but is primarily about miraculous cures. In *The Diving Bell and the Butterfly*, a priest invites Jean-Dominique Bauby to join a pilgrimage, and he remembers a prior, romantic weekend gone wrong in Lourdes before his stroke. He does not like the place with all the wheelchairs and trinkets including a red-blinking Maria statue that his girlfriend insists on having in their bedroom. The Bishop of Lourdes has regularly published miracle cures in multiple sclerosis, which is comparably common. No cure of MS has been certified from 1976 through 2006. See Francois B, Sternberg EM, Fee E. The Lourdes Medical Cures Revisited. *J Hist Med Allied Sci*. 2014;69:135–162.

may not lend itself to a full feature film unless the progression is dramatic. *A Certain Kind of Beauty* (2006) also involves a young patient with primary progressive MS with similar themes.

When I Walk invites viewers into the experience of a creative young man with progressive MS. It offers a compelling and realistic view into this rare form of MS and grappling with its challenges and limitations.[23] It focuses on one of the three main forms of progressive MS (primary progressive vs. relapsing-remitting and secondary progressive). Most people with MS have a relapsing-remitting form. Although many eventually go on to develop progressive MS, the primary progressive form only affects 10 to 20% of all patients with multiple sclerosis. It appears to be a type not responsive to therapy, but drugs are now available to improve symptoms. Currently, over 15 disease-modifying treatments (DMTs) are approved for MS with different efficacy and safety profiles.[24] Drug trials in chronic progressive MS also have shown efficacy in a number of immunotherapies.[25] The film shows some of the desperation and the desire to seek alternative therapies. Many undergo highly controversial, often plainly unsubstantiated interventions such as surgery to correct chronic impaired venous outflow of the central nervous system (shown by the latest studies to be flawed).[26] The documentary is effective in showing a progressive disease intertwined with the emotionality of having a supportive partner. It does exactly what a neurologic documentary should do—provide a valuable teaching resource.

Amyotrophic Lateral Sclerosis

Amyotrophic lateral sclerosis (ALS) was first characterized by Charcot (Chapter 3). One of his patients with hysteria had major spasticity (upper motor neuron sign), which at autopsy was found to be caused by involvement of the lateral tracts of the spinal cord (*la sclérose latérale*), and he distinguished it from multiple sclerosis (*sclérose en plaques*). It became known as Charcot disease in Europe and the United Kingdom. Here in the United States, it was known as Lou Gehrig's disease, for the famed baseball player who suffered from it (Chapter 7).

ALS usually results in progressive wasting of the shoulder and pectoral muscles, atrophy in hand muscles (mostly first interossei and thenar muscles), and features of spasticity. Much wasting may be misinterpreted as weight loss, some of which occurs because of major swallowing difficulties.

Noninvasive ventilation will eventually fail to help the patient, typically when oropharyngeal weakness becomes prominent. Impaired glottal closure impairs maintenance of large lung volumes, and pharyngeal weakness may lead to occlusion of the upper airway. Oxygen desaturation despite maximal noninvasive settings also indicates the need for a tracheostomy. Patients who choose a tracheostomy are typically young with families and may believe that holding on may buy them time until a cure is found. Tracheostomies are often performed emergently because no prior discussion has been entertained. This period of time is crucial for any ALS patient, and discussions are often postponed. If ventilation is not supported, most patients become unconscious or more unresponsive as a result of hypoxic-hypercapnic encephalopathy.[27]

---

[23] *When I Walk* argues for better access to public places and identifies the difficulty of finding accessible ramps. In one cartoon, a big, red, monstrous ramp is shown, and DaSilva drives home the point across that he cannot hail a taxi, cannot take the subway, and is markedly restricted in his mobility despite a scooter. He eventually develops a website for accessible places and an app helping persons with a disability.

[24] Khan O, Filippi M, Freedman MS, Barkhof F, Dore-Duffy P, Lassmann H, et al. Chronic Cerebrospinal Venous Insufficiency and Multiple Sclerosis. *Ann Neurol*. 2010;67:286–290.

[25] Koch MW, Cutter G, Stys PK, Yong VW, Metz LM. Treatment Trials in Progressive MS–Current Challenges and Future Directions. *Nat Rev Neurol*. 2013;9:496–503.

[26] Valdueza JM, Doepp F, Schreiber SJ, van Oosten BW, Schmierer K, Paul F, et al. What Went Wrong? The Flawed Concept of Cerebrospinal Venous Insufficiency. *J Cereb Blood Flow Metab*. 2013;33:657–668.

[27] See Brown RH, Al-Chalabi A. Amyotrophic Lateral Sclerosis. *N Engl J Med*. 2017;377:162–172; and Robberecht W, Philips T. The Changing Scene of Amyotrophic Lateral Sclerosis. *Nat Rev Neurosci*. 2013;14:248–264.

Three major documentaries on ALS deserve attention and close examination. *So Much So Fast* (2006) ✦✦✦✦ , directed by Steven Ascher, follows the progression of ALS in Stephen Heywood. The film is also about the founding of the ALS Therapy Development Institute, which currently operates in Cambridge, Massachusetts, testing hundreds of drugs on genetically engineered mice. The film discusses in great detail a wish to accelerate drug trials, and it alleges "slow" progress in academia. The film starts with an important statement. "Back then (1993), there was only one rule: there was nothing you could do, no treatment, no surgery, no drugs."

Heywood was diagnosed with ALS at the age of 29. His brother, Jamy, started a foundation to find a treatment and became an aggressive negotiator. ("For a family, a diagnosis like that stops time; for Jamy, time sped up.") The film shows them discussing their ideas at the annual meeting of the Society of Neuroscience. For Jamy, "It is a strange world. So many people obsessed with mice and rats." Jamy is determined to find ways to fight the establishment but also sees limitations. ("We are proposing ideas that can easily be shot down.") The documentary shows two parallel stories—the difficulty of making progress in the laboratory and the relentless progression of Stephen's ALS. His wife tells us she can deal with a wheelchair, but his losing his voice is the toughest blow. He is finally seen on a ventilator, virtually locked in. He died in 2006 before the film's completion.

Living with Lew (2007) ✦✦ , directed by Adam Bardach, is about Lew, a movie director diagnosed with ALS. The documentary opens with a Lou Gehrig clip: "I might have been given a bad break, but I got an awful lot to live for." (See Chapter 7.) The film shows an upbeat Lew who cracks cynical jokes—for example, showing a nasal CPAP ("just like a fighter pilot") and the pills he is taking ("this is Haldol, LSD, peyote nugget, marijuana, etc."). In addition, he is taking multivitamins and tamoxifen ("at least I do not get breast cancer"). He wears a Lou Gehrig New York Yankees shirt.

The film shows interviews with healthcare workers in the Forbes Norris MDA/ALS Research Center, and there is a very succinct explanation of ALS and its programs. It mentions 3- to 5-year survival and 10% long-term survival (showing Stephen Hawking as an example). The film shows Lew in an advanced stage of ALS, but this documentary does not have the gravitas of the other documentaries. Some viewers may be put off by the dark sarcasm.

I Am Breathing (2013) ✦✦✦✦ , directed by Emma Davie and Morag McKinnon, is a documentary about Neil Platt, a 33-year-old architect with a familial form of ALS (father and grandfather). He uses a voice-recognition computer. The film pushes the boundaries of documentary filmmaking and follows him into the terminal stages and just before hospice care. His case is somewhat unique; the familial form accounts for only 5% of all ALS cases. ALS is a relatively frequent neurologic disease with an incidence of 2/100,000. Platt died 14 months after the diagnosis (Figure 6.6). The title *I Am Breathing* refers to the constant sound of the mechanical ventilator heard when the film opens. Platt is diagnosed at the age of 33, and we get to know him after several unusual remarks. He explains that he is perusing coffin catalogs and is considering canceling his phone. Shockingly, he tells the clerk it is because he is dying. He challenges the viewer to try to fight an itch. This is all an introduction to what we are about to see—a young man struggling with a major illness while trying to keep up appearances and his sense of humor. Platt knows the cruel verdict all too well. The film shows him on CPAP and immobilized in a chair while being cared for by his young wife, Louise, whose bravery and compassion are extraordinary. Six months after his diagnosis, his hands stop working, followed by his legs three months later. His young child walks around in the room touching everything (including the power button of the ventilator).

The blog he started with his wife (a play on words called *The Plattitude*) becomes his only outlet, and he manages to dictate 100 blog posts.[28] The frustrating voice-recognition technology is notable here and becomes almost emblematic of the handicap he is facing. His blog is a long document that he has written for his son, Oscar, and he also ponders "the meaning of life and associated questions." ("I often ponder

---

[28] Platt N. Neil's Blog: www.iambreathing.com/introduction_plattitude

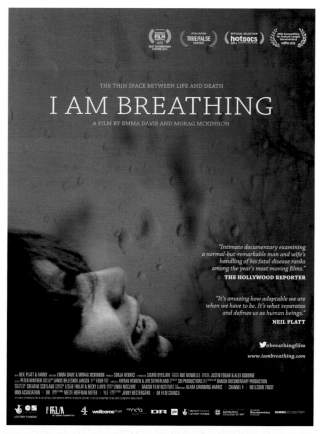

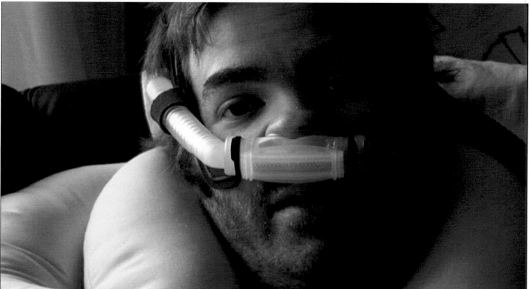

FIGURE 6.6   Film poster of *I Am Breathing*; Neil Platt on noninvasive mechanical ventilation. (Used with permission from Scottish Documentary Institute/SDI Productions Ltd.)

questions of such gravity and magnitude.") He is very clear that his advance directive is to forego more intervention or surgical procedures when his voice disappears. In his blog he writes,

> Just as the physical deterioration I have suffered is a result of motor neurone disease, so is the emotional deterioration of everyone touched by it. It pains me to think that the price being demanded by the disease is so high that not only does it reduce me to a talking head, but it eats away at the strong ties of family and friendship which ordinarily would withstand the most determined of attacks.

In an almost unbearable scene, Platt's airway obstructs, and he has a choking episode, resulting in his wife using urgent percussion. Here his dysphagia becomes notable. This defining moment inevitably becomes the saddest part of the documentary. Platt is shown dictating his last words before he goes to hospice: "The reason I have chosen to go to the hospice tomorrow is to draw the curtain over what has been a devastating, degrading year and a half." He made the decision to remove the ventilator when he could not speak or swallow. Neil Platt passed away on February 25, 2009. His son has a 50% chance of getting ALS. The film is a remarkable documentary on the rapid progression of young-onset ALS and perhaps of any neurologic disease.

These three documentaries show different courses but a similar ending. The outcome of ALS is an approximate 3-year survival in 50% of patients. The patient with onset in limbs seems to have less rapid progression than a patient starting the disease in the oropharyngeal region, and ALS starting in the legs has a slightly slower progression than early upper involvement of the arms. In Neil Platt's case, respiratory failure came relatively early, with largely preserved speech and no severe dysphagia. (He is seen eating fish and chips while supported on nasal CPAP.) In Stephen Heywood's case, dysphagia came with dysarthria—as is more commonly seen. After gastrostomy placement, survival is still variable, usually about a year.

As is shown in these documentaries, ALS with early respiratory involvement does not necessarily imply a more progressive disease. Once respiration becomes involved in progressive ALS, the patient has a high likelihood of demise within a year unless mechanical ventilation is provided, as was the case for Stephen Heywood. (We see him in a final scene, mostly locked in with a tracheostomy and a respirator.)

Management of respiratory symptoms remains the determinant of outcome. A gastrostomy is often inserted if the patient is unable to maintain body weight or if there is frank dysphagia. Hypoxemia or hypercapnia is an important indication for noninvasive ventilation, and most patients are able to tolerate noninvasive ventilation quite well. Noninvasive ventilation improves hypoxemia and hypercapnia, although it rarely normalizes these values.

ALS should be distinguished from primary lateral sclerosis (pyramidal signs only), progressive muscular atrophy (peripheral signs only), and progressive bulbar palsy (lower motor neuron involvement of speech and swallowing). Primary lateral sclerosis may have a median survival of 20 years, but the other disorders progress similarly to ALS. Outcome is also better in specialized clinics, largely due to much better symptom management. Weight loss also carries a poor prognosis, but even if gastrostomy placement leads to adequate feeding, it only improves quality of life.

This discussion has focused on three recent documentaries on ALS, each with a different perspective. Fiction films (see Chapter 4) have made a clumsy mockery of the disease. However, these documentaries present viewers with the effects of a devastating neurologic illness, and its progression is exceedingly difficult to watch.

Migraine

"One billion migraine sufferers" is one of the first stunning statistics presented in the film *Out of My Head* (2020) ◄◄◄ (Figure 6.7), directed by Susanna Styron. The film achieved its goal of increasing awareness of this disabling neurologic disorder with a tendency to become intractable. It was funded

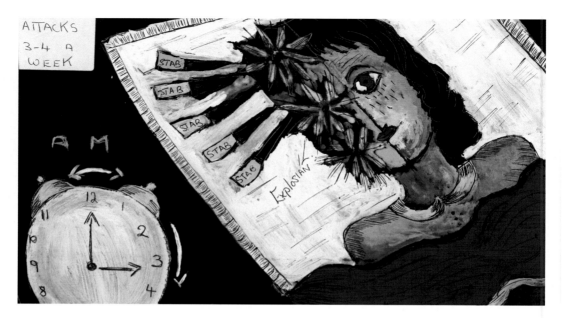

FIGURE 6.7   Drawing of a migraine attack in *Out of My Head*. (Kindly provided by the producer Jacki Ochs. Photo of artwork: Jacki Ochs. Artwork courtesy: Migraine Action UK.)

by the Association of Migraine Disorders, Migraine Research Foundation, among several others. At the end of the film, neurologist Peter Goadsby states that the funding of migraine disorders is "scandalous" and reveals a "complete lack of commitment." When a delegation goes to Congress to increase migraine awareness, the film shows its agenda. Migraine is presented as a horrible affliction with images of knife stabs or thunderstorms and lightning; the example of a patient with persistent visual symptoms, who sees "only shapes"; disability leading to major deterioration in daily activities and hygiene; patients who are largely bedbound; and frequent trips to the emergency department for "code blue." The language used by the experts is forceful and magnified; they tell us they are trying to change "unbearable pain to bearable pain" and warn that "there is no heat-seeking missile to turn it off." The initial impetus for the film came from Styron's own daughter, Emma Larson, who started experiencing migraines in college: "They kept coming every two weeks, nonstop, like clockwork, and I couldn't take it," "I felt betrayed by my body; I felt scared all the time. I never felt anxiety like that." She studied in Paris without attacks for 8 blissful months, but after her boyfriend visited, she had one attack after another and called her mother to say she was coming home.

The documentary very effectively shows how people wrongly dismiss migraine, see it as a female problem, and thus stigmatize the disorder. (Professional athletes with migraine, like Kareem Abdul-Jabbar and Dwyane Wade also get attention.) There is a delightful (but sad) section on how migraine sufferers were represented in the media as white upper-class women lying with a hand on their head and stretched out on a sofa, suggesting that migraine is a "lifestyle disorder" rather than a neurological disease. We see a segment of an episode of *The Dick Van Dyke Show* in 1964 entitled "Pink Pills and Purple Patients," in which Sally Rogers (Rose Marie) has a severe headache exacerbated by any level of noise. (The segment is about the mistake of taking pills prescribed for someone else and getting weird side effects.)

For years (and even up until the present day), migraine was considered a "psychosomatic" disorder. Migraine sufferers were accused of pretending or, as described by essayist Joan Didion, "For I had no brain tumor, no eyestrain, no high blood pressure, nothing wrong with me at all: I simply had migraine headaches, and migraine headaches were, as everyone who did not have them knew, imaginary."[29]

DIALOGUE

Out of My Head

Joan Didion
(from her essay, "In Bed")

Three, four, sometimes five times a month, I spend the day in bed with a migraine headache, insensible to the world around me. Almost every day of every month, between these attacks, I feel the sudden irrational irritation and the flush of blood into the cerebral arteries, which tell me that migraine is on its way, and I take certain drugs to avert its arrival. If I did not take the drugs, I would be able to function, perhaps, one day in four.

The complexity of migraine presentations are well discussed and explained ("all senses on alert"), but the film implies that all presentations involve major auras (normally, about a third or less) or major neurologic symptoms such as aphasia or hemiplegia (even less). Misattribution of specific triggers to migraine is well known. Contrary to popular belief, triggers play a very limited role.[30] The kaleidoscopic visual manifestations are shown. Others talk about "nausea and fatigue" centers in the brain and suggest opioids as an option. Fortunately, one neurologist in the film emphasizes that medications actually cause headaches. By now, the more perceptive viewers will get the impression that this is a trial-and-error medical practice. It is mentioned that in the United States, there are only ~500 headache specialists; that is, one expert for every 76,000 patients. The VA gets another bad rap and is accused of "passing off" post-traumatic headaches. (See also Chapter 4 on spinal cord injury and associated films.) The film gradually becomes a litany of concerns and mismanagement. Joan Didion writes about the wonderful feeling when a migraine ends: "I open the windows and feel the air, eat gratefully, sleep well. I notice the particular nature of a flower in a glass on the stair landing. I count my blessings." But that message is overshadowed in this film narrative of simplified personal and professional testimonies and distorted images and sounds.

Presumably, Lewis Carroll's own migraine attacks inspired *Alice in Wonderland*, but this is controversial.[31] Migraines also allegedly contributed to the creative efforts of Sigmund Freud, Georgia O'Keeffe, Virginia Woolf, and even Thomas Jefferson. The history of migraine is a bewildering mix of facts and speculations, some of which are mentioned in the film but not fleshed out.[32] In 100 years, we went from the discovery of ergotamine to first approval of a calcitonin gene-related peptide monoclonal antibody (the gepants) and from vasodilation and vascular, neurogenic, neurotransmitter, and genetic paradigms,[33] but classification remained a moving target. The ICHD-3 now provides diagnostic criteria

---

[29] Didion J. In Bed. *The White Album*. New York: Farrar, Straus and Giroux; 1979:168–172.

[30] See Hougaard A, Amin FM, Hauge AW, Ashina M, Olesen J. Provocation of Migraine with Aura Using Natural Trigger Factors. *Neurology*. 2013;80:428–431; and Lipton RB, Pavlovic JM, Haut SR, Grosberg BM, Buse DC. Methodological Issues in Studying Trigger Factors and Premonitory Features of Migraine. *Headache*. 2014;54:1661–1669.

[31] Some evidence exists that Lewis Carroll had visual manifestations of migraine when writing his landmark book, but others see it as "neuro-mythology." (The potential folly of neurologic interpretation of the arts is also discussed in Chapter 9.) For further discussion of Carroll, see Podoll K, Robinson D. Lewis Carroll's Migraine Experiences. *Lancet*. 1999;353:1366; and Blau JN. Somesthetic Aura: The Experience of "Alice in Wonderland." *Lancet*. 1998;352:582.

[32] Tfelt-Hansen PC, Koehler PJ. One Hundred Years of Migraine Research: Major Clinical and Scientific Observations from 1910 to 2010. *Headache*. 2011;51:752–778.

[33] Lipton RB, Croop R, Stock EG, Stock DA, Morris BA, Frost M, et al. Rimegepant, an Oral Calcitonin Gene-Related Peptide Receptor Antagonist, for Migraine. *N Engl J Med*. 2019;381:142–149; and Ailani J, Lipton RB, Goadsby PJ et al. Atogepant for the Preventive Treatment of Migraine. *N Engl J Med* 2021; 385:695–706.

for the three main categories of migraine: migraine without aura, migraine with aura, and chronic migraine.[34] Biobehavioral therapies (shown in the film) and acupuncture can be beneficial, but physical therapy, chiropractic manipulation, or dietary changes are ineffective. At the root of the problem is the unknown origin of migraine.[35]

Aphasia

Documentaries about stroke (in the dominant hemisphere) typically involve coping with aphasia.[36] Once a patient starts talking before the eye of the camera and the film demonstrates the impact of stroke on communication—something we take for granted—it invariably makes a strong impact on the viewing audience.[37] Aphasia can be an almost invisible disability, especially when not accompanied by hemiplegia. This is often the case in posterior (fluent) aphasias, which may spare the motor cortex, and in patients with primary progressive aphasias. The discussion here focuses on three recent major documentaries that address poststroke aphasia.

After Words (2013) ◄◄◄◄, directed by Vincent Straggas, includes the observations of several researchers who discuss the difficulties of living with an aphasic person. The documentary is notable for its comprehensive explanation of aphasia. There is an emphasis on therapy, recovery, and an especially effective focus on improving quality of life in patients with aphasia. *After Words* is a comprehensive look at aphasia caused mostly by stroke. It also briefly discusses primary progressive aphasia and presents one example of a patient with aphasia after a gunshot wound to the head. Patients, spouses, and other family members are interviewed, and each patient clearly explains marked difficulties with language (Figure 6.8). All aspects of aphasia are discussed. Several neurologists are invited to comment and explain in simple ways what aphasia entails.

Various types of aphasia, not all of which are depicted in this film, present different severity levels. The additional challenge with receptive (or fluent) aphasia is that it often includes considerable deficits

after words

"I got aphasia; what ya' gonna do? It's part of me now."

"He's still my father... We still have conversations; we still hang out."

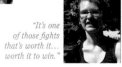
"It's one of those fights that's worth it... worth it to win."

"Speak no speak. I know it! But speak...no speak.

"Everything is not what I thought it was going to be like... Slowly but surely I will recover."

"It's hard for my husband to be the caregiver for everyone."

FIGURE 6.8 Patients with aphasia in scenes from *After Words*. (Kindly provided by Jerome Kaplan.)

---

[34] Headache Classification Committee of the International Headache Society (IHS) The International Classification of Headache Disorders, 3rd edition. *Cephalalgia*. 2018;38:1–211.

[35] Ashina M. Migraine. *N Engl J Med*. 2020;383:1866–1876.

[36] To date, documentary filmmakers have overlooked the other disabilities that can accompany a stroke, such as paralysis.

[37] The other major stroke-induced disability, neglect associated with the non-dominant hemisphere, which may be even more devastating, has not yet been discovered by filmmakers.

in comprehension, which complicate any effort to engage in meaningful dialogue. Dr. Marjorie Nicholas, Professor of Communication Sciences at the MGH Institute of Health Professions, provides an insightful description. Speech-language pathologists are interviewed in this film, notably those in the team led by Jerome Kaplan, founder of the Aphasia Community Group, one of the oldest groups of its kind in the country. They emphasize that patients with aphasia should be treated differently. Spouses (as well as other family members and caregivers) must figure out what their loved one is attempting to communicate. Some patients mention that perseveration associated with severe expressive aphasia can be exhausting, and it shows. The filmmaker Vincent Straggas recalls, "There is a struggle for them to communicate, and what one usually experiences is a more meaningful and thoughtful conversation. They are real and to the point, and don't waste time with idle chitchat."

DIALOGUE

After Words

Marjorie Nicholas

Imagine you are waking up in a foreign land, say Poland. They look around and everyone speaks Polish, and they do not understand the language; but they understand everything else about the world … and they cannot speak Polish.

After Words clearly dissects the abnormal components of aphasia and shows speech-language pathologists using a combination of music and speech therapy. (They demonstrate that singing often improves speech and can be used as a tool.) This documentary takes a slightly different turn when an attorney states that one of her clients (a patient) was assaulted by an aide in a nursing home and then was found to be incompetent by a judge. This scene points out the risk of stigmatization in aphasic patients. This documentary is a good resource for non-specialists because it explains and shows the challenges—and the sometimes devastating consequences—of aphasia.

Picturing Aphasia (2006) ⫻⫻ shows several patients explaining the medical event—usually a stroke but also a traumatic brain injury—that left them aphasic. The movie effectively combines interview-style filming with the stories interpreted into a sequence of drawings (hence, the title). This film also sought to raise awareness and understanding of aphasia, and it succeeds. The drawings provide visual symbols to improve communication. They help in understanding the spoken language and emphasize how aphasia is perceived and how patients with aphasia are disabled and cognitively impaired. The film also points to stigmatization and how difficult it is for patients when they cannot express themselves through words.

Aphasia (2010) ⫻ is acted and directed by Carl McIntyre and is used to support and promote his motivational speeches. Carl McIntyre was a theater actor who had a severe stroke, making it impossible for him to speak. The movie is also about errors in prognostication; he was assured that he would recover within 6 months to a year, but after 18 months, he had made little progress. A combination of speech and occupational therapy markedly improved his speech, and the documentary is largely about the will to overcome a major disability.

Produced in association with the University of North Carolina at Chapel Hill and the Division of Speech and Hearing Sciences, the film has McIntyre reenact his stroke and its adverse effects. The lighthearted approach here feels awkward. The film shows him having difficulty getting words out and understanding written language—all in a comedic way. The film starts when he falls on the floor and his wife thinks he is "joking around." He then summarizes the time it takes to get treated: "the stroke team had to be summoned from their secret hideout."

He "awakens" and sees blurred faces over his bed, "as if I am in a Charlie Brown Halloween special." The urgency of his stroke management is shown with shaky and blurred camera work. In the end, he feels he has transitioned into "second childlessness and mere oblivion." In addition to acting, McIntyre also worked as a salesman, two occupations now closed to him due to his stroke and inability to speak other than one- or two-word sentences. The documentary features several interviews with speech therapists—some serious, others with (somewhat lame) attempts at humor. ("Look at this guy. He is Mr. Aphasia.") The film, made 6 years after his stroke, shows him with a marked expressive aphasia. It shows the marked devastation of aphasia in a person who made his living through speech.

Aphasia may improve up to 6 months after a stroke, after which it reaches a plateau. Semantics and syntax may improve considerably up to 6 weeks; phonology and token test (measuring severity of the aphasias) may improve up to 3 months. In patients with global aphasia, speech output may improve, but verbal communication lags behind.

To a certain degree and depending on the severity of aphasia, the outcome may be influenced by speech therapy. There is some evidence that early daily aphasia intervention improves communication, but recovery from stroke-induced aphasia remains variable and unpredictable. There are major interventions available for aphasia, such as melodic intonation and constraint-induced therapy—all of which are technology based. Current concepts focus on inter-temporal lobe connectivity (with speech comprehension in the superior temporal cortex). Aphasic patients who retained this connectivity had notable improvement.[38]

Aphasia significantly disrupts people's lives, and quality-of-life studies in stroke have not always studied the additional factors including emotional distress and depression, the extent of aphasic impairment, the difficulty with communication, and productivity levels.[39] There is also a marked variability of recovery from aphasia, and apparently, improvement (i.e., changing from non-fluent to fluent) occurs within the first year. Factors that play a consistent role in language recovery have not yet been identified.

Poliomyelitis

As mentioned in Chapter 4, poliomyelitis is mostly a disease of the past—at least in the developed world. *A Paralyzing Fear* (1998) ◄◄◄◄ , directed by Nina Gilden Seavey, among other documentaries made over the years, is revealing because it touches on several major medical and sociologic themes. The documentary offers a glimpse into summers in the early twentieth century and fear that we really do not wish to revisit. The first-hand experience of patients is troubling in this film and brings us back to a time when every new summer brought the fear of poliomyelitis ("the crippler"). Patients described a "stiff neck, terrible pain, back pain, and every step I took would radiate through my body."

DIALOGUE

A Paralyzing Fear: The Story of Polio in America

Dr. Richard Aldrich

We admitted 464 proven cases of polio just at the university hospital, which is unbelievable. And this was a very severe paralytic form. Maybe two or three hours after a lot of these kids would come in with a stiff neck or a fever, they'd be dead. It was unbelievable.

---

[38] Dobkin BH, Dorsch A. New Evidence for Therapies in Stroke Rehabilitation. *Curr Atheroscler Rep.* 2013;15:331; Lazar RM, Antoniello D. Variability in Recovery from Aphasia. *Curr Neurol Neurosci Rep.* 2008;8:497–502; and Warren JE, Crinion JT, Lambon Ralph MA, Wise RJ. Anterior Temporal Lobe Connectivity Correlates with Functional Outcome after Aphasic Stroke. *Brain.* 2009;132:3428–3442.

[39] Hilari K, Needle JJ, Harrison KL. What Are the Important Factors in Health-Related Quality of Life for People with Aphasia? A Systematic Review. *Arch Phys Med Rehabil.* 2012;93:S86–S95.

The narration by Olympia Dukakis is serene and appropriate for the topic. The explanation of the complex immunology is very well done; it is simple and understandable. There were many phobias, including the fear of catching the disease, the fear of catching the worst kind, the fear of becoming ventilator dependent, and the fear of the vaccine itself, which—at least in the early developmental stages—was actually responsible for several hundred cases of severe poliomyelitis. When a case of poliomyelitis occurred, panic was evident, with neighborhoods emptying in the summer ("neighbor running away from neighbor") although to no avail (Figure 6.9). However, many children had only a mild form of the illness and were not affected by paralysis.

The documentary starts with the beginning of the polio epidemic in 1916. Infantile paralysis was known for many decades, but it was not understood like other epidemics such as cholera and diphtheria. Experts at the time felt that the 1916 epidemic was an aberrant event, and future upticks in infection "would never be as bad as this in the United States." The prevailing understanding was that it had to do with poor sanitation, and over one summer, officials killed hundreds of stray cats. Other sources were considered in New York City, and it did not take long for suspicion to fall upon the slums and the newly arrived Italian and eastern European immigrants. (See Chapter 4 on epidemic meningitis for a similar theme.) The 1916 epidemic eventually numbered over 27,000 cases, mostly children, with 6,000 deaths.

The most notorious epidemic occurred in Copenhagen in 1952. In the United States, Minnesota had the most cases of all the states. There were enormous challenges in managing a large number of patients with poliomyelitis at the same time. Negative-pressure ventilators were the only available ventilators, and their shortage during the zenith of the polio epidemic necessitated other methods of ventilatory support. Positive-pressure ventilation and tracheostomy became commonplace after the poliomyelitis epidemics. Early tracheostomy with bag ventilation and repeated suctioning and positioning could bring mortality down from 80% to 40%.[40]

The first shock in watching this documentary is the enormous number of children in braces, on crutches, and in wheelchairs. It is mentioned that "hospitals would see an emergency for weeks." It is shocking to see small children in iron lungs, and this gets a fair amount of attention in the film. (One patient recalls a "sea of beds and the sounds of bellows.")

The documentary also discusses the humanistic desire to help others under these circumstances and to proceed rapidly with fundraising. "Small fundraising" efforts such as dance marathons were typical ("dance so that others may walk"), but a major effort came with the March of Dimes ("send a dime"). Women became the backbone of this effort, and the documentary shows that "every mother—even busy—could spare an hour a day to help out." Other creative ways were found to solicit money. At 7 pm, sirens would go off, and women would knock on doors to solicit money. ("Turn on your porch light. Help fight polio tonight.") This charity raised millions.

The documentary also describes the academic struggles and cutthroat attitudes—the so-called Polio Wars—in some detail. The Salk (inactivated virus) vaccine reduced the number of cases by 80% in 2 years, and even in 1955, newspapers declared the polio epidemic conquered, but then came the Cutter incident (referring to the Cutter Laboratories of Berkeley, California). Some of the vaccine lots contained live virus and resulted in many infected children. In each case, paralysis occurred in the arm inoculated with a vaccine from Cutter Laboratories. The documentary does not mention that a jury found Cutter Laboratories not negligent but guilty of breaching an implied warranty. The Cutter incident reduced the willingness of pharmaceutical companies to make lifesaving vaccines.[41]

---

[40] For a comprehensive historical assessment of all aspects of poliomyelitis, see Oshinsky DM. *Polio: An American Story.* 1st ed. New York: Oxford University Press; 2005.

[41] For major works on vaccination development and unintended consequences, see Kluger J. *Splendid Solution: Jonas Salk and the Conquest of Polio.* New York: Berkley Books; 2006; Offit PA. *The Cutter Incident: How America's First Polio Vaccine Led to the Growing Vaccine Crisis.* New Haven, CT: Yale University Press; 2007; and Shell M. *Polio and Its Aftermath: The Paralysis of Culture.* Cambridge, MA: Harvard University Press; 2005.

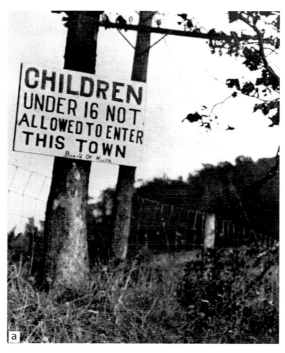

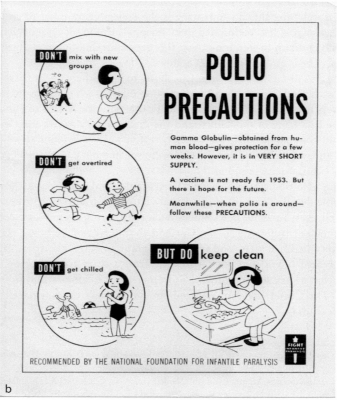

FIGURE 6.9 (a) Warning signs during the polio epidemic (b) A March of Dimes flyer distributed during the 1950s polio epidemic. (With permission of the March of Dimes.)

The documentary also calls out racial segregation in the South. Warm Springs in Georgia, the resort bought by Franklin D. Roosevelt to allow rehabilitation of polio patients, did not admit African Americans and possibly necessitated a separate polio building in Tuskegee but does not address the (inaccurate) assumption at the time that African Americans were somehow immune to the polio virus. It also shies away from the controversies surrounding the Sister Kenny approach (Chapter 4) and presents her method of treating poliomyelitis as an incontrovertible fact. The documentary also does not discuss one of the major reasons why polio has not been eradicated in the developing world and the role played by fundamentalist religious objections.[42]

In addition to documentaries presenting a historical assessment of the polio epidemics in the United States, there are personal accounts. Two documentaries present polio survivors and their long-term care in an iron lung. One is a documentary by Jessica Yu, *Breathing Lessons: The Life and Work of Mark O'Brien* (1996), which is also a subject of the feature film, *The Sessions* (2012), discussed in Chapter 4.

Martha Mason is the subject of another documentary film, *Martha in Lattimore* (2005) ◄◄◄. Lattimore is a small town with a population of less than 400. Martha was 71 when she died, after living for more than 60 years in an iron lung. She chose to remain in an iron lung for the freedom it gave her, to avoid a tracheostomy and more complex care, and possible future hospitalizations. She could stay home because the device took no professional skills to operate and was maintained by two aides. Martha bought a voice-activated computer that gave her access to e-mail and internet browsing, and this technological advance furthered her ability to communicate. It also allowed her to write her memoir, *Breath: Life in the Rhythm of an Iron Lung*. She took care of her own affairs, paid bills, and even arranged for her mother's care when she became demented and aggressive. Why would patients stay in the iron lung so long when there are better and more efficient solutions? One can only speculate it may involve becoming psychologically attached to the machine. Many iron lungs were decorated with paint or decorative magnets, to give them a personal touch. Many patients found it comfortable, and often these patients refused to be hospitalized unless the iron lung also came to the hospital when there was an intercurrent illness. Many patients simply felt that tracheostomy would kill them.

It is not known how many patients are still in an iron lung—the number may approach 50 in the United States. Many patients also use the so-called glossopharyngeal breathing—"frog" breathing. The technique was developed during the poliomyelitis epidemic. Patients used muscles of the mouth and pharynx to push air into the lower airways. Glossopharyngeal breathing is an emergency backup for patients with a malfunctioning iron lung, and this method can sustain ventilation for several hours.

The poliomyelitis epidemic has been a major topic of scholarly work, and good insight into this neurologic disease can be obtained by watching these documentaries. Poliomyelitis remains a major problem in the underdeveloped world, where healthcare workers administering a vaccine are at risk (and some have been murdered). Poliomyelitis only flares up in regions where there is conflict and war and where there are religious objections to vaccination. Elsewhere, poliomyelitis has largely been eradicated, although Spain recently saw an uptick.[43] The Global Polio Eradication Initiative (GPEI) continues to detect outbreaks in Somalia, Kenya, the Democratic Republic of Congo, and Nigeria.[44]

---

[42] Another documentary on poliomyelitis, *The American Experience: The Polio Crusade* by Sarah Colt, aired on PBS in 2009. This documentary has a similar subject matter and is based on Oshinsky's Pulitzer Prize-winning book.

[43] Lopez-Perea N, Masa-Calles J, Torres de Mier MV, Fernandez-Garcia A, Echevarria JE, De Ory F, et al. Shift within Age-Groups of Mumps Incidence, Hospitalizations and Severe Complications in a Highly Vaccinated Population. Spain, 1998–2014. *Vaccine*. 2017;35:4339–4345.

[44] Progress towards Polio Eradication Worldwide, 2013–2014. *Wkly Epidemiol Rec*. 2014;89:237–244; and Olufowote JO, Livingston DJ. The Excluded Voices from Africa's Sahel: Alternative Meanings of Health in Narratives of Resistance to the Global Polio Eradication Initiative in Northern Nigeria. *Health Commun*. 2021:1–12.

Traumatic Brain Injury and Neurorehabilitation

The Crash Reel (2013) ⫻⫻ , directed by Lucy Walker, is about snowboarder Kevin Pearce (Figure 6.10) and his major traumatic brain injury (TBI). The film shows Kevin through a combination of home recordings and promotional videos highlighting his tremendous skill in half-pipe snowboarding, his development into stardom, and his competition with and outperformance of his major competitors.

The film opens with footage of daredevil snowboarders demonstrating plenty of overconfidence. Kevin explains that a half-pipe with a 22-foot wall gives more "airtime" and also provides "more tricks." He adds that "people are going to be blown away with what they are going to see." This is during a training session in Park City, Utah, in 2009, a month before the 2010 Winter Olympics.

Two days before the accident, the documentary shows a night of drinking. Then we see the accident itself, when Kevin attempts a new "cab double cork," which is a double backflip with a twist. Without bracing himself with his hands, he lands with his face flat on the icy wall. He immediately becomes comatose with a marked orbital hematoma. Witnesses later tell us that he had to be intubated and was "shaking." Another bystander tells us that his left eye had a "blown pupil." He is helicoptered out to the neurointensive care unit, where he stays for 26 days. Shown on film is the family receiving notification of the accident—accompanied by a request to grant permission for a ventriculostomy. We get a glimpse

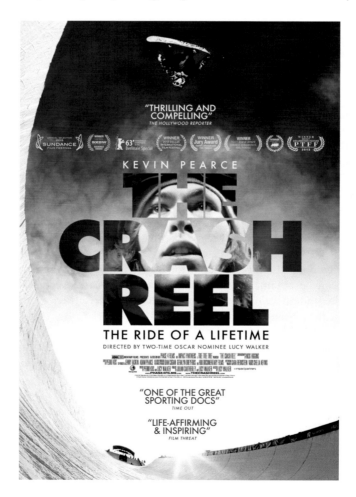

FIGURE 6.10   Film poster of *The Crash Reel*. (Used with permission from Prodigy Public Relations.)

of Kevin's MRI scan, which shows multiple, severe shearing lesions in the hippocampi and lesions peppered throughout the white matter. There is also an extensive intraventricular hemorrhage that likely prompted the ventriculostomy.

The documentary shows Kevin's slow recovery, and his brother explains the hospital course fairly well with his small incremental change, his inability to speak, Kevin's frustration ("constant new hurdles to get over"), and medical complications including a deep venous thrombosis. Nothing seems to change in the first months, but then he begins to make large strides, or what his brother calls an "amazing ladder of a progression." While we see him improve, the documentary contrasts Kevin's situation with his competitor Shaun White earning a gold medal at the 2010 Vancouver Winter Olympics. Now, Olympic medal contender Kevin Pearce, who was willing to push the boundaries to defeat Shaun White, has become a severely injured young man.

DIALOGUE

The Crash Reel

Mother	*I was so surprised they do see people with a second one [TBI] and a third one …. I thought if someone had one, why would they put themselves in a situation where they might have another one?*
Kevin	*It's really hard for you guys to know. It is unexplainable …. I just feel like no one else in this room has that feeling about anything.*

In an unprecedented way, the film shows the subtle but severe late consequences of TBI in elite athletes. Kevin takes antidepressants, two antiepileptic drugs, and struggles with his memory and attention. He has episodes of confusion, impulsivity, and what he calls "sensory overload." There is also surgery to correct his double vision, and he has to wear corrective glasses. However, Kevin is unfazed and wants to start snowboarding again, and the film turns into an important moral lesson. His parents feel understandable guilt that they did not stop Kevin from engaging in such a high-risk sport and that they gradually got caught up in the "branding and selling" of their son. The documentary shows multiple conversations around the kitchen table, with family members trying to discourage Kevin from going back to snowboarding. Kevin bluntly tells them that he feels that "there is no trust" in his family, and his father counters that he puts his family at risk. Clearly, his family feels that it is not fair to expect them to take care of him in the event of another injury. Kevin eventually returns to snowboarding, but it becomes apparent that he has lost his confidence and lacks sufficient coordination for the sport. Most of the documentary shows him becoming aware of this defeat. There is a delicate boundary over which it is hard to step. Athletes may want to go back after an injury, but very few have succeeded in elite sports.

This documentary offers a unique window into the significance of injuries associated with extreme sports. Some athletes have a more severe injury or death, such as Sarah Burke, a world-champion freestyle skier, who died as a result of a traumatic head injury sustained during a practice run—in the same half-pipe where Kevin Pearce had his injury. She is mentioned here too, and the documentary briefly touches on the substantial medical costs as a result of injury. Sarah Burke apparently was not insured, and her sponsors would only pay for medical costs incurred during events. (Her costs eventually were covered through fundraising efforts.)

The Crash Reel offers a unique view of the rehabilitation of traumatic brain injury and its long-term effects, particularly in young individuals who physically seem completely recovered. It shows the unstoppable drive to return to their original athletic prowess, only to find that it is no longer possible. It also emphasizes that, not surprisingly, accidents can be fatal and that a devastating traumatic injury can happen in a split second. For the youngsters who survive, the hospital course is endless, and the film shows the complex collaboration of rehabilitation physicians, psychiatrists, and ophthalmologists involved with Kevin's care.

Injuries among snowboarders are more frequent (two to three times higher) than in skiers; improper landing from high-altitude jumps is the most common accident among elite snowboarders. Studies have reported head and face injuries in approximately 1 of 10 elite snowboarders.[45] Additionally, over 1 in 4 skiers and snowboarders are at risk of a major traumatic head injury by not wearing a helmet or wearing an insufficient helmet. Snowboarders and skiers tend to wear ski hats underneath their helmets, causing improper fit and risk of displacement during sudden acceleration-deceleration impact.[46]

The documentary touches on the well-publicized, so-called second-impact syndrome. Usually, this controversial syndrome occurs soon after the incident while the patient is still symptomatic. The first minor concussion is followed by rapid fatal coma from brain swelling during the "second" impact. The main mechanism is impaired autoregulation of cerebral blood flow, with the first blow allowing massive cerebral edema and increased intracranial pressure after the second blow. The existence of second-impact syndrome has been accepted, but it is likely very rare and is seen shortly after a first injury.[47]

The film is also about recovery and recovery potential, showing other injured teenagers and optimistic rehabilitation physicians. ("He is going to get a lot better. Come see him in a year."). It may be farfetched to compare Kevin's brain injuries with other brain injuries ("your brain looks so much better than this guy"—referring to an NFL running back's MRI, which was affected with chronic traumatic encephalopathy). Kevin's injury should be set apart from chronic traumatic encephalopathy which is a neurodegenerative disorder showing diffuse accumulation of hyperphosphorylated tau. This disorder, in the past mostly connected to boxing ("punch drunk"), has been correlated with out-of-control, explosive, verbal, and violent behaviors, but the risks are not yet well defined and possibly exaggerated, and parkinsonism may not be present in many patients. (See Chapter 4.) Chronic traumatic encephalopathy injury should also be set apart from "concussions," defined by the American Academy of Neurology as grade 1: transient confusion resolving in 15 minutes ("the bell ringer"); grade 2: longer-lasting symptoms of transient confusion but no unconsciousness; and grade 3: a concussion with loss of consciousness.

TBI in freestyle skiers and snowboarders is not uncommon, and 10% of the 2,080 injuries during seven World Cup seasons were due to contusions (two were fatal). Some sports, such as half-pipe and snowboard cross, may be just too dangerous. Using new tricks that push the limits is necessary to win, and the winners are those snowboarders who are able to flip in three different planes. In Sochi 2014, Iouri Podladtchikov (also known as iPod) won with his impressive flip called the YOLO (You Only Live Once). Sadly, it was only a matter of time until he suffered a TBI in 2018. He retired from competition in 2020.

In addition, gear technology may not keep up with the major "advances" in highly competitive sports. Although helmets are compulsory, helmet standards are constantly changing, and there is active research in video analysis of injuries. There are also other pressing questions: Are goggles, which improve peripheral vision but reduce skull protection, too big? Are face-protection helmets needed, and how "uncool" is that? There are no answers to these serious concerns about where this elite sport is going. *The Crash Reel* confronts all of these questions but also has many other subtexts. It is an astounding

---

[45] See Steenstrup SE, Bere T, Bahr R. Head Injuries among FIS World Cup Alpine and Freestyle Skiers and Snowboarders: A 7-Year Cohort Study. *Br J Sports Med.* 2014;48:41–45; and Levy AS, Hawkes AP, Hemminger LM, Knight S. An Analysis of Head Injuries among Skiers and Snowboarders. *J Trauma.* 2002;53:695–704.

[46] Cundy TP, Systermans BJ, Cundy WJ, Cundy PJ, Briggs NE, Robinson JB. Helmets for Snow Sports: Prevalence, Trends, Predictors and Attitudes to Use. *J Trauma.* 2010;69:1486–1490.

[47] Wetjen NM, Pichelmann MA, Atkinson JL. Second Impact Syndrome: Concussion and Second Injury Brain Complications. *J Am Coll Surg.* 2010;211:553–557; and Cantu RC. Second-Impact Syndrome. *Clin Sports Med.* 1998; 17:37–44.

documentary about recovery from traumatic head injury in young athletes. The film is unique and important in showing the gradual, steady improvement of young individuals recovering from a TBI. It also shows what families have to face. The tremendous duress of the parents is obvious and well portrayed. How do parents cope with a child who now has a major handicap and lack of insight as a result of the brain injury? Kevin's father quotes an e-mail he received: "you need to be prepared for the Kevin who comes back not to be the same Kevin."

Coma Recoveries

Documentaries on rehabilitation in coma are virtually nonexistent. Filmed over the course of one year, *Coma* (2007) ◂◂ , directed by Liz Garbus, profiles four young patients with catastrophic traumatic head injury treated at the Center for Head Injuries at the JFK Medical Center in Edison, New Jersey. Though better than previous media portrayals of this topic, the documentary has shortcomings. The film shows hopeful families and friends deeply and compassionately involved with the care of their loved one. There is a surreal surfeit of pity, sorrow, and loneliness that continues for over 100 unrelenting minutes. One issue is that the mise-en-scène is essentially in the neurorehabilitation center. This is normally an unlikely setting because few centers see patients with catastrophic neurologic injury. In fact, only patients who have recovered qualify for a rehabilitation program.

The film starts with the statement, "The mystery of coma and brain injury has captivated America's imagination for decades." This is followed by snippets of newspaper and magazine articles, such as "What if something is going on in there?" "Twilight Zone," and with Senate leader and cardiovascular surgeon Bill Frist declaring that a minimally conscious state is "a tough diagnosis to make." The director primes us to expect ominous uncertainty with prolonged comatose states. (The use of the Terri Schiavo case is unclear, and this movie is not about her.) Some shots are filmed inside conference rooms and the intensive care unit. In allowing filming here, the staff and family opened themselves up for scrutiny including clever montages, camera angles, and close-ups.

DIALOGUE

Coma

Father	*I do not know what the worst thing is you want your doctor to say, but you hear it all the time, "Sean is unique; Sean is an enigma."*
Father	*I asked myself repeatedly, "What were these families told? Why the overwhelming incredulity and ambiguity? What were their expectations in the first place? Was there denial?"*

One could quibble with the neurorehabilitation team's approach and diagnostic accuracy. Their task is never easy. There is often confusion. Nowhere is this more evident than in a scene showing elated parents when they are told their son is not in a minimally conscious state. Next, they learn that word deafness is a major contributor to his condition. To see them recoil when his neurologic condition is not so good after all is unsettling. During the entire film, I kept hoping (in vain, as it turned out) for a neurologist to step in and offer clarification and insight. The director punctuates these heartrending stories with segments of unbridled optimism and healthcare providers mired in uncertainty. ("All brain injuries are different.") At the conclusion, we see one of the families providing home care for their son, who is in a permanent vegetative state. Disturbingly, the mother tries to spoon-feed him, which is a highly dangerous maneuver for a person in this state.

So, I thought, "What would I like to see in a documentary about coma, and what would best serve the public?" At the risk of being presumptuous, I would like to see a documentary that shows the entire spectrum of recovery from coma in intensive care units to neurorehabilitation centers.[48] Patients typically become comatose from a devastating traumatic brain injury, aneurysmal subarachnoid hemorrhage, fulminant encephalitis, or anoxic-ischemic injury after cardiopulmonary resuscitation.

Withdrawal of life support in patients who fail to awaken is a common outcome, often prompted by advance directives but also after extensive deliberation about realistic outcomes with family members. Film depiction of a family conference would show the complexity of these conversations. Perhaps such a documentary could also include a discussion of the benefits of organ and tissue donation after a comatose patient becomes brain dead, especially how it may prove lifesaving for someone else. An ideal documentary would also cover the wide range of possible outcomes from a catastrophic brain injury including the promises and limitations of neurorehabilitation.[49]

Most comatose patients and those in a minimally conscious state are cared for in a nursing home, but there are uniquely specialized centers, such as the JFK Medical Center, that admit patients for care and research. Disorders of consciousness, particularly when severe or prolonged, are artificially divided into minimally conscious state and persistent vegetative state, and physicians use several clinical tools to differentiate between the two. For families, discerning the different disorders is difficult, and there are moments when they think they see "more responsiveness." For physicians, the challenge is to judge these reactions accurately and not to easily dismiss them as "reflexes." Unfortunately, there are too many instances in which physicians have ignored families' observations. Then, when patients improve, there is much consternation and distrust. Prolonged observation by multiple healthcare providers skilled in this work is the only way to ascertain a lack of awareness or improved responsiveness.[50]

For the public, *Coma* offers an unprecedented look at the composure of some families suddenly struck with a disaster but who manage to see a silver lining. In depicting a bleak outcome for some patients, the director gets her point across. The film is less useful as a teaching tool for medical and nursing students or current healthcare providers. The director's suggestion that patients with a slow recovery may spend prolonged periods in rehabilitation centers is inaccurate. In addition, there is no discussion of current ethical, legal, and financial issues. I struggled to identify the purpose of this documentary because it is without context. Nothing here explains coma. The film does not address (a) the diagnostic certainty that exists in many instances based on the well-known prognostic indicators or (b) the questionable effect of pharmacologic interventions or so-called stimulation programs and the speculative nature of many of the newly introduced therapies. Rehabilitation physicians are divided on how to approach these unfortunate patients. The media (and documentary film) could do better in portraying the realities.[51]

---

[48] Giacino JT, Katz DI, Whyte J. Neurorehabilitation in Disorders of Consciousness. *Semin Neurol*. 2013;33:142–156.

[49] See Giacino JT, Katz DI, Schiff ND, Whyte J, Ashman EJ, Ashwal S, et al. Comprehensive Systematic Review Update Summary: Disorders of Consciousness: Report of the Guideline Development, Dissemination, and Implementation Subcommittee of the American Academy of Neurology; the American Congress of Rehabilitation Medicine; and the National Institute on Disability, Independent Living, and Rehabilitation Research. *Neurology*. 2018;91:461–470. This is a statement by a multidisciplinary group of rehabilitation physicians and neurology researchers. It involves a comprehensive summary of types of prolonged coma and neurorehabilitation options (and limitations): A warning not to give up too soon and to continue care in some cases.

[50] Wijdicks EFM. *The Comatose Patient*. 2nd ed. New York: Oxford University Press; 2014.

[51] Media reporting often ignores key limitations and evokes unrealistic visions of recovery. See Kitzinger J, Samuel G. Reporting Consciousness in Coma: Media Framing of Neuro-Scientific Research, Hope, and the Response of Families with Relatives in Vegetative and Minimally Conscious States. *JOMEC Journal*. 2013;(3).

End Credits

Although most films in neurocinema are fictional, we should not overlook the documentary genre. In all its aspects, these portraits differ from fiction film. None of the filmmakers attempt to "sugarcoat" the suffering of patients with (often progressive) neurologic disorders. We see it and believe it. We are closer than ever before. This is not how we would view a fiction film. We cannot indulge in remembrances of the actor's previous film roles or assessments of how convincingly he or she portrays a physician or a patient in this current vehicle. Some films unashamedly immerse us in the joyless states of disorders, occasionally interspersed with (dark) humor. But there is no redemption, and certainly, there are no happy endings. Documentary films have not yet shown the full spectrum of neurologic disease, but there has been a steady increase over the last two decades. There are films about disorders frequently seen by neurologists, but many important disorders have still not been subjected to a documentary treatment. Decline in cognition and memory from a dementing illness has been overrepresented, but that interest is expected in a world with a rapidly aging population. Often, young individuals recount athletic careers ended by neurologic disorders.[52] Many of these films describe how patients find dignity and meaning within their disability. We can certainly learn from them.

---

[52] Soon to be released is *A Day for Susana*, which showcases Brazilian swimmer Susana Schnarndorf, a six-time Ironman Triathlon winner who suffers from multiple system atrophy.

7

Neurocelebrities in Film

Bad news go away. I can't be bothered now.

Rhapsody in Blue (1945)

Who are these people?

Glen Campbell... I'll Be Me (2014)

He was just sort of off.

Robin's Wish (2020)

Main Themes

Another thematic question in this book is why persons with a celebrity status and neurologic disease are cinematically interesting. Celebrities create a major business attraction when it pertains to the endorsement of products, but it is different in disease where they would like to stay incognito as much as feasible. They quickly become very important persons (VIPs) in hospitals with all the necessary and unnecessary services provided. Doctors may unconsciously (or consciously) behave differently with celebrities, and caring for celebrities is generally distracting, potentially taking time away from other patients. Some physicians worry that their decisions will be scrutinized by the press and public, and this fear has a basis in reality. Public relations policies differ greatly among hospitals, but VIPs deserve privacy and protection as much as anyone else. None of these challenges are found in any of the films.

Frequently, foundations, professional journals, and periodicals approach celebrities with requests to share their story. The Academy of Neurology has *Brain and Life* (formerly known as *Neurology Now*), which features stories of actors suffering from neurologic disease (e.g., multiple sclerosis, Parkinson's disease, spinal cord injury, stroke, aneurysmal subarachnoid hemorrhage, and dementia). Some actors have received Public Leadership Awards by the American Academy of Neurology; for example, Cuba Gooding, Jr. (*Jerry Maguire*), because of his work to raise public awareness of multiple sclerosis, and Emilia Clarke (*Game of Thrones*), for raising awareness of surviving brain injury after a ruptured brain aneurysm. (Thomas Sherak, former president of the Academy of Motion Picture Arts and Sciences, also received the award for his fundraising for multiple sclerosis research.)

Some actors have been diagnosed with a neurologic disorder. There is no evidence that any of the early symptomatology has impeded their acting, but some actors have used their neurologic disability in a movie (e.g., Rene Kirby with spina bifida walks on four limbs in the film *Shallow Hal* [2001]). Michael J. Fox has Parkinson's disease and had a Golden Globe-nominated TV show making light of his dyskinetic movements and his Parkinson's disease in general. Michael J. Fox reportedly has said, "I can play anybody, as long as the character has Parkinson's disease." As an example of how actors can contribute significantly to various neurologic causes, Michael J. Fox started a foundation that has raised millions for Parkinson research. In 2012, Bob Hoskins, best known for his award-winning role in *Mona Lisa* (1987) and his feature role in *Who*

DOI: 10.1201/9781003270874-7

Framed Roger Rabbit (1988), retired from acting because of Parkinson's disease. Other examples of neurologic disease, and leading to an early demise, are David Niven, who developed amyotrophic lateral sclerosis (ALS). The late actor and comedian Richard Pryor suffered from severe disability due to multiple sclerosis and multiple bouts of depression. The late actor Dudley Moore was impaired by the devastating effects of progressive supranuclear palsy (PSP), which resulted in his demise from pulmonary infection. His final role was in *The Mirror Has Two Faces* (1996), but during filming he was fired for forgetting his lines. His role as a happy-go-lucky drunk in *Arthur* (1981) may have wrongly suggested he was drunk when he developed symptoms of bulbar dysarthria, which mimicked intoxication. Moore has said: "It's amazing that Arthur has invaded my body to the point that I have [started] to become him. That's the way people looked at me. But I want people to know I am not intoxicated and … that I am going through this disease as well as I can. But I'm trapped in this body and there's nothing I can do about it." He started to develop his symptoms one year after heart surgery in 1998—a known but odd association—and his health rapidly slid into decline.[1]

On the other end of the neurology severity scale is Katharine Hepburn, who was known to have essential tremor that significantly worsened over the years. (Note the profound voice tremor and head bobbing in *On Golden Pond* [1981].) Many actors have recovered from Bell's palsy, except for Sylvester Stallone and Joe Mantegna, which may explain their crooked smiles.

Neurocelebrities

The films on celebrities are a whole new ballgame. The stories of the "neurocelebrities" differ from the non-celebrities among us—for sure, most had good outcomes, and their story of survival is potentially inspiring for others. Do any filmmakers want to make a film on the long-lasting, devastating effect of severe aneurysmal hemorrhage or traumatic brain injury in celebrities? Their illness attracts attention when it impacts their career. In others, the uncompromising downhill course of a neurodegenerative disease—the dementias in particular—may make them forget why they were celebrities in the first place, and that is the tragedy of suffering. Untimely death, particularly when it does not occur because of bad behavior, is also revelatory and sad. Exaggerating the heroism of the person is a serious threat to each of these films. Few of us can hardly fathom that, yes, non-self-inflicted disease is a random event and can affect anyone, famous or not. Even longstanding drug abuse with celebrities often comes to light late (disclosed by the coroner) and as a surprise for many.

Despite biopics since the beginning of cinema,[2] films featuring celebrities with neurologic disease have been sporadic since the very first neurocelebrity film, *Pride of the Yankees* (1942). It can hardly be called a genre within a genre. There has recently been a renewed interest in documentary film, but over many years, several "celebrities" have been the subject of fictional "biopics."

Documentaries tell a different picture; recent ones have featured a scientist, actor, and musician. Some documentaries create opportunities to promote awareness and fund research on their disease. Some charity foundations consider these films useful (and participate actively), while others see them come and go without a lasting impact. Some biopics only transiently show neurologic disease; this was evident in *A Quiet Passion* (2016) about American poet Emily Dickinson, who was diagnosed with Bright's disease and had recurrent seizures. *Iron Lady* (2011) depicts the final dementia of Margaret Thatcher (Meryl Streep), who hallucinated conversations with her late husband (Jim Broadbent) until the end of the film, when she asks him to leave, and the illusion disappears.

---

[1] C Reed. Now Dudley Confronts His Demons. *The Guardian*. November 21,1999. Despite "kiss-and-tell" books alleging drug use, there was never evidence that Moore abused alcohol. See also Fruchter R. *Dudley Moore: An Intimate Portrait*. Ebury Press; 2005 For a possible PSP and heart surgery association, see Tisel SM, Ahlskog JE, Duffy, et al. PSP-Like Syndrome after Aortic Surgery in Adults (Mokri Syndrome). *Neurol Clin Pract*. 2020;10:245–254; and Park KW, Choi N, Ryu HS, et al. Post-Pump Chorea and Progressive Supranuclear Palsy-Like Syndrome Following Major Cardiac Surgery. *Mov Disord Clin Pract*. 2019;11:78–82.

[2] See listings of films on Wikipedia since the 1906 film on the Kelly Gang https://en.wikipedia.org/wiki/List_of_biographical_films

These films deserve a separate chapter because they tell us a story we may need to verify and put into context.[3] But we also must ask ourselves why they are made in the first place. I have a hunch it is because the plight of a celebrity seems more emotionally charged, their manner of coping demonstrates their bravery, and in the end, we are always drawn to triumphs and tragedies. I will mostly concentrate on the biopics—from athletes to scientists—and highlight recent documentaries.

Lou Gehrig

Without doubt, the most well-known celebrity with neurologic disease is Lou Gehrig, famous first baseman for the New York Yankees. (ALS is commonly referred to in the United States as "Lou Gehrig's disease," but most of the world calls it "Charcot's disease.") He was diagnosed at Mayo Clinic by Department of Neurology Chair Henry Woltman. He was seen earlier by Dr. Harold Habein, who was an internist rather than a neurologist. Habein immediately recognized the characteristic muscle wasting and fasciculations, mostly because his mother died of ALS a few years earlier. Gehrig's diagnosis was obviously clear already on inspection.[4] Gehrig befriended Dr. Paul O'Leary, a dermatologist also known as "Mayo's usher," who often facilitated care and provided additional explanations of complex medical issues. Later, Dr. Bayard Horton gave him high-dose Vitamin E shots, which were in vogue at the time but later discounted as ineffective. Gehrig, a major lefty hitter with incredible durability, shattered many records and contributed immensely to the Yankees' winning reputation, which earned him his nickname, "The Iron Horse." (He played 2130 consecutive games in 14 years.) Gehrig's hitting streak ended in 1939, when he missed 19 straight fast balls during practice.[5] Later, he took himself out of the lineup, stunning both players and fans, after which he was unable to perform due to a loss of strength. He did attend games in the dugout. He retired at age 36 and died two years later. His farewell to baseball after his (in his own words) "bad break" was capped off by his iconic 1939 "Luckiest Man on the Face of the Earth" speech at Yankee Stadium. This famous speech is prominently shown at the end of the film the *Pride of the Yankees* (Figure 7.1). *Pride of the Yankees* (1942) stars Gary Cooper and was directed by Sam Wood. It shows him telling his manager, Joe McCarthy, that he should bench himself. The film is remarkably short on baseball (Gary Cooper allegedly hated the sport) and has one tearjerker of a medical theme (he promised a boy in the hospital to hit two home runs for him). The film has nothing to say about the progress of his disease, and the diagnosis is never told. When asked what the doctor said, he says: "some little thing with some long name, something with an itis." In the movie, Mayo Clinic becomes the Scripps Clinic, a result of the guarded relationship Mayo Clinic maintained with the entertainment industry.

The physician displays a bunch of (wholly irrelevant) X-rays with him when he tells Gehrig the news in hidden terms.

DIALOGUE

Pride of the Yankees

Gehrig:	*Is it three strikes, Doctor?*
Doctor at the Clinic:	*It's three strikes.*
Gehrig:	*If I learned one thing, I know that all the arguing in the world can't change the decision of the umpire.*

---

[3] There is uncertainty if Emily Dickinson had epilepsy and if it influenced her work. In the film *A Quiet Passion*, she is diagnosed with renal disease (called Bright's disease at the time), and she has several seizures, which could be due to hypertensive emergencies. The film does not address how the seizures affected her life. See also Gordon L. *Lives Like Loaded Guns: Emily Dickinson and Her Family's Feuds.* New York: Viking, June 10, 2010.

[4] Eig, J. *Luckiest Man: The Life and Death of Lou Gehrig.* New York: Simon & Schuster, March 1, 2005.

[5] Ibid.

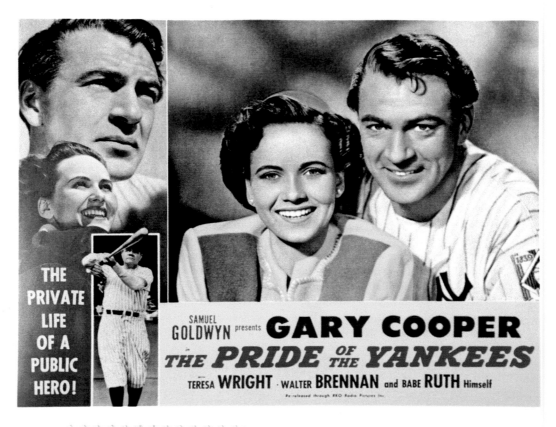

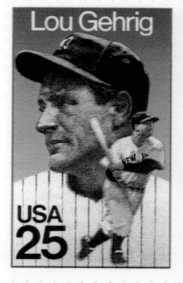

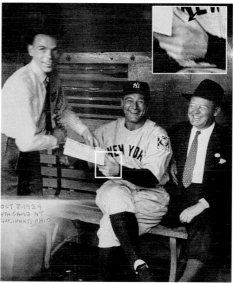

FIGURE 7.1 Lou Gehrig. Gary Cooper as Lou Gehrig in *Pride of the Yankees* (Everett Collection, Inc.). Commemorative stamp and photo of Lou Gehrig with Dr O'Leary showing the markedly atrophic left interosseous muscle (insert). The photo was also featured in *USA Today* questioning the authenticity of 24-year-old Frank Sinatra asking for an autograph. (Kindly provided by Gehrig's biographer, Jonathan Eig.)

This closely reflects Habein's Mayo Clinic press release, who unfortunately called it "a form of chronic poliomyelitis" (infantile paralysis).[6] The diagnosis of ALS was later discovered by a reporter. The movie received nine Academy Nominations and was a box office success.[7] Several studies have been published attempting to pinpoint visible atrophy, including a recent review of the film *Rawhide* shot in 1938, where Gehrig plays a retiring baseball player telling reporters that he is "through with baseball," and he wants the "peace and quiet" of the cowboy life. No atrophy or speech difficulties were found after close analysis.[8] However, a photo with Dr. O'Leary shows left-hand atrophy (Figure 7.1).

Pride of the Yankees connected Gehrig's acceptance and bravery with the soldiers at war. The film opened with "He faced death with that same valor and fortitude that has been displayed by thousands of young Americans on far-flung battlefields." Many consider the film to be one of the greatest baseball films, although some prominent critics (e.g., Manny Farber[9]) disagreed and felt Gary Cooper was miscast.

Muhammad Ali

In the promotional material of his biography the legendary boxer was acclaimed as follows, "He was the wittiest, the prettiest, the strongest, the bravest, and of course, the greatest (as he told us himself)."[10] Muhammed Ali is considered one of the major heavy weight boxers of all time and for his biographer Jonathan Eig "as perfect a boxer as the world had ever seen"—56 wins, 5 losses, and 37 knockouts. He received the Presidential Medal of Freedom.

For many, Muhammed Ali represented redemption through suffering but also the cycle of defeat and triumph. Ali's rise to stardom also came during cultural change in the United States, and he became connected to the civil rights and antiwar movements. He became a moral authority after taking an unpopular stand against the Vietnam War. The 2001 upbeat biographical sports drama film *Ali* with Will Smith in a feature role did show his struggles and activism, but there was absolutely nothing about his neurologic decline. When Ali died on June 3, 2016, Will Smith was one of Ali's pallbearers.[11]

He has been subject to a number of documentaries, but far more detail is found in *Muhammad Ali*, an 8-hour TV documentary (2021), ⬥ , directed and produced by Ken Burns and David McMahon; it is an American story viewed through the prism of racism in America and concentrates on his personal history and phenomenal fights. Unfortunately, it also superficially addresses Muhammed Ali's Parkinson's disease, which started at the young age of 35. We see footage of a gradual decline, slowness, slurring, and despite that, his commitment to continue boxing in major, well-publicized contests. The documentary does not ignore the dark side of boxing and shows the unrelenting bloody brutality of head punches (Figure 7.2) with boxers staggering back to their corners after a few rounds ("punch drunk"). Burns and McMahon missed an opportunity to explain why Ali was preferentially affected whereas many other boxers were not. For sure, Ali kept on boxing even with clear signs of Parkinson's disease. Because the autopsy was refused, we will never precisely know. (Was it young-onset Parkinson's disease, which often has more dyskinesia rather

---

[6] The original Mayo Clinic letter by Dr Harold Habein, dated June 19, 1939, To Whom It May Concern, can be found on the National Baseball Hall of Fame website.

[7] Eig, Ibid.

[8] Lewis M, Gordon PH. Lou Gehrig, Rawhide, and 1938. *Neurology*. 2007;68:615–618.

[9] Polito R, ed. *Farber on Film: The Complete Film Writings of Manny Farber*. Paperback ed. New York: Library of America; 2016.

[10] Eig J. *Ali: A Life*. 1st ed. Boston: Mariner Books; 2017:640.

[11] Mann M. *Ali*. United States: Sony Pictures; 2001.

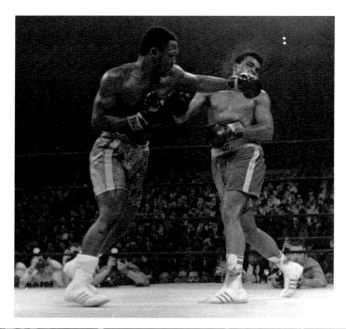

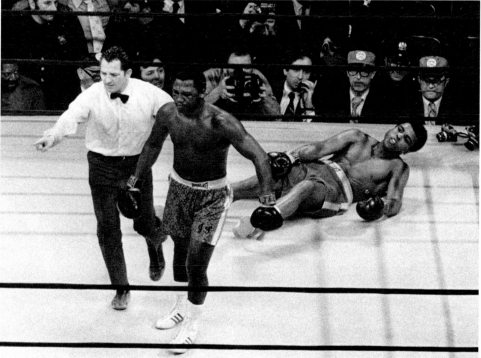

FIGURE 7.2   Joe Frazier vs Mohammad Ali, March 8, 1971 ("The Fight"), at Madison Square Garden in New York City. Frazier took 15 rounds to win. Two other fights followed, Super Fight II (1974) and Thrilla in Manila (1975), both won by Ali (AP Photos).

than rigidity, or severe chronic traumatic encephalopathy, which involves major mood disorders?)[12] It has been wildly speculated that autopsy was not performed to avoid giving the boxing federation a bad reputation. In 1998, Ali worked with actor Michael J. Fox, who also has Parkinson's disease, to raise awareness and fund research.

Stephen Hawking

Errol Morris is an accomplished documentary filmmaker, and his style includes re-enactment.[13] Morris's film *A Brief History of Time* (1991) ◄◄◄ uses the same title as Stephen Hawking's best-selling book (Figure 7.3). The film notably highlights Hawking's struggles. Morris, in an interview on the Criterion issue, pointed out that he had no intent to produce "a primer on science" or to explain Einstein's relativity for a movie audience, although the film does go into complex theoretical physics. Those expecting an elaborate explanation of Hawking's theories, which some feel is the major responsibility of a documentary filmmaker, will be disappointed. Indeed, the documentary confuses. Hawking always claimed that the basics of the cosmos can be stated without mathematics, but this is a challenge for less-gifted minds. Although the visual imagery is very attractive (watches floating into dark holes), it remains more cinematic than scientific and, of course, oversimplifies Hawking's theories. Morris was fascinated by Hawking's connection to the world around him through the mouse of a computer. ("The clicker is the essence of the entire movie" and a metaphor for "the fine line between communication and expression and nothing.") Morris wanted to create a dreamscape while having Hawking explain his theories on the expanding universe.[14]

It has been said that Hawking was "thinking the unthinkable" and on a great academic path. His diagnosis of motor neuron disease at the age of 21 is very unusual, but progression is not typically slower than other types of ALS, mostly occurring between 50 and 75 years of age. The documentary illustrates revealing the diagnosis with a photo of a myelogram and uses a Ken Burns-type panning-movement effect over the picture. The documentary makes use of several medical tropes and devices that are unrelated to the diagnosis of ALS. After spilling beer due to difficulty holding a mug, Hawking told his friend, straight and flat, that "he had been diagnosed with a progressive neurologic illness and would lose use of his body" and "eventually he would have essentially the body of a cabbage, but his brain would be still in perfect order." In the documentary, Hawking reveals a dream of being executed after leaving Addenbrooke's Hospital in Cambridge. (His voice box speech is illustrated by images of an [out-of-context] anesthesia bellows and a dripping IV). One commentator says "he flatly accepted his diagnosis instead of asking 'why this, why now, why me?'" He nevertheless became badly depressed and disinclined to continue work, knowing he could not finish his PhD. Then, he claimed that the disease slowed down; this is unlikely, given his subsequent progression. When he became the Lucasian Professor of Mathematics (adding that it was the same chair held by Newton), it was the last time he signed his name, and a shaky but still readable signature is shown. He was placed on the ventilator and received a tracheostomy. Communication with a plastic board is also shown. (A similar use is demonstrated in *The Diving Bell and the Butterfly;* see Chapter 4.)

His condition demanded complex care for decades. The multiple nurses needed for his care were not fully covered by NHS, and at the end of his life, after 5 decades of progressive motor

---

[12] Autopsy in other boxers revealed multiple microhemorrhages in brain and brainstem parenchyma. Given his very long career and the considerable number of head punches, Ali may have suffered from this syndrome. (See Eig J. *Ali: A Life.* 1st ed. Boston: Mariner Books; 2017. The author claims that Ali sustained ~200,000 blows to the head and body during his boxing career.) With every major blow to the head, a quick rotational movement from front to back of the cerebral hemispheres occurs with the immobile brainstem.

[13] Resna D. *The Cinema of Errol Morris.* Illustrated ed. Middletown, CT: Wesleyan University Press; 2015. Resna described the film as a portrayal of "Hawking's diminishing control of his body, down to the mere functioning of his mind is like a star's collapse to a singularity."

[14] Errol Morris on Stephen Hawking. In. *Criterion.* Vol 2021. New York: Criterion; 2014.

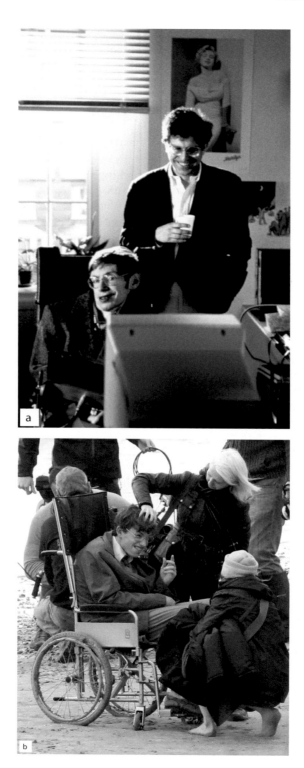

FIGURE 7.3 (a) Stephen Hawking with Errol Morris during filming *A Brief History of Time* (Everett Collection, Inc.). (b) Eddie Redmayne playing Stephen Hawking in *The Theory of Everything*.

neuron disease, he seemed to be chronically short of money despite millions of royalties from his best-selling book and financial help from other foundations. He was frequently admitted to hospitals for respiratory infections. In the final decade of his life, he married his nurse Elaine Mason after he divorced his wife Jane (who featured prominently in the fiction film *The Theory of Everything*). He suffered multiple injuries and hip fracture. Allegations of abuse surfaced and were investigated but dropped. (He vehemently denied these despite his children's serious concerns.) His biographer Charles Seife said that religion (Jane devout–Stephen atheist) did not end his marriage, which was a major contention in the movie *The Theory of Everything*). The many nurses needed to care for him and his growing celebrity status, which was not fully understood by Jane, have been accepted as the major reasons for the divorce.

Hawking became well known after the no-boundary proposal, black hole radiation, and discarding the black-hole theory, a theory that few understand; even fewer understand how it was debunked.[15] Most of his original work was done in the 1980s. He was unable to use his hands or write complex formulas. His calculations were visual in his "geometric mind."[16] He was known to repurpose previous sentences, particularly when his typing speed declined to less than 15 words per minute. Many of his talks were cut-and-paste jobs from previous work, a not-uncommon practice of older scientists, and it was obvious that he stole the limelight away from other, more introverted scientists[17]—another common phenomenon in the academic sciences. There has been evidence of patch writing by his assistants (a form of plagiarism where text is changed but with identical phrasing and copied ideas).[18]

A Brief History of Time, based on his book, achieved a major deceptive twist by using the same computer voice box (provided by *Words Plus,* Lancaster, CA), entering texts said by Hawking, and then altering what was previously said. The documentary does not delve deeply into his illness but used his locked-in state by showing a single muscle twitch on a mouse-operated computer that would be his motor replacement. (Later, he twisted his cheek to control it.) Hawking's brain compensated for his bodily inadequacies and eventually uselessness; for all other motor neuron disease sufferers, it is a far different story. Errol Morris had little to say about that in his multiple commentaries.[19]

Hawking was also part of a major fictional film, *The Theory of Everything* (2014) ◄◄◄ directed by James Marsh, which significantly minimized the challenges of his care, and this remained his wife's major criticism of the film.[20] Eddie Redmayne's imitation of Hawking's collapsed posture and facial mimicry won him an Oscar for Best Performance by an Actor in a Leading Role (Figure 7.3). Inquisitive about the nature of the decline, he obtained information from the Institute of Neurology in London and observed ALS patients and families. As a result of working with a vocal coach, Redmayne effectively displayed lost clarity of speech and progress to full inarticulate speech. His progression to a near-locked-in state is shown extraordinarily well. *The Theory of Everything* (2014) has Redmayne trying to show the progression of the disease. He starts with tremor and difficulty holding chalk. Later, he has difficulty running for a train, followed by mimicking of a clawed hand, then unilateral followed by bilateral dragging of his feet, and a gait that seems to come straight out of Monty Python's "The Ministry of Silly Walks." He uses a cane followed by two canes, and finally, he sits in a wheelchair and acts out severe bulbar dysarthria—well done, Eddie Redmayne! He has several choking bouts, leading to tracheostomy. He develops pneumonia and was placed on a ventilator (never seen). Withdrawal was suggested, but his wife adamantly refused and pushed a French doctor to keep fighting. The film failed to show the tremendous complexity of care required for a patient in a motorized wheelchair with a ventilator, except that it was difficult to haul upstairs.

---

[15] Dobson R. An Exceptional Man. *BMJ*. 2002;324:1478.

[16] Seife C. *Hawking: The Selling of a Scientific Celebrity*. New York: Basic Books; 2021.

[17] Ibid.

[18] Ibid., p. 90.

[19] Butler I. Errol Morris on His Movie—and Long Friendship—With Stephen Hawking. In *Slate*. Brooklyn, NY: The Slate Group, a Graham Holdings Company; 2018.

[20] Shoard C. Stephen Hawking's First Wife Intensifies Attack on *The Theory of Everything*. *The Guardian*. 2018. Published October 3. Accessed June 17, 2021.

Hawking's later years and celebrity status were more tactical than high-minded. Some considered him a deft self-promoter, and his computer voice became legendary. His monotonic electronic voice was even used in the Pink Floyd song "Talking Hawking." After he died, his wheelchair was auctioned off for nearly half a million dollars. Hawking speculated (probably correctly) that most buyers of his best-selling book, *A Brief History of Time*, never read it.[21] The publisher Bantam also came under fire for accusations of exploiting Hawking's illness to get a bestseller.[22] At the height of his celebrity, Hawking offered opinions on areas of science far outside his expertise, e.g., "Today we are on the brink of a new age in medicine. An age where we will be able to heal our bodies of any illness."[23] He opined on artificial intelligence, space travel, and other aspects of astronomy with no proven expertise, but his musings were tolerated due to his iconic status. Nonetheless, he was an admirable spokesman for disabilities and the struggle of so many for acceptance. The *Los Angeles Times* called him the "Mandela for the disabled."[24]

A *Brief History of Time* and *The Theory of Everything* remain the most serious attempts to show both Hawking's work and his disability. Morris's documentary does that through several cinematic tricks (or, in film critic Richard Schinkel's words, "metaphorical richness"). He invariably shows Hawking in his wheelchair. A 360-degree view of his dark office emphasizes his loneliness. Showing his hand barely moving to activate his computer also illustrates how "locked in" he had become. Some have suggested that Morris juxtaposes ALS with a "death of a star."[25] The film ends with Hawking in his wheelchair floating in space.

George Gershwin

There are several hundred biographical works[26] on George Gershwin's life. Gershwin died of a brain tumor at the age of 38, but *Rhapsody in Blue* (1945) ◄, his one and only major biopic, only hints at it. *Rhapsody in Blue*, directed by Irving Rapper, stars Robert Alda (Figure 7.4) as George Gershwin (and Paul Whiteman, Al Jolson, and Oscar Levant playing themselves). In the last 15 minutes of the 141-minute film, he complains of a headache and is told he is overworked and should slow down for 6 months.[27] While playing one of his piano works, he misses some notes and then drops a carafe of water and tells his friends "my fingers would not obey" and that he has "pain between the eyes." In the next scene, he collapses at the piano and dies. Here, the film partially reenacts an actual event at a concert on February 11, 1937, during the performance of his "Concerto in F." With hindsight, some physicians interpreted the attack as a complex focal seizure because he missed several bars of his piano solo for 10 to 20 seconds.[28] After the concert, Gershwin told his friend, pianist Oscar Levant, that he had also smelled something like burning rubber or garbage and that this had happened a number of times before.[29] These "uncinate fits" or olfactory hallucinations are common in glioblastoma. The epigastric aura, which can be symptomatic of temporal focal seizures without loss of consciousness, was also linked to his brain tumor.[30]

[21] Oulton C. Cosmic Writer Shames Book World. *Sunday Times*. August 28, 1988.

[22] Blum D. The Tome Machine; Hawking the Great Unread Books of Our Time. *New York Magazine*. New York: Vox Media; 1988.

[23] Sharp G. Stem Cell Universe with Stephen Hawking. Science Channel. February 3, 2014.

[24] Simply Human: Science: Wheelchair-Bound Physicist. *Los Angeles Times*. June 6, 1990.

[25] Resna 2015, op. cit.

[26] Leffert M. The Psychoanalysis and Death of George Gershwin: An American Tragedy. *J Am Acad Psychoanal Dyn Psychiatry*. 2011;39:421–452. Mark Leffert, M.D., Training and Supervising Analyst, the New Center for Psychoanalysis, Los Angeles, California, reviewed the entire body of work on Gershwin's illness, which he calls "this lengthy narrative of dusty events," and shows the wild speculation about when Gershwin's symptoms started and if he could have been saved.

[27] Paradoxically, while overlooking the illness of the protagonist, *Rhapsody in Blue* spends considerable footage on the medical condition of Gershwin's father, who died of leukemia, starting with tests and ending with his death bed.

[28] Kasdan ML. The Final Days of George Gershwin, American Composer. September 26, 1898–July 11, 1937. 50th Anniversary. *J Ky Med Assoc*. 1987;85:649–652.

[29] Leffert 2011, Ibid.

[30] Ibid.

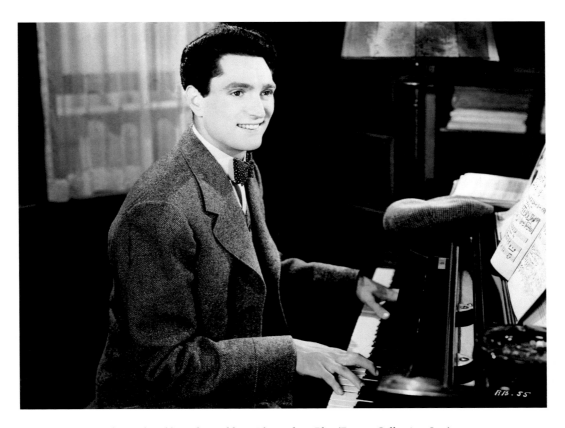

FIGURE 7.4   Gershwin played by Robert Alda in *Rhapsody in Blue* (Everett Collection, Inc.).

Gershwin's brain tumor (and delayed diagnosis) has been researched extensively. He attributed his headaches and dizziness to an extremely overextended songwriting schedule, and the film shows exactly that. Delays in recognizing a real medical concern may have been compounded by his being in analysis with Dr. Gregory Zilboorg, a psychoanalyst, from the spring of 1934 to the end of 1935 at a frequency of up to five sessions per week for several somatic problems such as dyspepsia.[31] After his headache became more troublesome, he saw several psychiatrists, but the Los Angeles-based psychiatrist and psycho-analyst Ernst Simmel suggested "organic disease." After admission to Cedars of Lebanon (now known as Cedars-Sinai Medical Center), he was seen by neurologist Eugene Ziskind, who was not convinced anything was wrong. Gershwin agreed and refused a lumbar puncture because he was worried it would worsen his headaches. The final note in his chart was "most likely hysteria."[32] However, he continued to decline. Prominent neurosurgeon Walter Dandy was urgently summoned but could not make it in time from a yacht off the Atlantic coast; neurosurgeon Howard Naffziger (later known by his syndrome related to cervical rib compression) was also on vacation but in nearby Lake Tahoe, and he was picked up by helicopter. Upon arrival, because Gershwin was already unconscious, Naffziger performed emergency surgery and found a large cystic tumor. Gershwin remained comatose, dying later that day (July 11, 1937). A coincidence should be mentioned. Something similar happened with composer Maurice Ravel, who also died of a brain tumor soon after surgery by the founder of French neurosurgery Clovis Vincent.

---

[31] Bagatti D. Music and Medicine: The Tragic Case of Gershwin's Brain Tumor and the Challenges of Neurosurgery in the First Half of the 20th Century. *World Neurosurg.* 2016;85:298–304.
[32] Leffert 2011, Ibid.

In an era with very limited diagnostic tools, Vincent operated on the wrong side. Both composers died in the same year several months apart.

Iris Murdoch

Dame Iris Murdoch, previously a tutor in Philosophy at St. Anne's College at Oxford, became a full-time writer producing more than two dozen novels. *Iris* (2001) ◄◄◄◄ , directed by Richard Eyre, accurately tells the story of one of the most gifted novelists of the twentieth century. Her dementia became apparent in 1995 after her last book, *Jackson's Dilemma*. She attributed major problems writing this novel to "writer's block," but in retrospect, there were early red flags.[33] That is the underpinning of this film. *Iris* is about Murdoch's courtship with John Bayley (played here both by Jim Broadbent and Hugh Bonneville), who would himself write several memoirs. The movie shows the early beginnings of other manifestations of dementia that, in retrospect, were early signs. During a TV interview, she loses her train of thought, is lost for words, and comes home confused and agitated, not remembering details about the interview.

DIALOGUE

Iris

| Neurologist | *What is the name of the prime minister?* |
| Iris | *Are you asking me? I do not know. Surely it does not matter. Ask John. Someone will know.* |

The film introduces circumlocutory errors ("It is the man who brings the mail") and the inability to name the prime minister. In her cluttered office, she seems to agonize over words ("puzzle is a funny word," to which John answers, "All words are like that when you take them by surprise, aren't they?"). When the general physician arrives, she tells him that writing her new book is very tiring and difficult. She is shown wandering within and outside the house, and this restlessness is a common theme in all films involving dementia. A significant deterioration in sanitation is shown, culminating in a nursing home placement. A scene showing her sitting on the beach trying to write notes is allegoric (Figure 7.5). She won the Man Booker International Prize for her novel *The Sea, The Sea* (1978). Her diary entries after 1993 were indicative of a marked decline. John continues to remind her she wrote "novels—wonderful novels."

Glen Campbell

Glen Campbell—the "golden boy," as he was called—is a country music legend. In 2011 Campbell was diagnosed with Alzheimer's disease, after which he released the album *Ghost on the Canvas*. This studio album had the following coda "*Some days I'm so confused, Lord, my past gets in my way. I need the ones I love, Lord, more and more each day.*" Glen Campbell released his final studio album, *Adiós*, in June 2017. He died the same year from advanced Alzheimer's disease.

Glen Campbell no longer knew it, but he sold millions of records, was a brilliant guitarist who sat in with major bands, and even authored several instructional books on guitar performance. In his autobiography, *Rhinestone Cowboy* (1994), named for one of his biggest hits, he noted that already in 1963, his playing and

---

[33] Garrard P, Maloney LM, Hodges JR, Patterson K. The Effects of Very Early Alzheimer's Disease on the Characteristics of Writing by a Renowned Author. *Brain.* 2005;128(Pt 2):250–260.

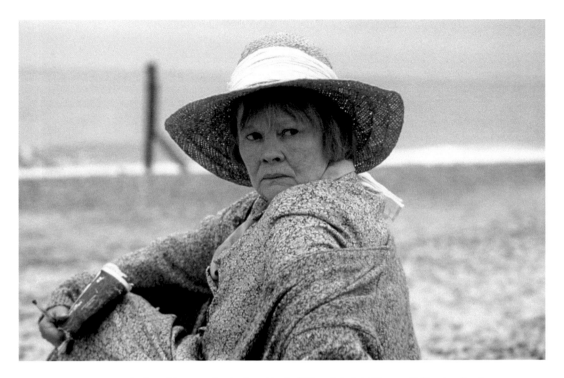

FIGURE 7.5   Iris Murdoch and her note book played by Judi Dench in *Iris* (Everett Collection, Inc.).

singing had been heard on nearly 600 songs recorded songs. He gave up alcohol and drugs and became a born-again Christian, although a fall off the wagon in 2003 led to a brief jail sentence for drunk driving.

In *Glen Campbell … I'll Be Me* (2014) ≪≪≪, directed by James Keach, we see Campbell sitting on a couch with his current wife, Kim. They watch old Super 8 home movies, and Kim identifies the family members for him. He does not recognize them, although, granted, the films are decades old. It is sad to see his disconnect; in many ways, Keach's documentary records the unfolding of one of the great medical tragedies. When Glen was told he had Alzheimer's disease, his failing memory was obvious to his family members. Surprisingly, Glen and his band (with three of his children) decided to go on tour to promote his new studio album (Figure 7.6). This documentary captures the immediacy of pulling it off. We follow Glen Campbell closely and sense at each moment the contrast between his musical virtuosity and his major cognitive deficit. Most of all, the documentary is about procedural (non-declarative) musical memory in dementia—the learned motor skill from countless hours of practicing, which remains intact longer than any other intellectual skill. Patients with Alzheimer's dementia may sing a tune correctly but are unable to name the title. Still, the right hemisphere remains important when playing an instrument, and once that area of the brain becomes affected, musicians may lose mastery altogether.

The tour starts off great. The teleprompter is a godsend and even cues him when to play a solo. He may not always know the key, but he knows the melody and rhythm perfectly. Initially, he plays without any fault, comes in with the band when he needs to do so, and his solos rock the house. He jokes about his memory loss when he introduces the band, "pretending" he does not know them. He is visibly enjoying the moment, and as expected, his emotional response to music is fully preserved. When later asked whether he got a lifetime achievement award at the Grammys, he answers, "Did I?"

The film also shows he can be out of character. At one point, he probes a knife in his mouth when he has a toothache, but in a burst of forceful denial, he refuses to go to the dentist. He has episodes of scary anger and, during the tour, wanders around in hotel hallways. Gradually "the frequency of bad

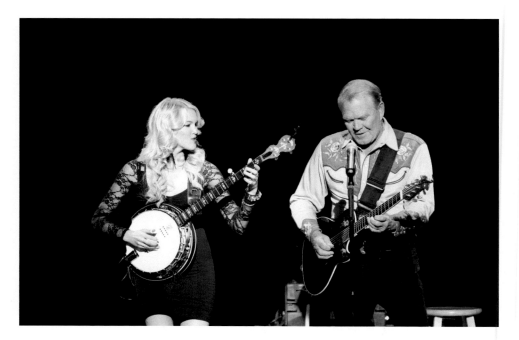

FIGURE 7.6   Glen Campbell and his daughter during his last tour in *Glen Campbell … I'll Be Me* (courtesy of PCH Films).

shows increase," and the tour comes to a stop. He is repeating songs, talking too much, missing notes, losing the rhythm, and becoming visibly agitated. One poignant scene shows his extreme vulnerability when he complains about his guitar sounding terrible ("too thin"). In another scene, he struggles to keep up with the teleprompter ("who runs this thing? I have to have that thing on me"). During one show, his loss of decorum seems apparent when he opens his shirt and shows off contracting pectoralis muscles. Glen has word-finding difficulties and semantic substitutions. His introductions during concerts seem to become truncated. "I am Glen Campbell … I am … God bless you." His family members feel that "working seem to stimulate his mind," and despite all the haziness, "he becomes himself again." His music-making is now a necessity. Those in charge continue the concerts knowing that all bets are off. His fans seem to accept his slip-ups.

For Glen Campbell, dementia meant forgotten lyrics and unusual tempo changes, which the band manages to follow. Most remarkably, the film captures his effortless playing and singing onstage while offstage he cannot tie his shoes. *Glen Campbell… I'll Be Me* is a celebration of his family's compassion. His wife made admirable efforts to keep him from injury and spiraling into self-neglect, but inevitably, because of his relentless decline, she loses control of the situation. Metaphorically, we see the rhinestone cowboy riding off into the sunset, and the audience is right there with him. It is an important, well-made documentary on the ravages of Alzheimer's disease in a legend. It is also about the disappearance of a great past.

Robin Williams

A more recent documentary showed another type of dementia. *Robin's Wish* (2020) ⚞ featured Robin Williams and was directed by Tyler Norwood (Figure 7.7). What was his wish—in his own words, to reboot his brain? *Robin's Wish* is based on experiences gathered from secondary sources and attempts to show how Robin Williams's brain could have been working—and, in this interpretation, it is a horror-freak show. Scenes have the camera snooping through empty hallways, snaking around corners, going in and out of focus, and showing tilted images (and all set to minor-key spooky music). The filmmaker

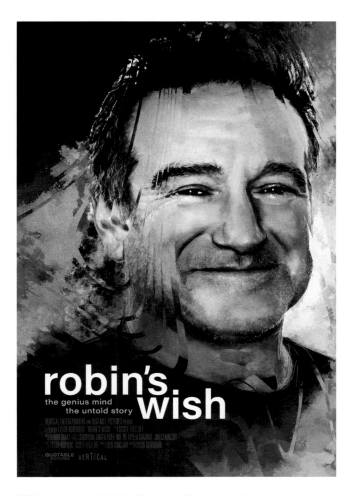

FIGURE 7.7   Robin Williams in *Robin's Wish* (Everett Collection, Inc.).

employs these tropes to show the problems Williams may have endured.[34] The documentary hypothesizes that his diagnosis was missed and that he was treated for Parkinson's disease rather than Lewy body disease. The documentary has little to say about his use of antidopaminergic drugs, which could have exacerbated his symptoms. Lewy bodies are aggregations of misfolded proteins in the cell, formed when the protein degradation system of the cell is overwhelmed and thought to be responsible for 10% to 15% of dementia cases. People with Lewy body disease experience anxiety, memory loss, hallucinations, and insomnia, and these symptoms are generally accompanied or soon followed by Parkinson's symptoms. Robin Williams knew something was not right, but nobody could pin it down.

We cannot know how the anxiety is really experienced in dementia or Lewy body disease. (Often, bursts of anxiety are quickly forgotten.) The documentary also shows that Williams could not remember his lines, which frustrated him greatly. (Robin Williams was good at reciting rapidly and frequently.) While watching the film, I constantly wondered how his diagnosis could have been missed by several neurologists. It could be the basic difficulty in diagnosing real disease in someone known for his quirks. His

---

[34] See Chapter 4 for a review of *The Father* (2020), in which the film maker also attempts to delve into a demented mind but without sensationalism or horror.

second wife of 7 years wrote an essay entitled "The terrorist inside my husband's brain" in *Neurology*. The main theme is her surprise at learning he had Lewy body disease and how everything he did or complained about was an eye-opener for her. In this essay, she describes "paranoia, delusions, looping, insomnia, memory, and high cortisol levels – just to name a few – were settling in hard."[35] Panic attacks were frequent, and he even asked if he was "schizophrenic." Ms. Schneider Williams pulls out all the stops to promote recognition of Lewy body disease. But, it was a case of a wild comedian becoming rapidly "zanier."[36] Her interpretations of her "brilliant husband" are after the fact but seem factually correct. The film shows the funny Williams as a standup comedian ("he drained every scintilla of laughter out of the crowd") and showing compassion as exemplified by his performances for troops overseas and his long friendship with actor Christopher Reeve, who was paralyzed in a riding accident.

Robin Williams died by suicide. The film implies his death could have been prevented if the diagnoses had been established and if family and friends had understood his struggles. One neighbor says, "I felt remorse and guilt. I could have done more. I should have done more." Neurologists are not so sure.

Jacqueline du Pré

Two films are based on the late cellist Jacqueline du Pré, her family, and her relationship with her sister (see also Chapter 4). This film is based on Piers and Hilary du Pré's memoir entitled *A Genius in the Family. Hilary and Jackie* (1998) ⚊ is directed by Anand Tucker and stars Emily Watson (Figure 7.8), Rachel Griffiths, James Frain, and David Morrissey with an Academy Award for Best Actress (Emily Watson) and for Best Supporting Actress (Rachel Griffith). Jacqueline du Pré married Daniel Barenboim, and both became prominent musicians. The two sisters, both musicians, had a lifelong rivalry with bitter words exchanged between them, but then one of them was struck down by MS. "I have a fatal illness," Jackie says. It was another film dealing with how a progressive neurologic disease could impact a musician's career. "Would you still love me if I couldn't play?" Jacqueline asks her husband. "You wouldn't be you if you didn't play," he replies, and that response gets to the heart of the problem with a progressive disease, which could immediately affect the coordinated artistry of the cello technique. The film is mostly about the two sisters' close relationship, and Jackie's diagnosis of MS does not emerge until 90 minutes into the film. No discussion with a physician is seen. Complaining of cold hands is one of the first premonitory signs presented here, but there is otherwise an accurate portrayal of rapidly progressive MS. Jackie (Emily Watson) first notices her inability to grasp the bow followed by tremor, incontinence, and being unable to rise from a chair after performing a concert; then her hearing disappears, canes appear, she cannot roll over in bed, and she ends up in a wheelchair. This all plays out in the last 20 minutes of the film, likely to achieve grand effect. Most prominently displayed by Jackie are her emotional mood swings and her euphoric outlook.[37]

DIALOGUE

Hilary and Jackie

Jackie

I have got a fatal illness, but you must not worry. I got it very mildly.

I am so relieved it is only MS. I know it is serious, but I thought I was going mad.

---

[35] Williams SS. The Terrorist Inside my Husband's Brain. *Neurology.* 2016;87:1308–1311.

[36] A consummate actor, he could also shine in serious roles, notably *Dead Poets Society* (1989), *One Hour Photo* (2001), and, of course, *Awakenings* (1990).

[37] Corona T, Poser C. Jacqueline Du Pre. Talent and Disease. *Neurologia.* 2004;19:85.

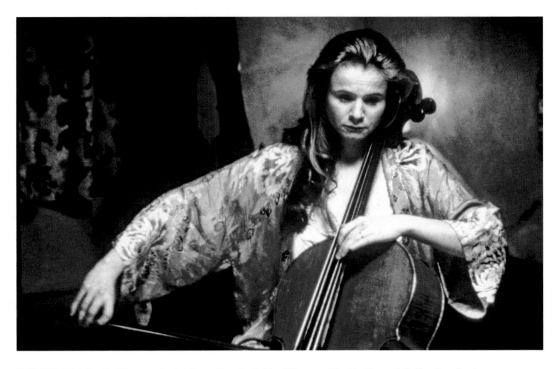

FIGURE 7.8   Emily Watson playing Jaqueline du Pré in *Hilary and Jackie* (Everett Collection, Inc.).

These affective states are well known in MS ever since Charcot's original description. Uncontrollable laughing and crying, however, are not shown. Jackie strived to be a happy-go-lucky person, although that often did not reflect her true mood. The film shows spastic ataxia and dystonic (tremor) posturing, all consistent with primary progressive MS. In the early stages, there is a brief mention of "pills" to allow her to play her instrument, but no specific treatment is mentioned.

Hilary and Jackie is based on medical reports and witness reports. A review of MS portrayal in the movies has been published and found mostly correct portrayal.[38] Sensational contextualization was absent in most films. The mean age of diagnosis of multiple sclerosis is 32 years—a time when artists are building careers. The impact of the diagnosis on affected individuals and their families can be profound. Now, there are costly, effective, disease-modifying treatments that can reduce the disabling effects ascertainably but not likely for artists who are dependent on fine manual skills. (See Chapters 4 and 6 for more details on multiple sclerosis and questionable treatments.)

End Credits

Stargazing or celebrity worship is, of course, nothing new. We identify with someone who seems to lead a perfect life, and many are shamelessly eager to hear about their vicissitudes. Tellingly but deliberately, human interest journalism of celebrities and actors has been selective. Actors such as Ronald Reagan (Alzheimer's disease) and Michael J. Fox (Parkinson's disease) received more attention than David Niven (ALS) and Cary Grant (stroke). David Niven is also featured in this book as a presumed epileptic in *A Matter of Life and Death* (Chapter 4). David Niven's decline from ALS[39] with rapid muscle wasting

---

[38] Karenberg A. Multiple Sclerosis On-Screen: From Disaster to Coping. *Mult Scler.* 2008;14:530–540.
[39] See Munn, M. *David Niven: The Man behind the Balloon.* JR Books; 2010 and Morley, S. *The Other Side of the Moon: The Life of David Niven.* Paperback ed. London: Dean Street Press; 2016.

and mostly loss of speech was again misjudged as drunkenness (Niven previously sold and enjoyed whiskey) His disease progression been recounted in multiple biographies, and he bravely accepted his illness with unusual humor using military metaphors and other comparisons ("my right arm now has gone over to the enemy" and "my Gandhi body"). Just like Lou Gehrig, he was diagnosed at Mayo Clinic in 1982 but at the more typical age of 71 and after a prior misdiagnosis.

Few know that Cary Grant had a fatal intracerebral hemorrhage ("one side paralyzed and dilated pupils" and severe hypertension of 210/130 mmHg).[40] Biopics on celebrities with neurologic disease are few and far between. The most famous American poliomyelitis patient, Franklin Roosevelt (FDR), never merited a biopic, although the most recent film came close. However, *Hyde Park on Hudson* (2012) inaccurately shows FDR (Bill Murray) walking with crutches or walking unassisted with two canes.

With increased awareness of neurologic disease, we will see more documentary films on neurologic disease in celebrities. However, these documentaries are important; not only do they explore the intersection between neurologic disease and profession, but they also provide more insight into personal experiences—albeit filtered by the surviving members of the family.

Filmmakers may have accepted that their disease-themed films may become banners for disease-based charities, and this promotion even may show up (at least for some viewers) unexpectedly. For example, in *Still Alice* (2014), Alice (Julianne Moore) gives a major speech explaining her experiences at an Alzheimer's Association event. Even if they focus on celebrities, we should not overlook the fact that these films will bring disease information to a wide audience, and thus, they undeniably have merit.

---

[40] The otherwise superb biography on Cary Grant (Eyman S. *Cary Grant: A Brilliant Disguise.* New York: Simon & Schuster: 2020) has some details on Grant's stroke but concentrates more on whether he could have been saved in a tertiary center with a neurology ICU (not likely without leaving him acutely and severely devastated) but then peculiarly concludes "it was his time."

8

Neuropsychiatry in Film

It is not showing up on the tests

Safe (1995)

New discoveries are made all the time. Things we never dreamed possible. To cure someone of blindness by having her lie on the couch and talk about her childhood. I mean, who'd have thought?

Magic in the Moonlight (2014)

Main Themes

Placed in historical context, psychiatry and neurology have always been sinuously intertwined. Why would diseases of the mind differ from diseases of the brain? That was clearly obsessing many pioneering physicians in these specialties—and honestly, it still is. Attempts to establish a biologic foundation for psychiatry (scouting for abnormal neuroimaging and other biomarkers) continue to this day and, at first glance, would be far preferable to explaining psychiatric disorders fallaciously as a consequence of motherhood deprivation or some other traumatic event.[1] The so-called "organic causes" of psychiatric disease (e.g., brain injury-induced mental disorders) obscured the clear dividing line between the two specialties because, for example, syphilis could invade the brain and spine, presenting with both paralysis and insanity. To be sure, there are at least two stories. One is the history of psychiatry seen through neurosyphilis (a disease of the brain eventually causing megalomania), and the other is the story of hysteria (a disease of the mind causing paralysis, blindness, and abnormal movements).[2] At least in the United States, much of this dichotomy was a consequence of psychiatry ceding to psychoanalysis after Freud came on the scene. But there is no clear separation between psychodynamic principles explaining neurosis and neurobiology explaining psychosis, and splitting neurology and psychiatry is sort of artificial. Psychiatrists have understandably struggled with the diagnosis and classification of mental illness because of their inability to confirm anatomical abnormalities with MRI and autopsy. On the other hand, abnormally complex emotions cannot easily be localized in the brain. Some psychiatrists are convinced that much of what we see in the major psychosis entities is a chemical imbalance rather than a structural defect. Our understanding, however, is more primitive and inferential (drug X works, so it must be this neurotransmitter). A consequence of this reasoning could be that drugs are prescribed for dubious indications (i.e., something many of us would consider within the margins of a normal adaptive response). Psychiatry cannot be poles apart from neurology; this has become more apparent in the modern age, where we see well-known

---

[1] For years, the real culprit of a later mental disorders was the "seductive and smothering mother." For a discussion of these outrageous theories see Harrington A *Mind Fixers*. New York: Norton & Company; 2019.

[2] Ropper AH, Burrell B. *How the Brain Lost Its Mind: Sex, Hysteria and the Riddle of Mental Illness*. New York: Atlantic Books; 2020.

DOI: 10.1201/9781003270874-8   187

psychiatric disorders, such as malignant catatonic states, caused in some previously mentally healthy patients by a neuroimmunologic disorder that responds to immunosuppressive agents.

The history of psychiatry from asylum to shock therapies, lobotomies, and anti-psychotic drugs is vastly interesting to filmmakers, has spawned some scholarly work, and begs the question of whether these movies have a deeper meaning.[3] Cinema also investigated mass hysteria in films such as *The Witch* (2015) and *The White Ribbon* (2009), but these topics are not considered here and will be addressed in a forthcoming work.

In this book on neurology in the movies, we find significant overlap in illnesses seen by both specialties. It is not always so clear to filmmakers, who have a broad definition of psychiatry, and that includes any murderous mind. Mostly, we will find these so-called functional diseases previously labeled conversion disorders or, plainly, hysteria, and autoimmune encephalitis presenting with mental illness also recently received a cinematic treatment. In Chapter 4, we already encountered the catatonic state with encephalitis lethargica (*Awakenings*) and the sleepwalking side effects of an anti-depressant (*Side Effects*), but these themes were incidentally used and did not return. Moreover, cinema continuously churns out horror-and-slasher flicks for the dubious joy of scaring ourselves witless, but we will let that pass this time. Even so, with all the richness of cinematic convergence of neurology and psychiatry, it goes without saying we are still in for a treat.

Functional Neurology

Functional neurology is diagnosed in patients who have neurologic-type symptoms (inability to speak, move, or feel or a persistent muscle contraction) but without brain tissue or physiological change. The incidence is comparable to many known neurologic illnesses and is a very common observation in neurology clinics and epilepsy monitoring units. Preceding stressors are no longer a requirement in the diagnostic criteria for functional neurologic disorder, but with hindsight, it can be linked to a triggering event in many patients. Before "functional neurology" became the accepted term, Charcot started the diagnostic inquiry into functional symptoms and diagnosed "hysteria" if there were convulsive crises with the characteristic poses such as *arc-en-cercle* or if patients presented with persistent neurologic deficits without an identifiable substrate. Charcot divided hysteria into four phases—epileptoid, clownism (i.e., contortions and acrobatic postures), postures indicating passion and desire ("*délire érotique*"), and delirium-hallucinations, which he called "*Grande Hystérie.*" Numerous labels have been applied over the years for more specific manifestations such as seizures, ranging from "hystero-epilepsy" in the 19th century to "non-epileptic attack disorder" in the late 20th century. For Charcot, hysteria was primarily a hereditary disorder. (Freud later added sexual abuse fantasies in females.) Charcot knew too well that hysteria was distinct from malingering. He also recognized physical trauma could cause "hysteria" and more in males, often in muscular, virile men of the working class with only a minor visible injury (e.g., a burn on the hand causing a permanent contracture). Charcot is featured in *Augustine* and discussed in Chapter 2. Augustine has a functional hemiparesis that requires treatment (Figure 8.1). Charcot could not possibly film his patients, and we only have descriptions and drawings of the attacks (Charcot and Richer's *Les Démoniaques Dans l'Art*). Some of his patients were photographed in a studio (*Service Photographique de la Salpêtrière*). A spell followed a breath-holding pallor followed by redness, neck engorgement, and upward eye deviation. Foam appeared on the lips, usually early and not during the resolution phase as in a true seizure. Initially, the muscles were completely limp, and then "acrobatics" began. Sometimes, the patient curved forward with the head and feet touching the bed, but the patient could also lie on the side. Charcot also described bizarre movements (as

---

[3] Wedding D. *Movies and Mental Illness: Using Films to Understand Psychopathology.* 3rd ed. Boston: Hogrefe Publishing; 2009.

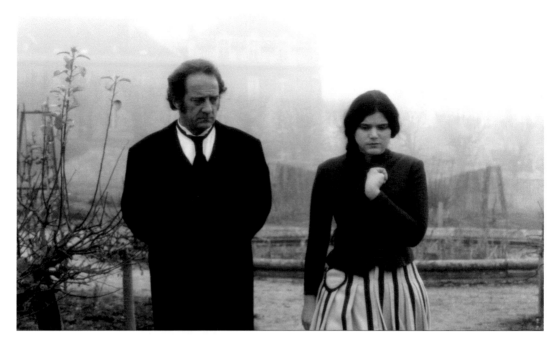

FIGURE 8.1 Vincent Lindon as Charcot and Stéphanie Sokolinski as Augustine in *Augustine*. (Note the functional flexed arm posture) (Photos provided by courtesy of Music Box Films: Charcot © Dharamsala Photo. J.C. Lother Charcot and Augustine: © Dharamsala Photo.).

if wrestling with an imaginary being) and savage cries. Hissing respiration would be interrupted by hiccups, and the mouth would droop open with tongue protrusion. Charcot often described these contortions as "being possessed." Later, in 1899, the Romanian Gheorghe Marinescu filmed a single case of "hysterical hemiplegia" cured with hypnosis (see Chapter 2). In the next century, hypnosis received more serious attention, and movie cameras allowed us to view functional disease in soldiers returning from World War I.

Damaged Homecoming

During wartime, as part of post-traumatic stress syndrome, hysteria had other names such as "nostalgia" and "war neurosis." Many labels suggest faked or deliberately manufactured symptoms.

The first cinematic presentation of these neurologic symptoms appeared in a short educational film by Arthur Hurst. a neurologist at the Royal Victoria Hospital, Netley. *War Neurosis* was filmed in Seale Hayne Military Hospital in 1917 and 1918 and showed several abnormal movements, postures (dystonia), and gaits in 21 soldiers (Figure 8.2). One soldier with receptive aphasia does not respond to questions, except that the sudden introduction of the word "bomb," would suddenly cause the soldier to dive under his bed. Hurst used intertitles to explain the best approach to their problems, which he postulated as "education," followed by "persuasion" and "re-education," combined in most cases with "manipulation"—all rather vague descriptions of interventions that seemed to have originated in his mind. Cures could be rapid; one example showed an abnormal gait at 2 pm that was "cured" by 3 pm. In another, a patient with functional paraplegia for 18 months was "cured after a quarter of an hour's suggestion and re-education." Sudden recovery of memory after 8 months of complete amnesia was described. Eighteen patients (86%) had partial or complete recovery, two were not shown in the film, and one had no benefit.

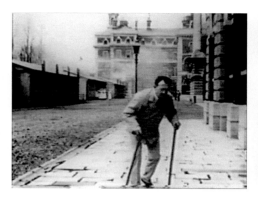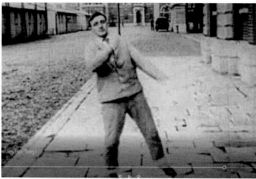

FIGURE 8.2   Abnormal gaits (dragging with two canes and swaying) as part of functional neurology in Hurst film *War Neurosis*. (Courtesy of Edgar Jones and Jon Stone.)

Hurst also championed the use of physiotherapy in the context of re-education.[4] He offered a more complete description in an article in the *British Medical Journal* in 1917.[5] He described the emotions produced by a horrible incident in the trenches that would cause "stupor and amnesia, psychasthenia, and hysterical symptoms." Concussion or toxins were obviously considered as main causes but rapidly dismissed. Hurst also provided a great neurologic insight into the phenomenon of overlay and how a structural lesion could change into a functional manifestation:

> When one side of the brain has been chiefly affected by the concussion, an initially organic hemiplegia merges into hysterical hemiplegia. I have watched several cases, in which all the physical signs of organic paraplegia or hemiplegia were at first present but have gradually disappeared in the course of a few days or weeks, although the paralysis has remained, until by suggestion or persuasion it has been cured in a few minutes. Sometimes, however, some organic signs remain, and suggestion then can only produce an, incomplete cure, a slightly spastic gait or some slowness and lack of accuracy in the first movements of a limb being left as the permanent result of the shell shock.[6]

Hurst's film was a dramatic demonstration of functional weakness but with extraordinary results after the intervention, and one can rightly question the veracity of these clips. As with so many other documentaries, re-enactment was likely. Despite Hurst's report of dramatic cures, others discovered major relapses in the patients seen in this hospital. Hurst later acknowledged the possibility of relapse and, despite early cures, felt that once these soldiers presented with functional disease, they could never return to active service.[7]

No other contemporary films appeared at this time, nor did the topic appear in a fictional film. But after the end of the Second World War, British and American military psychiatrists also began seeing soldiers with speech difficulties, tics, weakness, amnesia, and other signs and symptoms mimicking

---

[4] For a recent detailed discussion on Hurst's film, see Jones E, Stone J. Hurst Rehabilitated: The Treatment of Functional Motor Disorders by Arthur Hurst during the First World War. *J R Coll Physicians Edinb.* 2020;50:436–443. The authors postulated that Hurst should be considered one of the foremost pioneers of multidisciplinary treatment for functional movement disorders. See also Moscovich M, Estupinan D, Qureshi M, Okun MS. Shell Shock. Psychogenic Gait and Other Movement Disorders-A Film Review. *Tremor Other Hyperkinet Mov* (N Y). 2013;3:1–7.

[5] Hurst AF. Observations on the Etiology and Treatment of War Neuroses. *Br Med J.* 1917;2:409–414.

[6] Hurst, 1917, Ibid.

[7] See Wright MB. Treatment of psychological casualties during war. *Br Med J.* 1939;2:615–617; Tippett JA. Psychological casualties in war. *Br Med J.* 1939;2:742; and Jones E. War neuroses and Arthur Hurst: A Pioneering Medical Film about the Treatment of Psychiatric Battle Casualties. *J Hist Med Allied Sci.* 2012;67:345–373.

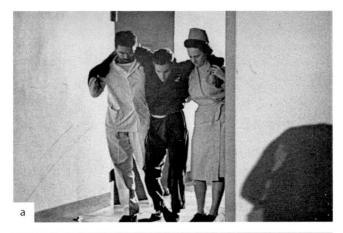

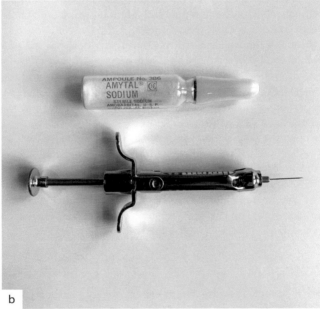

FIGURE 8.3   (a) Functional paraparesis in Huston's *Let There Be Light* (United States Army Signal Corps/The LIFE Picture Collection/Shutterstock). (b) Sodium pentothal was commonly used at the time in the treatment of these manifestations. (Courtesy of Dr. Jonathan Beary.)

neurologic disease. The U.S. Army assigned famed filmmaker (and then U.S. Army Major) John Huston to produce and direct the documentary *Let There Be Light* (1946) .[8] Most strikingly, the film shows the effect of sodium amytal-induced hypnosis in removing psychologic barriers in a soldier who cannot walk (Figure 8.3). Remarkable also is the instantaneous recovery of a patient with a functional stutter. The soldier is unable to speak except for a few stuttering words, but then, soon after a sodium-amytal injection, he loudly proclaims, "I can talk! I can talk! I can talk!" A man with total amnesia is brought under hypnosis by Colonel Benjamin Simon and, under hypnosis, is taken back to the battlefield to try

---

[8] Huston J. *Let There Be Light*. U.S. Army. 1946.

to remember each moment of explosions and to visualize fellow soldiers taken away wounded. A snap of psychiatrist Simon's finger brings him back, now with a restored memory.

Huston famously said that making the documentary (a re-enactment would be more accurate) was "an extraordinary—almost a religious—experience." Huston also admitted in his memoir that hours of footage were shot, but he selected the more unpredictable exchanges. Despite commissioning it, the Army suppressed *Let There Be Light*. (The reasons given were concerns with patient confidentiality, and it remains highly dubious whether consenting signatures ever existed.) It remained banned and was only released for restricted viewing by vice-presidential order 35 years later.

The Army followed up with John Henabery's *Shades of Gray* (1948) ◄◄◄◄ .[9] This refocused documentary with redacted and re-acted scenes introduced a psychodynamic explanation. *Shades of Gray* uncompromisingly stated that the manifestations were a result of the sufferer's upbringing, lack of athletic ability, and inability to stand up to bullying. More offensively, some psychoanalytical psychiatrists interpreted these manifestations as a response to arousal of (repressed) homosexuality in the company of men. The film narrator states that "shades of gray" refers to their common observation that most men are not "100% perfect - nobody has pure white mental health" and we are all in a gray zone. *Let There Be Light* and *Shades of Gray* both prominently show how functional neurology was concealed in what we now known as post-traumatic stress disorder or PTSD. *LIFE Magazine* claimed that the US Army admitted to its hospitals thousands of neuropsychiatric patients for treatment as and that "more than 40% of all Army medical discharges have been neuropsychiatric cases."[10]

Functional paralysis also returned a year later in the film *Home of the Brave* (1948) ◄◄◄◄ , directed by Mark Robson, about a black soldier unable to walk after his best friend died in his arms in the South Pacific. The army doctor takes a history, uncompassionately yells at him, and tries to have him recall the event, which, parenthetically, he can remember exactly. ("Why can't you walk? You weren't shot, were you? You ran through the jungle, didn't you? So, your legs were alright!") Then, the army doctor tells him that he will walk out of the hospital but adds that is not enough. ("You got to be cured!") The army physician now introduces feelings of guilt but also introduces a racial element. He emphasizes he is no different than everybody else and orders him to get up and walk. ("I can't!" "Try!") Only when the doctor uses a racial slur does he stand and walk—out of anger. Subsequent fiction films on PTSD would be much different and concentrate on current symptoms of depression, suicidal daydreams, and angry outbursts (often to spouses).[11]

Something Is Wrong

Given all the grandiosity the topic provides, functional neurology also emerged in fiction film, and the key film to see is *Safe* (1995) ◄◄◄◄ directed by Todd Haynes. Carol White (Julianne Moore) gradually develops inexplicable symptoms. Her life as a homemaker consists of domestic routine with errands, luncheons, and visits to the gym. (Immediately, the film cleverly creates a sense of doom when we overhear a radio discussion on the ethics of withdrawing support in sick patients and a discussion about the end of the world on a Christian channel.) She lives comfortably in a gated mansion with her husband, who is denied intimacy because of her headache. ("I still have this head thing.") Carol's husband, Greg, expresses anger and frustration at his wife's inability to meet his sexual demands. ("Nobody has [expletive] headache every night of the [expletive] week!") The next morning, Carol initiates an embrace only to draw away convulsively as she retches and vomits. (His excessive use of hair spray may be responsible.) Next, exhaust from the car in front of her leaves her choking, and a perm induces a nosebleed.

[9] Henabery J. *Shades of Gray*. U.S. Army. February 6, 1948.

[10] Hersey J. A Short Talk with Erlanger: The Army Is Using a Dramatic Treatment Called Narco-Synthesis to Help Psychiatric Casualties. *LIFE*. New York: Time Inc.; 1945.

[11] See Wijdicks EFM. *Cinema, MD*. New York: Oxford University Press; 2020, Chapter 6, for examples. The most accurate fiction film based on a true story is *American Sniper* (Eastwood C. Warner Bros. Pictures. December 25, 2014).

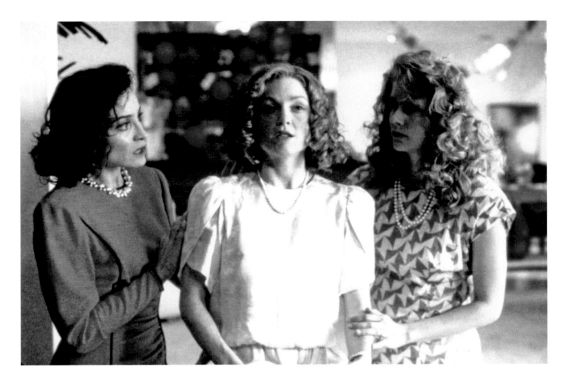

FIGURE 8.4 Dazed Carol (Julianne Moore) in *Safe* (Everett Collection, Inc.).

The physicians she consults are baffled and become increasingly impatient. The family physician insists that there is nothing physically wrong with her; an allergist finds a major reaction (hyperventilation) after subcutaneously injecting milk. She develops major swallowing difficulties, and the film shows her in an impressive seizure with blood from a tongue bite. Carol also wanders on her front lawn in a midnight fugue and has other blackouts (Figure 8.4). Carol is convinced something is wrong; after all, one does not just spasm on the floor of the local dry cleaners or have a panicked choking spell at a friend's baby shower for no good reason. The men around Carol, including Greg, all but declare this a case of "female hysteria," insinuating that whatever ails her is in her head. Her last physician hands her husband a psychiatrist's card, but in the next scene, the psychiatrist remains nebulous behind his desk and tells Carol she must talk about herself without depending on him to ask questions. An alternate answer emerges when she spots a flier at the gym that reads: "Do you smell fumes? Are you allergic to the twentieth century?" Through support groups, she learns of multiple chemical sensitivity (MCS) or environmental illness, and to avoid these exposures, she ends up in a windowless porcelain dome breathing through a facemask with oxygen tank.[12] Haynes said," In *Safe*, you find this woman who's almost a cipher, even though she lives the American Dream and this life of luxury. She has the lifestyle and material things that are valued in our world, but in many ways, her encountering of illness is the thing that triggers her worry that maybe something is not quite right in her life."[13] The film resonates in the age of COVID-19, when there is constant fear that an invisible killer virus is "loose and at prey, and that anyone could become susceptible to it."[14] *Safe*, in its portrayal of a woman alienated from the people

[12] Haynes T. *Safe*. Sony Picture Classics. January 25, 1995. Carol's illness, although unidentified, serves as an analogy for the 1980s AIDS crisis, a largely unspoken "threat." Haynes in interviews has said that AIDS was on his mind. (See Sneak Peaks: Julianne Moore and Todd Haynes on Safe. In *The Current*. Vol 2021. Criterion; Sony Pictures Home Entertainment; 2014.)

[13] Roth D. Todd Haynes's Masterpiece "Safe" Is Now a Tale of Two Plagues. *The New Yorker*. New York: Condé Nast; 2020.

[14] Roth D., 2020, Ibid.

surrounding her, indeed, has an eerie resonance. Carol, in today's parlance, is "socially distanced." She might also have been a victim of a new, or newly recognized, illness caused by the growing environmental load of chemicals in the modern world. In the past, it has also been named, environmental illness or 20th-century illness. The symptoms are usually headaches, confusion, depression, dizziness, rashes, watery eyes, asthma, nasal congestion, fatigue, and nausea—symptoms that are also physiologic manifestations of anxiety and fear. It is a malady that baffles physicians. They disagree over whether the disease is real, and they disagree over its definition, cause, and treatment. And the diagnosis of MCS or environmental illness is not recognized as an organic, chemically caused illness by the World Health Organization or the American Medical Association. The sociologist Gaye Naismith said, "we might identify Carol's illness as an instance of the body speaking when Carol cannot, much like in the case of the nineteenth century hysteric."[15] Certainly, Carol presents with inexplicable medical and neurologic symptoms (blackouts, choking, convulsions) frequently seen in any neurology clinic.

There have been several other portrayals of functional neurology. Functional seizures are most prominent in *Drugstore Cowboy* (1989) ⫷⫷. Here, the pseudoseizures are deliberate, and in the film, the "seizing" person takes Alka-Seltzer to fake foaming at the mouth. The attention to the "seizing" person allows others to steal prescription drugs in the drugstore. The functional seizure is surprisingly accurately done, with thrashing movements, moaning, and tightly closed eyes. When it is over, she suddenly walks away with bystanders asking, "Are you okay?" A pseudoseizure is also seen in *The Intouchables* (2012), where it also is intended as a deliberate deceit — and thus more malingering than functional.

Functional blindness appears in *Hollywood Ending* (2002) ⫷⫷. Woody Allen plays a director with a somatic symptom disorder and, when he gets to direct a major film, becomes blind and tries to fake his way through the picture. The completed film in *Hollywood Ending* is panned by every American critic but is hailed as a masterpiece in France. It is unclear why Woody Allen thought portraying blindness, which has a stigmatized history, was such a funny idea.[16] He used it with greater metaphorical significance in *Crimes and Misdemeanors* (1989). In this film, the rabbi goes blind and cannot see the evil done by Judah, the ophthalmologist, who has been complicit in murder and seems to get away with it. The rabbi's blindness may also be symbolic of his detachment from real-world villainy when he lives a life devoted to God.

Ingmar Bergman used functional mutism twice. *The Magician* (1958) ⫷⫷ revolves around the mesmerist Vogler, who becomes mute when his tricks are exposed. His throat examination is normal, and his physician concludes there is nothing wrong and states that the mesmerist represents "something I abhor – the unexplainable." In *Persona* (1996) ⫷⫷, Elisabet becomes mute during her performance of Elektra, but again physicians can find nothing wrong with her. (Bergman devised a complex psychoanalytic explanation.)

Finally, functional unresponsiveness shows up in the Spanish film *The Spirit of the Beehive,* directed by Victor Erice in 1973. In a remote village in the 1940s, two little girls attend a viewing of James Whale's *Frankenstein* (1931), which fascinates and terrorizes them. Later, one of the girls is found unresponsive. When her sister tries to wake her up, she is limp. When her arms are lifted over her head and released, they do not fall on her face but slide sideways and fall, in a surprisingly similar manner to what we see in a patient with functional unresponsiveness.

Functional or psychogenic amnesia is harder to find in cinema (see also Chapter 9.) Impaired recall of autobiographical events is the most prominent symptom of psychogenic amnesia, deficits in retrieving personal facts. Many functional amnesias are diagnosed without a background of psychological factors.

---

[15] Naismith G. Contamination and Quarantine in Todd Haynes's *Safe*. In: Treichler P, Cartwright L, Penley C, eds. *The Visible Woman: Imaging Technologies, Gender, and Science.* New York: NYU Press; 1998:360–388.

[16] Ironically, the film was a bit of a flop. Woody Allen was mystified "it is a funny picture with a funny idea, executed funny. I was amusing in it." (Cited in Eric Lax. *Conversations with Woody Allen. His Films. The Movies and Movie Making.* New York: AA Knopf; 2007.)

Functional amnesia may affect memories from across the whole lifespan or just those from a specific time period or with a specific content. For instance, some patients "forget" events that happened within the last five years before the critical incident. With respect to content, the amnesia may affect all autobiographical memories or just specific autobiographical material. (*The Vow* in Chapter 4 is a good example.) Patients may forget their personal identity, resulting in fugue with sudden, unexpected travel away from home and an inability to recall the past (e.g., *Paris, Texas*).

A Tortuous Diagnostic Process

For many years, neurologists knew that antibodies from cancer attack the brain and change behavior and memory. But one of the "new" discoveries is that a vigorous immune response can attack specific brain structures without a known cause and out of the blue. This so-called autoimmune encephalitis can present with dramatic symptoms first, suggesting to physicians that a major psychiatric disorder (i.e., schizophrenia, bipolar disease, catatonia) is at play. There still is a great need for detailed descriptions of psychiatric syndromes in patients with autoimmune encephalitis, which will better characterize the psychiatric features of this disease, but overall, most manifestations are due to involvement of the limbic system (i.e., hippocampus, amygdala, and hypothalamus). This limbic encephalitis is also comprised of psychiatric features such as depressive syndrome, behavioral abnormalities, and anxiety in addition to seizures and impaired consciousness. Most patients develop more than one neuropsychiatric symptom; the encephalitis rarely presents as an isolated psychiatric syndrome. Psychiatric and cognitive changes mostly consist of paranoid thoughts, agitation, personality changes, and auditory or visual hallucinations. In anti-N-methyl-D-aspartate receptor (anti-NMDAR) encephalitis, the major neuropsychiatric features are epilepsy, dystonia, psychotic agitation, refractory agitation, followed by cognitive sequelae, such as executive dysfunction. The association between catatonia and psychiatric features (hallucinations, delusions, mood disorder, and cognitive regression) is a red flag for a possible underlying autoimmune disorder. The response of autoimmune catatonia to treatment further supports the existing literature for both early and aggressive immunosuppressive treatments.[17] The disorder is one of the more recent entities in which psychiatry and neurology overlap.

While it is still a rare disorder, anti-NMDA receptor encephalitis already had its own feature film, mainly due to the success of the 2012 book by Susannah Cahalan called *Brain on Fire: My Month of Madness*. The feature film *Brain on Fire* (2017) was directed by Gerard Barrett with Chloë Grace Moretz playing Susannah Cahalan. Cahalan was an investigative journalist at the *New York Post*. She is listed on her Wikipedia page as person #217 to be diagnosed with anti-NMDAR encephalitis. Cahalan has no full memory of what happened to her but describes her symptoms, as told by others, as follows:

> I slurred my words. I drooled. I didn't have proper control over my swallowing … I kept my arms out in unnatural poses. At one point, I was like the Bride of Frankenstein—I kept my arms out rigidly. I was slow. I could hardly walk, and when I did, I needed to be supported … I started [acting] very psychotic. I believed that I could age people with my mind. If I looked at them, wrinkles would form, and if I looked away, they would suddenly, magically get younger. And I believed that my father had murdered my stepmother. I believed all these incredibly paranoid—a huge, extreme example of persecution complex. And then as the days went on, I stopped being as psychotic, and I started entering into a catatonic stage, which was characterized by just complete lack of emotion, inability to relate, or to read, or hardly to be able to speak.[18]

---

[17] See Hansen N, Timaus C. Immunotherapy in Autoantibody-Associated Psychiatric Syndromes in Adults. *Front Psychiatry.* 2021;12:611346. Also, Schieveld JNM, Strik J, van Kraaij S, Nicolai J. Psychiatric Manifestations and Psychopharmacology of Autoimmune Encephalitis: A Multidisciplinary Approach. *Handb Clin Neurol.* 2019;165:285–307.

[18] A Young Reporter Chronicles Her "Brain on Fire" [Internet]: National Public Radio; November 14, 2012. Podcast.

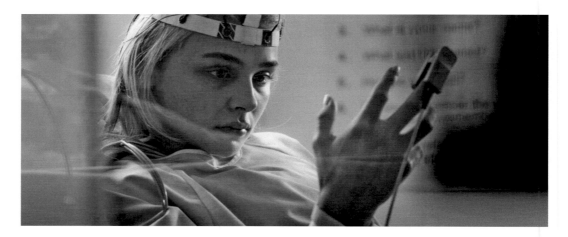

FIGURE 8.5 Surprised Susannah (Chloë Moretz) finding herself in the hospital in *Brain on Fire* (Everett Collection, Inc.).

Both book and film emphasize the tenacity of the neurologist who finally diagnoses her.[19] As neurologist Souhel Najjar cryptically describes it to Cahalan's parents, "her brain is on fire."

The film opens with Susannah finding herself restrained in a hospital bed while looking at her pulse oximeter (Figure 8.5). The room appears out of focus (a common trope of filmmakers to show disorientation). This realization leads to a severe agitation, screaming, "Help Mom, God, Dad! "The film then moves more chronologically to show Susannah's distress at her deteriorating mental state. At a confusing birthday picnic, 24-year-old Susannah first notices that something is wrong. She has a brief spell of zoning out (cleverly done by fading out voices with sounds rapidly ramping up again). Soon, she hears voices, feels disoriented in the city, and steps in front of taxi cabs. Mounting paranoia follows, and she feels persecuted by a drippy faucet in her apartment and screams at it: "What!? Do it again!" It is not much better at work, where she climbs on cabinets and shrieks at her colleagues. Susannah feels that her "sense of self" is disappearing. (High-pitched ringing, skewed camera angles, and overlapping voices are used for emphasis.) She sees a psychiatrist and bluntly tells him she has bipolar disease. (After he challenges her, she responds, "I looked it up on Google.") He has no difficulty prescribing medication to see if it makes a difference. A defining moment is when she has a seizure. Despite this, she is told by one nurse that it is "all in your head" and repeatedly by a physician that she has simply been "partying too hard" and has alcohol withdrawal symptoms. Her frustrated, aggressive father, Tom (Richard Armitage), explodes: "find out what is wrong with my daughter!" However, her mother (Carrie-Anne Moss) is more quietly assertive: "Dr. Ryan, why don't you do further testing before you send her to a psychiatric hospital?" Eventually, Dr Najjar shows up and makes a plan after he discovers spatial neglect with the clock-drawing test, which indicates to him that one part of the brain is not functioning and also rules out schizophrenia.[20] In the hallway, he tells the parents that the best way to treat her is to do a brain biopsy and to confirm the diagnosis, adding with some coercion, "I would do it if it were my child."

The film certainly captures the relatively protracted prodromes of anti-NMDA receptor encephalitis ("Feels like my head is fuzzy all the time," "numbness in her arms"), and Susannah is finally admitted to

---

[19] See his work on the link between psychosis and NMDA encephalitis: Najjar S, Pearlman DM, Alper K, Najjar A, Devinsky O. Neuroinflammation and Psychiatric Illness. *J Neuroinflammation*. 2013;10:43; and Najjar S, Steiner J, Najjar A, Bechter K. A Clinical Approach to New-Onset Psychosis Associated with Immune Dysregulation: The Concept of Autoimmune Psychosis. *J Neuroinflammation*. 2018;15:40.

[20] This is yet another example of the "genius" neurologist finding something other have not even considered and something screenwriters love (See Chapter 3.) This symptom is a very unusual presentation in a disorder that typically presents with pressured speech, faciobrachial dyskinesia, dystonic postures, and seizures. See Dalmau J, Graus F. Antibody-Mediated Encephalitis. *N Engl J Med*. 2018;378:840–851.

a hospital at her family's insistence. Both the memoir and the film were created in the hopes of educating the public about anti-NMDA receptor encephalitis. From instantaneous mood swings to seizures that felt truly genuine, Moretz grasped the right emotions and physical expressions as well as the histrionics. The film is an accurate depiction of autoimmune encephalitis. At the time of Cahalan's diagnosis, approximately 200 patients had been described by Dalmau and co-authors, and the diagnosis was still quite new. The link with psychosis was largely unknown. At the time, performing a brain biopsy in unexplained encephalitis was not unusual but now is largely abandoned due to the ease of diagnosis with CSF for antibody study. In several invited talks, Cahalan has explained her disorder (and, not unexpectedly, received an endorsement from the Encephalitis Society). In addition, she has become interested in "misdiagnosed psychiatry,"[21] has denounced the stigmatization of mental illness, and highlights what she perceives as the flaws of the discipline of psychiatry. Also, following the publication of her book, she has implied—rightly or wrongly—that people have been diagnosed because of what she wrote.

End Credits

Psychiatry has inspired many films including films where agitation is misdiagnosed and quickly treated aggressively without a clear diagnosis. Some shocking examples have been shown, such as *Bigger Than Life* on cortisone-induced psychosis with use of cortisone, and *One Flew Over the Cuckoo's Nest*,[22] which implied that ECT was administered as the ultimate punishment for bad behavior, and, more definitively, that lobotomy was an option for permanent behavior modification.

Films on the intersection of neurology and psychiatry are far less common but no less of interest. It began by filming soldiers back from battle and diagnosed as deeply suffering from some mental problem ("the psychoneurotic" or "hysterics"). Malingering was always on the mind of the brass but much less on the mind of military psychiatrists and interested filmmakers such as the neurologist Hurst and the amateur hypnotist, psychoanalysis enthusiast, and filmmaker John Huston. The suggestion that it takes very little to be thought of as mentally ill is, of course, a great story to tell, and so Cahalan's story was quickly picked up.

Be that as it may, functional disease is of interest to some filmmakers. Patients with functional neurologic disease may present acutely to the emergency department with symptoms similar to epileptic seizure, stroke, or other neurological conditions.[23] After the diagnosis is made, few clinical neurologists and psychiatrists want to manage patients with these functional symptoms. Not only was little known about the treatment and origin (and still is), but for many patients, the symptoms persisted for months or progressed to other symptoms, eventually leading to a state of disability. Functional disease cannot be associated with a reproducible, observable pathophysiological mechanism. Treatments such as hypnosis, electrical stimulation, and barbiturate injections have all been rightfully abandoned. Specialization in medicine separated areas of expertise, and functional neurology was stuck in the middle, even though it stayed as a subcategory in the DSM classification[24] as somatic symptom disorder. There is now some willingness to accept a possible disconnection syndrome in the brain, but psychosomatic medicine, clinical psychology, and medical specialties all have their own monolithic views, which unfortunately have important consequences for patients. Neurology may indeed be guilty of calling these disorders "not my problem," but there is now a new international multi-disciplinary and multi-perspective group (the FND Society) with an ambitious agenda. It starts with accepting that there is a problem with the

---

[21] Cahalan S. *The Great Pretender: The Undercover Mission That Changed Our Understanding of Madness*. New York: Grand Central Publishing; 2019.

[22] Forman M. *One Flew over the Cuckoo's Nest*. United Artists. November 19, 1975.

[23] Finkelstein SA, Cortel-LeBlanc MA, Cortel-LeBlanc A, Stone J. Functional Neurological Disorder in the Emergency Department. *Acad Emerg Med*. 2021;28:685-696.

[24] Perhaps one of the more important developments was the reclassification of diseases. After many years of synonyms for psychiatric diagnosis, a widely recognized classification appeared. *The Diagnostic and Statistical Manual of Mental Disorders* (DSM) named and classified the main psychiatric disorders and personality disorders.

functioning of the nervous system—a brain-network problem or a problem with the brain's "software" rather than its "hardware." But in modern parlance and the movies, "hysterical" symptoms are easily interpreted as the result of a strong emotion. In *The Godfather* (1972) Michael Corleone (Al Pacino) blurts out, "She is hysterical,"[25] when his sister Connie goes after him, linking the word hysteria to female nervous breakdowns.

And the film director's point? It may be the deceit they are after, mocking physicians making mistakes and blaming it all on them. As long as the perception remains that physicians misdiagnose, misjudge, and mistreat psychiatric disorders with mind-numbing drugs, and a belief that psychiatry cannot get its act together in terms of categorizing mental illness (i.e., inventing new afflictions as they go along and crossing ethical lines), filmmakers will have no lack of material. But we all know the current practice of psychiatry has evolved significantly from its early history, and psychiatrists, psychologists, and many other allied healthcare providers admirably treat the entire spectrum of mental health needs.

---

[25] Of course, she was irate because she was certain that Michael had ordered the execution of her husband.

9

Neurofollies in Film

Leave me alone. My brain is torturing me. I cannot seem to control it.

Crimson (1973)

Main Themes

Some screenwriters worship at the altar of folly and let their imagination run wild. Without taking oneself too seriously, one could question whether neurology is an appropriate topic for entertainment. Although we may condemn the practice, exaggerations and absurdities by scriptwriters proliferate in the film industry. In fact, screenplays may be more compelling to the audience when there is novel, creative exaggeration and silliness, which I mean in the best possible way. The rebellious filmmaker Jean-Luc Godard famously said, "Cinema is the most beautiful fraud in the world." Some may protest this contention, but isn't it ironic that absurdly cunning films showing minimal regard for the major neurologic disorders are sometimes highly appreciated? One only must turn to *Extreme Measures* and *The Death of Mr Lazarescu* to make this point.

Historically, from the very first moment that silent film came on the scene, absurdism has been held in high esteem, and early plots were pure fantasy. Later, a considerable amount of neurologic nonsense emerged in horror movies involving the brain (*The Brain Eaters* [1958], *Brain Damage* [1988]) but these films are a particular genre. There is a renewed interest in zombie and vampire themes. Epidemics of scavenging undead appear to have become an industry, often specifically related to rabies encephalitis or some fictional infection of some mutated rabies virus. The *Resident Evil* game and later movie series started it all by proposing a rabies-like virus as a catalyst of zombies, which spawned multiple horror flicks. In *I am a Legend* (2007), a genetically engineered measles virus is responsible for a plague that produces zombie-like creatures. In addition, the exceedingly rare psychiatric disorder called Cotard's syndrome supposedly causes people to "act like zombies." The syndrome is characterized by nihilistic delusions ranging from denial of parts of the body to the delusion of being dead and decomposing. Moreover, the psychoactive drug Spice (an herbal mixture sprayed with synthetic cannabinoids) has been called the "zombie drug." All these attempts to link psychiatric and neurologic manifestations to a pop-culture phenomenon are a cheap way to attract attention.[1]

Some films in this "folly" category are classic, just plain ridiculous comedies. For example, *The Man with Two Brains* [1983] features Steve Martin as Dr. Hfuhruhurr, famous for the so-called cranial screw-top brain surgery, who falls in love with the brain of a young woman. Sadly, her brain has been preserved in a jar in a Vienna laboratory.

---

[1] For the link between rabies and zombification See Verran J, Reyes XA. Emerging Infectious Literature and the Zombie Condition. *Emerg Infect Dis.* 2018;24:1774–1778 Also Berrios GE, Luque R. Cotard's Syndrome: Analysis of 100 Cases. *Acta Psychiatr Scand.* 1995;91:185–188 and Pintori N, Loi B, Mereu M. Synthetic Cannabinoids: The Hidden Side of Spice Drugs. *Behav Pharmacol.* 2017;28:409–419.

DOI: 10.1201/9781003270874-9

Other films may just have a single "funny" scene. The John Landis-directed slapstick *Kentucky Fried Movie* (1977) has a scene in a "headache research center." Patients are shown with their heads being slammed against the wall, hit by reflex hammers, and struck with glass bottles—all to test the painkiller "Sanhedrin Extra Strength."

Neurologic absurdity also extends into science fiction. We should not be surprised to see mind control, brain stimulation, "entering" the mind, and other far-out stories such as the murderous monomaniacal epileptic. Another nifty concept is a neurologic injury that gives the villain an advantage, such as *The World Is Not Enough* ⋏⋏⋏ directed by Michael Apted. In this film, the villain, a KGB agent turned terrorist, takes a bullet through the medulla oblongata, "killing off his senses," which enables him to "push himself harder than any normal man."

Futuristic neurology may seem very real to some, close to home and not at all implausible or preposterous; that is where partly the interest lies. A perceptive analysis of science fiction and neurology may be of widespread interest without revealing much because neurology in science fiction is sparingly represented.

I see no room for absurdist horror in this book, and there is significant use of neurosurgical procedures in these body-horror films that are gradually entering mainstream cinema.[2] I have selected films that present an absurd theme creatively, effectively, and with enough plausibility that the viewer can almost suspend disbelief; we can all cite many others done poorly.

So, it all becomes swirling speculation ungrounded in evidence. But, let's enjoy the fine irony, smirk at the sweet folly, and laugh at these nonsensical films.

Is That So? Finding "Hidden" Neurologic Disease

Medicine in art can be cataloged in different ways, and it depends on how much an interpreter wants to add general humanistic elements to the subject matter (e.g., places of care, showing suffering, healing, and death beds.[3]) Another popular diversion is to find previously unknown connections. This intellectual exercise may range from foolishness to seriousness. Neurology in the Art has been studied from different aspects. It may have started with figurines on Greco-Roman pottery and medieval statues. Interpretation of anomalies of body anatomy in several art forms is a fascinating game.

Paintings and painters can be interesting to check out. A painter with progressive neurologic disease may change his style, or a painting may suggest neurologic disease. It may require a closer look at their brushstrokes over time (Manet, Dalí and de Kooning). Neurologists have published on the Babinski's sign in Renaissance paintings. Babinski's sign (spreading of toes and upgoing big toe in babies) was found in one out of three paintings. It remains unclear why, and sometimes it appears the sole is inadvertently touched. Other epochs offer few examples of Babinski's signs, particularly in DaVinci's work. More recently, attention was drawn to Andrew Wyeth's iconic painting, *Christina's World*. It portrays a woman in the grass in the barren landscape of coastal Maine, seen from behind, wearing a pink dress and with probable Charcot-Marie-Tooth disease. (This hereditary neuropathy was first suggested by the neurologist and neuromuscular disease expert Robert Pascuzzi.) Christine Olson often moved across her family property by crawling. Wyeth painted her after he observed her dragging her body across the field. The painting reveals visible atrophy of her arms and legs. The diagnosis is also plausible because photos

---

[2] The Palme D'Or winner *Titane* (2012), directed by Julia Ducournau, shows the placement of a titanium mesh cranioplasty and suggests that it causes (or enhances) extreme love for metal and even sexual intercourse with a car resulting in pregnancy and birth of a bionic baby.

[3] Bordin G, Polo D'Ambrosio L. *Medicine in Art (A Guide to Imagery)*. English, Paperback ed. Los Angeles, CA: Getty Publications; 2010. In this magisterial collection, the authors have grouped medicine in painting into a number of categories; from physician consultation at the bedside to autopsies as well as depictions of pain and surgical interventions. Diseases are mostly representations of scourges in the Dark Ages (plague, scrofula, leprosy).

and descriptions of Christina Olson's disability are widely available.[4] However, another paper on neuromuscular disease was criticized for its loose interpretations of claw hands in ulnar neuropathies.[5]

Similarly, an occasional enthusiast may comb films for neurologic themes even when there was never an obvious intent by the filmmaker or even an allegory. These tantalizing interpretations generate interest—and publications—but we all know it can be misdirected. Physicians and other health care workers, particularly observant neurologists, have the innate urge to speculate about which disease, which symptom, and which sign indicates a neurologic disease concealed in the plot.

Finding neurology in the arts (and film) is a type of iconology, and trying a diagnosis becomes "icono-diagnosis." An iconological investigation looks at the sociohistorical values that the artist might not have consciously considered but are nevertheless present. Films can also be willfully misinterpreted by those scouting for clues, and once found, these interpretations can stick tenaciously if they lend an aura of scientific authority. We should not forget that deep readings often cover up a simpler explanation, and this definitively applies to cinema. Don't expect a filmmaker to go too deep in the complex field of neurology diagnosis and neurologic disease. The thought that early filmmakers would greatly research neurologic disease and spend inordinate time to get the neurologic picture right through consulting specialists may be a little foolhardy.

In Chapter 4, we saw icono-diagnosis in *A Matter of Life and Death*, where Peter's symptom of smelling fried onions was interpreted as uncinate hallucinations. Hogan, who first found the association, was followed by Friedman (Chapter 4), who admits she had only partial answers and used a "flood of associations" to make her point.[6] This film's original intent was to serve as an ode to the brotherhood of mankind, showing statues of historically prominent men on the stairway to heaven and a pro-American trial by a heavenly tribunal. It emphasizes the remarkable diversity of Americans, their openness, and their opportunities, all with the intent to smooth post-war tensions between Britain and the United States. (Powell reminisced in an interview that he was asked by Jack Beddington, head of the Ministry of Information's film commission, to make this original film because "when we were losing the war, our relationships with the Americans were very good, but now we're winning the war they are not so good"). Peter (David Niven) experienced spells with vivid and detailed hallucinatory worlds, but these were just a clever ploy to create a parallel story and two worlds. It is inconceivable Powell and Pressburger wanted to highlight the intricacies of neurosurgical procedures, the esoteric manifestations of some brain tumors, or the complexity of neurology in general. But by collecting neurologic material (or something that looked neurological such as brain paintings on the wall), they worked hard to make it all look plausible—and what fun it must have been to reveal later that the brain surgeon is the judge of the tribunal (i.e., God).

We may see icono-diagnosis in films in which the protagonists have spells. For example, in *Beanpole* (2019), the protagonist has blackouts that strongly resemble complex partial seizures (now called focal onset impaired awareness seizures). She stares into space and has episodes in which her body freezes

4 See Sellal F, Tatu L. The Babinski Sign in Renaissance Paintings-A Reappraisal of the Toe Phenomenon in Representations of the Christ Child: Observational Analysis. *BMJ.* 2020;371:m4556. See Pascuzzi RM, Brooks JO. Neurology in the Art Museum: Andrew Wyeth's Christina's World. *Semin Neurol.* 2000;20:255–259 and Patterson MC, Cole TB, Siegel E, Mackowiak PA. A Patient as Art: Andrew Wyeth's Portrayal of Christina Olson's Neurologic Disorder in Christina's World. *J Child Neurol.* 2017;32:647–649.

5 See Vein AA, Mouret A. Claw Hand in a Renaissance Portrait. *Lancet Neurol.* 2018;17:742 and Charlier P, Lippi D, Perciaccante A, Appenzeller O, Bianucci R. Neurological Disorder? No, Mannerism. *Lancet Neurol.* 2019;18:135.

6 Hogan DB. Temporal Lobe Epilepsy in the Cinema. *Arch Neurol.* 1982;39:738 and Friedman D. *A Matter of Life and Death. The Brain Revealed by the Mind of Michael Powell.* Bloomington: Author House; 2008. See Criterion Edition and visual essay on why film was made—https://www.criterion.com/films/28833-a-matter-of-life-and-death

up and she mumbles incoherently. The filmmaker used these spells as a brief metaphor for the shell-shocked Russian populace struggling to find a purpose after the Second World War.[7]

Some have interpreted the inability of the main character in Stanley Kubrick's satire *Dr Strangelove* (1964) to control his right arm as an alien hand syndrome. Dr. Strangelove's mechanical right hand has a life of its own.[8] Neurologists know that an alien hand/limb syndrome can result from callosal and parietal lesions, but it almost invariably affects the opposite left arm! But, quite frankly, Kubrick modeled this arm after the metal prosthesis of the genius scientist Dr. Rotwang (Rudolf Klein-Rogge) in Fritz Lang's *Metropolis* (1929). Rotwang lost his hand after some unnamed incident in his laboratory full of boiling chemicals, induction coils, and other puzzling machines. In a key scene in *Metropolis*, Rotwang has his stretched-out right arm in front of him, where he talks to it. He wants everyone to believe losing a hand is a price only great scientists may have to pay. Kubrick used the same idea and changed it into a nuclear incident. However, there is nothing alien to Dr Strangelove's body and mind, and most scholars agree he (not only his arm and hand) was a former Nazi. In a final scene, he rises from his wheelchair miraculously healed by a Hitler effigy ("Mein Führer, I can walk!"), ready to implement his plan to create a new breed ("a nucleus of human specimens") after the Bomb falls. Dr. Strangelove, as a symbol of fascism (and eugenics) infiltrated into military thinktanks, was always part of Kubrick and Terry Southern's screenplay, but when Peter Sellers donned the black glove, he was reminded of a stormtrooper.[9] Again, the hand (and possibly arm) was mechanical and mended to his body and not part of Strangelove's flesh and blood. Further ad-libbed and worked out by Peter Sellers, the immobile arm hangs next to him, and he "reboots" it by pouncing on it. Then, in a moment of excitement, it shoots up in a Nazi salute. Strangelove pushes it down, but it keeps popping up until he bites it, and then the prosthetic hand attempts to strangle him. (Lang, who fled Nazi Germany, surely would not have appreciated having his Dr. Rotwang re-imagined as the Nazi Dr. Strangelove.) This is, of course, far removed from the neurologic interpretation of an alien/anarchic hand syndrome when antagonistic (opposite to what they are supposed to do) movements occur in a limb.

Staying within the oeuvre of Kubrick, we can find what may well be the epitome of icono-diagnosis. *The Shining* (1980) ends with a shocking photo of a 4th of July gala party in 1921 at the Overlook Hotel, and we suddenly realize that Jack Torrance (Jack Nicholson) was in the Overlook Hotel before. Kubrick suggested in an interview that he was reincarnated as a monster. The original photo of the man who was taken out of the photo (and replaced by Jack Nicholson for the film) is now known. The authors carefully looked at the original photo of this man, and based on frontal baldness, hollowed cheeks, drooping mouth, and ptosis, and declared that this erased man could have the genetic disease myotonic dystrophy, type 1. Furthermore, the authors also suggest that Kubrick deliberately chose the picture to demonstrate "a clue to the deep connection which links together the past and present inhabitants of the cursed hotel in almost a genetic way."[10]

Interested readers may seek out *Cleopatra* (1963). Julius Caesar's late-onset epilepsy has intrigued many writers including Shakespeare. Epilepsy was common throughout history, and the Romans

[7] Balagov K. *Beanpole*. MUBI. May 16, 2019. Director Kantemir Balagov's major themes are the trauma of the injured Soviet soldiers and class disparity in the post-Second World War Soviet Union.

[8] Murdoch M, Hill J, Barber M. Strangled by Dr Strangelove? Anarchic Hand Following a Posterior Cerebral Artery Ischemic Stroke. *Age Aging*. 2021;50:263–264. And Biran I, Chatterjee A. Alien Hand Syndrome. *Arch Neurol*. 2004;61:292–294. For the Rotwang-Dr Strangelove connections see the *Stanley Kubrick Archives* by Alison Castle Taschen (2008) and Rotwang and Sons in *Mad, Bad, Dangerous The Scientist and the Cinema* by Christopher Frayling. London: Reaktion Books; 2005. The gloved puppet idea was mentioned in *Roger Lewis and Peter Sellers. The Life and Death of Peter Sellers Applause Theatre & Cinema Books (2000)*. For the Nazi connection see Krämer P, *Dr Strangelove*. (BFI Classics) 2014.

[9] The screenwriters also toyed with a possible link to Sooty, the gloved bear puppet bear created by puppeteer Harry Corbett for BBC's *The Sooty Show*, a long-running children's television series.

[10] Oh, come on! Let me up the ante. How about the lady next to him with drooping eyes and the man behind him with a very long jaw? Might they have, respectively, congenital myasthenia and mitochondrial or congenital myopathy? For additional entertainment, see Brigo F, Igwe SC, Bragazzi NL. Kubrick's *The Shining* and the Erased Myopathic Face. *Neurol Sci*. 2017;38:2227–2228.

recognized it. Most medical historians accept the diagnosis of epilepsy in Caesar, and debate focuses on possible causes. This issue has sparked wild speculation including one neurologist who suggested a neuroinfectious cause—another example of icono-diagnosis.[11] Others still debate whether he even had seizures.[12] In *Cleopatra*, Caesar (Rex Harrison) proclaims, "One day it will happen where I cannot hide, where the world shall see me fail … I shall foam at the mouth, and they will tear me to pieces."

Many of the "symptoms" of vampirism (again) suggested rabies encephalitis infection with light sensitivity, heightened senses, unusual food and drink cravings, fatigue, headaches, and altered sensorium.[13] Others have seen acute porphyria or lead poisoning in Count Dracula (neuropathy) and myasthenia gravis as a graft-versus-host disease in Boris Karloff's portrayal of Frankenstein's monster.[14]

Filmmakers derive considerable amusement from these interpretations. Many may have physician friends and may enjoy hearing them "talk shop,"[15] but little recorded communication between them has surfaced. In Erasmus' words, should we praise folly? I consider much icono-neurology in films to be purely nonsensical, and that is putting it mildly. The main motivation may be to get attention by introducing an unusual angle and a stunt. It often feels more flippant than considered. And remember, when movies are mentioned, people notice.

Does Implausible Neurology Look Plausible?

The main purpose of this chapter is to discuss films with potential plausibility, films with a high degree of implausibility, and to explore how these fantastic ideas could have originated. The themes I found are— prepare yourself—how to enter the mind, a psychic mind after coma or a brain tumor, a pill to stimulate the mind, and brain transplantation. The following ten representative films are presented in detail.

Mine the Mind

The brain and mind: how far can our fantasies go? Here are some examples. *Donovan's Brain* (1953) ᚻᚻᚻ is directed by Felix Feist and has become a cult classic of science fiction. It stars Lew Ayres, Gene Evans, Nancy Davis (Reagan), and Steve Brodie. Dr. Cory ("Kildare" Lew Ayres) experiments with monkey brains by placing them in solutions, applying electrodes, registering brain waves, and imaging these with an oscillograph. When he is called to assess a plane crash, he steals the brain from the corpse of a well-known businessman. Unbeknownst to Dr. Cory, the man indulged in questionable business practices. Dr. Cory preserves this human brain with the same methods used for monkey brains. Electrodes pick up activity, and the brain glows and pulsates. ("It looks like a beta frequency … oh it is … the brain must be

---

[11] McLachlan RS. Julius Caesar's Late Onset Epilepsy: A Case of Historic Proportions. *Can J Neurol Sci*. 2010;37:557–561.

[12] See Cawthorne T. Julius Caesar and the Falling Sickness. *Proc R Soc Med*. 1958;51:27–30; Galassi FM, Ashrafian H. Has the Diagnosis of a Stroke Been Overlooked in the Symptoms of Julius Caesar? *Neurol Sci*. 2015;36:1521–1522; Montemurro N, Benet A, Lawton MT. Julius Caesar's Epilepsy: Was It Caused by a Brain Arteriovenous Malformation? *World Neurosurg*. 2015;84:1985–1987; Hughes JR. Dictator Perpetuus: Julius Caesar–Did He Have Seizures? If So, What Was the Etiology? *Epilepsy Behav*. 2004;5:756–764; and Bruschi F. Was Julius Caesar's Epilepsy Due to Neurocysticercosis? *Trends Parasitol*. 2011;27:373–374.

[13] Rabies can spread rapidly through a vampire bat colony. See Johnson N, Arechiga-Ceballos N, Aguilar-Setien A. Vampire Bat Rabies: Ecology, Epidemiology and Control. *Viruses*. 2014;6:1911–1928 and Wilkinson GS. Vampire Bats. *Curr Biol*. 2019;29:R1216–R1217.

[14] Pascuzzi RM. Pearls and Pitfalls in the Horror Cinema. *Semin Neurol*. 1998;18:267–273. The author cites bilateral "wrist drops" and photosensitivity as arguments to consider acute intermittent porphyria. The author claims the atypical ptosis worsens with light exposure in Frankenstein's monster supporting myasthenia gravis. The paper is pervasively tongue-in-cheek and amusing. The author closes with "Wishing not to offend the readers of Seminars, I shall not print the collective reaction of my respected neurologic colleagues!"

[15] Ingmar Bergman, for example, had many friends who practiced medicine, which may explain why Bergman featured so many physicians in his films and definitively more than other filmmakers.

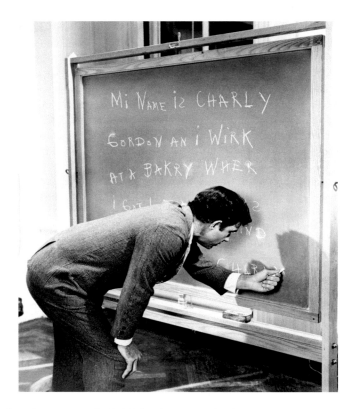

FIGURE 9.1   The absurd writing in *Charly* (Cliff Robertson is Charley; Everett Collection, Inc.).

thinking systematically.") Through telepathy—and here it becomes even more dicey—"the brain" makes Dr. Cory act out the businessman's bad intentions.[16]

Of course, this must stop, and in the final scene, "the brain" gets shot—but to no avail. Only after connecting it with electrical wires to a lightning rod during a storm is "the brain" destroyed by incineration. Dr. Cory is saved and confesses that things got out of hand. It is suggested that he may even survive a medical board examination into his ethics. If that happens, he floats the idea of coming back as a "country doctor," to which his wife (Nancy Davis) responds, "No, dear, you are a scientist and always will be."

Charly (1968) ∿∿∿, directed by Ralph Nelson, stars Cliff Robertson, Claire Bloom, and Leon Janney. Charly (Cliff Robertson) has a disability: an IQ of only 59 ("retardate"), and at his work, he is often the butt of jokes. Testing shows that he has difficulty writing and often writes in mirror images (Figure 9.1). When Charly is subjected to a maze test identical to one traversed by a mouse, the mouse beats him consistently. Charly wants to be smarter and undergoes (unspecified) brain surgery, which improves his cognition. He becomes highly intelligent and suddenly has a good grasp of abstract theoretical metaphysics. His IQ now approaches genius category. He is now also serious marriage material and develops a relationship with his former schoolteacher, Alice Kinian (Claire Bloom), but emotionally he remains a child. Unfortunately, his intelligence fades, and because of this decisive turn, he is unable to marry Alice—even when she insists. The film ends on a sad note. The movie *Charly* was adapted from the novel *Flowers for Algernon* (the name of the mouse). It is difficult to grasp why (in

---

[16] See Naci L, Monti MM, Cruse D, et al. Brain-Computer Interfaces for Communication with Nonresponsive Patients. *Ann Neurol.* 2012;72:312–323 and Owen AM, Hampshire A, Grahn JA, et al. Putting Brain Training to the Test. *Nature.* 2010;465:775–778.

the 1960s) brain surgery was suggested to improve intelligence. The film is more about the limitations of living with a disability and being out of touch, which may have explained its great success. A personal favorite of many baby boomers, the film was commended by the Presidential Committee for Mental Retardation, although one could argue that it exploited intellectual disability. Cliff Robertson, in the title role, won an Academy Award for Best Actor.

BrainWaves (1983) 〽〽〽, directed by Ulli Lommel, is a science fiction film starring Tony Curtis, Keir Dullea, Suzanna Love, and Vera Miles. The theme is the replacement of defective areas of the brain with new (presumably positive) brain activity. The head neuroscientist, Dr. Clavius (Tony Curtis), extracts neuronal activity from the brains of fresh corpses and loads it into a computer. (The assumption here is that although the body is dead, the brain still has electric activity.) This is how it works. First, Dr. Clavius maps the brain of a comatose patient and identifies the "defective areas." He then uses this map to replace damaged neuronal activity with new electrical activity he has previously stored on a computer, as if he is simply replacing parts. Everyone in the film seems impressed. There is a discussion in which one of the neurosurgeons' remarks about this neuroscientist, "Dr. Clavius's methods can be unusual, but his work and his results are extraordinary." Then a traffic accident puts the leading female character into coma. To help her regain consciousness, Dr. Clavius—looking deadly serious—plans to awaken her with the neuronal pattern of someone else. The film shows her brain being "fed" brainwaves, and she awakens and gradually recovers all function. However, she begins to have night terrors, and it appears that she has been given the "neuronal pattern" of a young girl who was murdered. She not only sees images of this girl's murder but eventually is able to recognize the identity of the girl's killer. *BrainWaves* suggests that not only can EEG activity be captured, stored, and transplanted but also that EEG represents thought and memory. There is not a sliver of accuracy in this dark film.

Phenomenon (1996) 〽〽〽, starring John Travolta, Kyra Sedgwick, and Robert Duvall and directed by Jon Turteltaub, is about George Malley (John Travolta), who looks up and sees a bright light from the sky that knocks him unconscious. This is a life-changing event. He now reads more than two books a day, effortlessly completes difficult crossword puzzles, and notes that everything seems "clearer" to him. But there is more: George now "feels" pre-earthquake activity and develops levitational and telekinetic abilities. With his super intelligence, he can decode top-secret signals. The film becomes more preposterous when his unusual symptomatology is attributed to a brain tumor, and this constitutes a surprise ending. Apparently, this malignant astrocytoma does not cause impairment, but, in fact, its "tentacles" stimulate parts of the brain. This attracts the attention of the medical community, and George is admitted for observation. One neurosurgeon suggests performing awake surgery "to understand his brain better," and he hopes he will be "science's greatest teacher." When George realizes that this surgery will likely be fatal, he escapes. He dies suddenly and peacefully in the arms of his lover, with his last words being "It's happening." The film represents a gross misrepresentation of the progression of a malignant brain tumor. The film also grossly misrepresents medical science and suggests there is an inclination of neurosurgeons to experiment on unusual cases.

The Cell (2000) 〽〽〽, starring Jennifer Lopez, Vince Vaughn, and Vincent D'Onofrio and directed by Tarsem Singh, suggests that future advances might enable a person to enter the mind of another. This is a complex thriller that involves a schizophrenic killer named Stargher (Vincent D'Onofrio), who lapses into a catatonic state after a recent crime and after he notices he is being tailed by the FBI. (To be fair, we see a very good representation of catatonia here, with what appears to be a rigid composure, a fixed gaze, shivering, and sweating.) Without giving away too much of the plot, it becomes clear to the investigators that the only way to solve the main character's crime is to enter his mind. Using sophisticated technology ("Neuromed"), child psychologist Catherine Deane (Jennifer Lopez) accomplishes this. The film is cinematically spectacular, and scenes show Stargher's early memories and traumas as a child as well as fantastical gothic worlds. The film suggests that our memories are simply boxed-in stories that we can revisit. The brain of this psychopathic killer is full of violent, vivid imagery and simmers with anger. The "Neuromed" technology shown in this film will immediately remind neurologists of a functional MRI, and "Neuromed" seems like the next advancement in MRI technology. There is no question that MRI technology has contributed greatly to our understanding of brain activity; it has already demonstrated that certain brain areas become activated by motor tasks and emotions. In recent studies of unresponsive patients, communication has been established through complex pathways in one or two patients, but there is not yet a reproducible way of doing that. For many rehabilitation physicians, it is unclear whether a consistent response can be generated that would allow a brain–computer interface to function. In its defense, this film suggests how to "communicate" with unresponsive patients and may have a kernel of truth. Of course, to "enter" a mind is unfathomable.

In *Limitless* (2011) ⌐, which stars Bradley Cooper, Abbie Cornish, and Robert De Niro and was directed by Neil Burger, Eddie (Bradley Cooper) has writer's block and is told that a pill can improve his brain function. Eddie further learns that "typically, we only access 20% of our brain" and his brain will work much better by taking a small, colorless pill containing a neurostimulant. When he does, his senses drastically improve, and this is cleverly depicted by suddenly changing the scene hues from dark blue into gold yellow. His eyes now have a light blue color. He starts writing his book. The neurotropic drug is called NZT48. Eddie also uses his dramatically improved brain function to play the stock market and become wealthy.

The film poses an interesting question: can drugs improve brain function, assuming that there are dormant areas (apparently 80% according to this script) that need to be stimulated? The unfortunate fact is that no drug can.[17] Many stimulants (amphetamines, cocaine, and ecstasy) change the senses temporarily, but none improve productivity, artistic ability, or intelligence. Similar statements have been made about alcohol and writers, but there is no evidence that there has ever been a consistent positive effect. Stimulants have major side effects, including hallucinations and behavioral changes, and the sad truth is that drug use by artists (writers, composers, actors) often leads to addiction and sometimes death.

The question of how much brain we actually use fascinates screenwriters. According to them, it may not amount to much (20% according to the creators of *Limitless*), and in *Lucy* (2014) ⌐, the active part of the brain is set even lower at 10%. Neurons may indeed take up only 10%, but guess what? We use 100% of the brain most of the time.

Awakening in a Strange New World

The Dead Zone (1983) ⌐⌐⌐, starring Christopher Walken, Brooke Adams, and Tom Skerritt and directed by David Cronenberg, is adapted from a novel by Stephen King. The protagonist Johnny (played by Christopher Walken) wakes up in a skilled nursing facility. His physician, Dr. Weizak, explains that he has been in a motor vehicle accident. ("You have been our guest here for a while.") Johnny looks confused and finds he has no bandages or visible injury and asks why he is in here. His parents arrive and tell Johnny that he has been unconscious for five years. ("The Lord has delivered you from your trance.") Dr. Weizak, visibly irritated, corrects them, "No, he has been in a coma, not in a trance." As a rehabilitation physician, Dr. Weizak proclaims, "Your therapy will be long and painful, but you will walk."

Johnny discovers he has "extrasensory perception." When he touches a nurse, he has a vision that her daughter is in a fire. (This vision turns out to be true, and she is saved as a result.) When he touches Dr. Weizak, Johnny has a vision of violent Second World War scenes of people fleeing Poland. (Johnny tells Doctor Weizak his mother is still alive, and it turns out that this, too, is true.) It is now clear that Johnny has become psychic. He cannot only see the future but can also change it by altering events. These premonitory signs are a major plotline in the movie.

Most viewers will understand that premonitions do not occur after a severe traumatic brain injury (and certainly not after a 5-year vegetative state). However, severe traumatic brain injury leading to prolonged coma may be followed by a post-traumatic stress disorder involving night terrors. Receiving visions (or even a sense of coming doom) is not a manifestation of severe brain injury. However,

---

[17] McDaniel MA, Maier SF, Einstein GO. "Brain-specific" Nutrients: A Memory Cure? *Nutrition*. 2003;19:957–975.

personalities can change after a traumatic brain injury—and imaginative screenwriters may ask why not for the good? A similar theme arises in the film *Regarding Henry* (Chapter 3).

The Dead Zone is emblematic of Cronenberg's catalog of films with hallucinatory surreal worlds, and it remains a classic Stephen King novel. Recovery from a vegetative state is not common. It is virtually impossible after 5 years, by which time patients lose all cognitive function and, most certainly, do not acquire pre-cognition. But the act of awakening after many years continues to fascinate and inspire writers.

One recent film seems to top them all. *Isn't It Romantic (2019)* ⋔, directed by Todd Strauss-Schulson, stars Rebel Wilson. Her character gets mugged and, while running away, hits her head against a metal pole. She awakens from coma in a lovely emergency room ("this is not an emergency room; this is Williams and Sonoma"). When she leaves the emergency room, she enters a sugarcoated wonderland called New York, a far cry from the dilapidation she remembers—and she dates the perfect boyfriend! But then it turns out she was in a drug-induced coma, and the wonderful new life was merely a dream. Once she wakes up, she is instantaneously cognitively intact, shows an unprecedented energy and sparkle, and intimately connects with her boss. The film suggests that everything is possible after a severe traumatic head injury but also a newly found romance can be a byproduct of brain damage.

One comedy on traumatic brain injury can probably be ignored. *Post Concussion* (1999) ⋔ deals with a person with a concussion who is unable to go back to work and has a lot of headaches. He is tested for personality and recall. He has a virtually impossible line to repeat: "Though they had bad disguises, it was their inscrutable style that allowed them to escape the dogged policemen." Then he is blindfolded and performs a round-hole test. The narrator comments that "the medical profession does not understand the psychological ones." After these tests, he is declared unfit for work. There is little substance in this film; testing of brain-injured patients is ridiculed, and much of the script is objectionable.

When Amnesia Actually Helps

We can expect that any type of amnesia to be concocted by a screenwriter. They are not necessarily amnesias that could be interpreted as functional amnesia. Whatever the cause, amnesia usually debilitates; in these films, however, there is humorous advantage.

The Penalty (1920) ⋔, directed by Wallace Worsley, stars Lon Chaney as Blizzard. The neurosurgeon Dr. Ferris mistakenly amputates both legs of a child with polytrauma and a traumatic brain injury. Grown up, he becomes the leader of the criminal underworld (Blizzard) and plans a revenge. He forces Ferris to reattach new legs, but while Blizzard is under anesthesia, Ferris also manages to do brain surgery to make Blizzard forget what has happened to him and which makes him a better person.

50 First Dates (2004) ⋔⋔ stars Adam Sandler, Drew Barrymore, Rob Schneider, and Dan Aykroyd; it is directed by Peter Segal. After a motor vehicle accident, Lucy (Drew Barrymore) forgets every day or, as her family friend says, "It's like her slate gets wiped clean every time she sleeps." The film is a screwball comedy. Every day, Lucy wakes up thinking it is October 13—the day of the accident—and all her days are similar. The whole family plays along. Eventually, she discovers, by seeing a newspaper with a different date, that she has been deceived. She sees a neurologist (Dan Aykroyd), who tells her that the condition is known as the "Goldfield Syndrome," named for a brilliant Lithuanian psychiatrist, which leaves her unable to convert short-term memory into long-term memory. The neurologist points to her parietal lobe and proclaims, "I see that your sense of humor is intact. You have a magnificent amygdala as well." Because Lucy's memory loss is a surprise and major disappointment for her, the neurologist introduces her to "Ten-Second Tom," who apparently forgets everything every 10 seconds and, in one scene, repeatedly introduces himself to others. There is some truth to the existence of this type of amnesic syndrome, and it reminds us of the film *Memento* (2000). There is a detailed discussion on this type of amnesic syndrome in Chapter 3.

The amnestic theme appears in other films. In *Clean Slate* (1994) 🎬🎬, the protagonist has no problems with his memory during wakefulness but loses his memories during sleep. Inability to memorize is well documented but losing all memories during sleep is not.

Another noteworthy movie is *Groundhog Day* (1990) 🎬, in which all of the actors forget prior events, allowing the leading character (Bill Murray) to correct—and that is the point—his previous blunders in courting his colleague.

Memory is a highly complex, wondrous brain function. Our worlds shrink when we lose it. We may have to conclude that accurate dramatization of acute amnesia is rare, although imaginative and artistic.

The Violent Epileptic

Adapted from a novel by Michael Crichton,[18] *The Terminal Man* (1974) 🎬🎬 stars George Segal, Joan Hackett, Richard Dysart, and Jill Clayburgh; it is directed by Mike Hodges. The film opens with a dinner-table discussion between psychiatrists and neurosurgeons about the merits of a new operation for violent seizures.[19] The surgery had been tried in animals, but Harry Benson (George Segal) is the first human patient. The surgeons implant an electrode to control the seizures electrically. Harry has violent seizures of which he has no recollection. One of the physicians says, "Nobody thinks of these people as physically ill. They are predisposed to violence, aggressive behavior, hypersexuality, pathological intoxication." Because Harry has uncontrollable rages but not physical seizures, the physicians decide to stimulate the structures of the limbic system (involved with emotion and behavior) and to proceed with "limbic brain pacing." Apparently, a computer connected to the grids will fully control the seizures.

Before the surgery, the patient and treatment proposal are presented in a conference to a group of physicians. One of the physicians stands up and starts to rail against psychosurgery and the wrongs that lobotomy has done. (He is informed that what is proposed here is not a lobotomy.) Harry undergoes an awake stereotactic operation. In the post-operative phase, each of the electrodes is stimulated, causing different sensations each time. One stimulus makes him feel that he has eaten ham sandwiches; another one induces an urge to urinate. Yet another electrode causes uncontrollable laughing while one induces him to make sexual advances to the investigator. Another stimulated electrode makes him behave "like a 5-year-old." When he describes his aura, he says he smells "pig shit and turpentine." He further describes the seizure as feeling angry and being on a rollercoaster that he cannot stop. ("There is no feeling like that in the world.") Initially, treatment seems successful, but then seizures return and are even more severe than before. Eventually, the seizures take control, and he starts killing, which is preceded by a spell shown as eyes turning up and an angry grimace (Figure 9.2).

Limbic stimulation and control of seizures with implanted electrodes that, when stimulated, cause very specific responses are the stuff of fantasy. The film does touch on reality with a partly accurate description of temporal lobe epilepsy, and the literature on violence in temporal lobe epilepsy is abundant. Most epileptologists have seen postictal violent automatisms or a verbal intermittent explosive disorder. When Michael Crichton wrote his book in the 1970s, he drew upon several actual court cases for inspiration. In his book, he justifies the plot by adding a table on the therapy of "psychomotor" epilepsy. His book is filled with neuro-images and an extensive, annotated medical reference making it all look very real. However, there have been very few acquittals of persons with epilepsy based on criminal insanity and murder because the link with temporal lobe epilepsy has not been proven. (Also, see Chapter 3 on violent sleepwalking.) The film may also refer

---

[18] Crichton wrote the screenplay and also directed *Coma* (1978), a film on organ trafficking based on the best-selling novel by Robin Cook.

[19] See Fazel S, Philipson J, Gardiner L, Merritt R, Grann M. Neurological Disorders and Violence: A Systematic Review and Meta-Analysis with a Focus on Epilepsy and Traumatic Brain Injury. *J Neurol*. 2009;256:1591–1602 and Treiman DM. Epilepsy and Violence: Medical and Legal Issues. *Epilepsia*. 1986;27(Suppl 2):S77–S104.

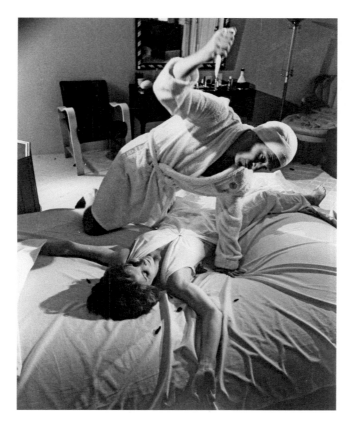

FIGURE 9.2   The killing epileptic Harry Benson (George Segal) in *Terminal Man* (United Artists / Zuma Press, Inc. / Alamy Stock Photo).

to the Klüver–Bucy syndrome, which may develop after a right temporal lobectomy to treat epilepsy and is characterized by hyperphagia and hypersexuality.

All the elements are here, and they superficially mimic the current state of treatment of intractable seizures (i.e., a vagal nerve stimulator). In the end, it does not add up, although it all seems deceptively real. It fits well in Michael Crichton's body of work with books on topics with plausible medical authenticity. When asked about the film, neurologists, epileptologists, or neurosurgeons have a lot to say and most of it is not good. For obvious reasons, epilepsy societies and epilepsy support groups found the book and film objectionable.

Brain Transplantation

The Brain That Wouldn't Die (1959) ⋀⋀⋀, starring Jason Evers, Virginia Leith, and Eddie Carmel and directed by Joseph Green, is about bringing the dead back to life and preserving a full head. In this film, Dr. Cortner (Jason Evers) is a plastic surgeon who dabbles with transplantation in his country home. The film opens with an operation performed by father and son, but the patient unfortunately dies on the table. The son asks his father if he can do an experiment because, really, "He is dead; I cannot do any harm." His father agrees. "Very well, the corpse is yours. Do what you want to do." Dr. Cortner then stimulates the brain with electrodes while his father performs open heart massage to bring the patient back. Despite this success, the father warns, "The line between scientific genius and obsessive fanaticism is a thin line." Indeed, the patient becomes a hideous creature.

In the next scene, we see Dr. Cortner driving his car with his fiancée, Jane Compton (Virginia Leith). The car careens into a ditch, and the girl is decapitated. Dr. Cortner runs away with her head to his country home/research laboratory, where he connects it to several tubes. The revived head remains fully awake, although her voice is a bit hoarse. The film ends with him trying to drug a model and to connect her perfect body to the head of his beloved. However, he fails and is killed by the monster he previously created. At this point it is nothing more than a "Franken" film.

Another brain transplantation film is *Crimson* (or *The Man with the Severed Head*) ⚡⚡ directed by Juan Fortuny.[20] A jewel heist goes awry, and the jewel thief needs a brain transplant to survive. The transplanted brain of a criminal called The Sadist takes control of his body. The film also rips off *Frankenstein* except this time as a sexploitation film. The interesting twist is that the protagonist awakens as himself but still realizes his brain is from someone else, resulting in getting tortured against his will.

It all seems ridiculous, right? Well, surprise—in 1970, the head of one monkey was transplanted on the body of another monkey, and the monkey lived for a week.[21] That might have been the end of it, but recently a proposal for the first human body-to-head transplantation has been published—the donor a brain-dead person, the recipient unclear—but the author suggested a young individual with progressive muscular dystrophy or genetic and metabolic disorders. Whether such a procedure could ever pass an institutional research board is not even a question—it is impossible.[22]

End Credits

We must avoid too much seriousness in films that are, of course, funny or tear-jerkers. Neurofollies give us the delightful absurdity of comedy and the captivating technology of science fiction. Revisiting these films shows us that screenwriters have picked up on certain pieces of neurologic knowledge, repurposed and exaggerated them, turned them upside down for entertainment, and made them science fiction. These filmmakers, I suspect, tried to imagine how the whole fantastical tale could work and how to maximize the fun. Some films are based on books by renowned authors of science fiction[23] and thrillers. Some have become cult classics and have even won Academy Awards. Some are giddily awful. However, the introduction of psychosurgery in film may signal some blurring of the lines between current clinical practice and science fiction. Science fiction takes it a step further, attributes more and more, and goes beyond parody. In a way, cinema has always been about something else. It is the same old song:

> *And Swanson and Keaton and Dressler and William S. Hart -*
> *No-one pretended that what we were doing was art.*
> *We had some guts and some luck,*
> *But we were just making a buck.*
> *Movies were movies were movies when I ran the show![24]*

---

[20] Fortuny J. *Crimson (or The Man with the Severed Head)*. Bonus Features (1973).

[21] White RJ, Wolin LR, Massopust LC, Jr., Taslitz N, Verdura J. Primate Cephalic Transplantation: Neurogenic Separation, Vascular Association. *Transplant Proc*. 1971;3:602–604.

[22] Canavero S. HEAVEN: The Head Anastomosis Venture Project Outline for the First Human Head Transplantation with Spinal Linkage (GEMINI). *Surg Neurol Int*. 2013;4:S335–S342.

[23] See Cameron J. *James Cameron's Story of Science Fiction* (2018). For some time science fiction was not considered worthy of attention. James Cameron defined the major themes of science fiction as time travel, space exploration, dark dystopian futures, time travel, and intelligent machines. However, he omitted medicine of the future and grand cures. Science fiction has become much more respected.

[24] "Movies were movies" from *Mack & Mabel*, music by Jerry Herman, lyrics by Michael Stewart.

10

Come and See: What to Get Out of Neurocinema

No form of art goes beyond ordinary consciousness as film does, straight to our emotions, deep into the twilight room of the soul.

Ingmar Bergman

I go into the movie, I watch it, and I ask myself what happened to me.

Pauline Kael

Have you noticed the emotionally charged descriptors of towering praise used by some film critics? To name a few: "engrossing," "exalting," "stunning," "riveting," "transforming," "astonishing," "thrilling," "intense," and even "mind-blowing" and "hallucinogenic." Do we all share these extreme feelings, or are some of us left wondering what there is about a particular film that could have possibly engendered so much excitement? Certainly, the darkened cinema has been perceived by some as a "place of our wondering."[1] As a matter of fact, some of us may wonder what actually happens deep in our brain and consciousness. This final chapter is a collection of miscellanies of factual odds and ends. It is also about how to best make use of these films—incidentally in a forum or formally in a structured curriculum and why there often is discovery.

Bending the Mind

It is possible to argue that movies with medical themes tend to upset the unprepared audience and rarely provide a sense of relief. When do we feel off-kilter? Why are we anxious as we try to process what we see? What happens in the brain with all this bewilderment? Be that as it may, neurologists have a superficial interest in how films affect the brain and what watching a film could "do" to you—as a matter of fact, the field is being developed by cognitive psychologists. I will not attempt a detailed exposition here, but, by its nature, film impacts emotion and thus by implication memory also, which requires the involvement of certain parts of the brain. We remember scenes best when emotions are strongly displayed. Emotional narratives filled in with music activate certain parts of the brain. Altogether, functional brain MRI—a technique that records activity and information processing—has shown that watching movies activates the amygdala, a structure known for providing emotional rewards. This is particularly apparent when the musical soundtrack works to convey happiness or sorrow.[2] Actively trying to empathize with another's emotional state intensifies amygdala activity. Film-induced anxiety (e.g., through horror movies) moves brain activity to the frontal lobe (the anterior

---

[1] Thomson D. *A Light in the Dark: A History of Movie Directors*. New York: Knopf; 2021.

[2] Pehrs C, Deserno L, Bakels JH, et al. How Music Alters a Kiss: Superior Temporal Gyrus Controls Fusiform-Amygdalar Effective Connectivity. *Soc Cogn Affect Neurosci*. 2014;9:1770–1778.

DOI: 10.1201/9781003270874-10

cingulate cortex) and thalamus, suggesting increased arousal (a primitive guarding or fight response). Others showed that witnessing other people in pain boosts activity both in the insula and the anterior cingulate cortex and may be loosely interpreted as an emotional desire to do something about it and have it stop.[3] Brain activity is far less localized with humor, and many brain areas are involved. Prefrontal and temporal areas are involved mainly in humor perception, and the temporoparietal junction plays an important role in understanding jokes.[4]

We do not know exactly which element of the moving picture stimulates the brain and where; we deal with the light, the dark, the cuts, the shots, and the sound, and there is likely more than one stimulus. Neither do we know with precision how a problematic storyline affects an abnormal or immature mind, and this has remained a central point of interest for psychologists (e.g., exposure to extremely violent movies). Why a tense scene can disturb sleep remains a mystery. Why we cannot forget what we saw or try to unsee certain disturbing images is also less understood. We may speculate about deep brain stimulation to erase memories or wait until Dr. Howard Mierzwiak, the founder of Lacuna Inc, comes along.[5] But all these emotions—primal or moral—make cinema dramatically interesting and often unforgettable. Our engagement with modern film is influenced by rapid cuts and pacing and changes in luminance patterns, which heighten the narrative impact and enhance the viewers' tendency to get "lost in the story."[6] This is also known as "narrative transportation." Chatting with reporters in 1956, Alfred Hitchcock phrased it even more succinctly: "Drama is life with the dull bits cut out."

There is another irony. Some actors are deeply affected by their work. A great actor gives a natural and sincere impression and assumes the role. During the filming of *Dark Victory*, Bette Davis strongly empathized with the protagonist and reportedly sobbed constantly during the filming of the last scene.[7] Peter Lorre played a vile psychopathic pedophilic serial killer in *M* and was often cast as a villain. Speaking figuratively to a reporter, Lorre once said, "You know, I can get away with murder. The audience loves me." However, Lorre suffered multiple setbacks and morphine addiction and often felt he could not get away from his horrid screen persona. He often complained that filmmakers always offered him the same type of roles, and he could not escape it ("I am stamped"). When playing a paraplegic in *The Men*, Marlon Brando recalled that he "went through all these things" and that he was depressed and cried. "I reached down into the depth of myself."[8] More recently, the 84-year-old Anthony Hopkins told interviewers he was, at times, overwhelmed during the filming of *The Father* because it reminded him of his own mortality.

Have you ever watched other moviegoers while sitting in a theater? Or when entering a large multiplex late, after the movie has started? Have you seen their faces? Filmmakers do it occasionally in their own films. The pivotal scene in *The Spirit of the Beehive* (Figure 10.1) occurs when horrified young children in a small Spanish village attend a screening of the original *Frankenstein*,[9] and this experience

[3] Meffert H, Gazzola V, den Boer JA, Bartels AA, Keysers C. Reduced Spontaneous but Relatively Normal Deliberate Vicarious Representations in Psychopathy. *Brain*. 2013;136:2550–2562.

[4] Sawahata Y, Komine K, Morita T, Hiruma N. Decoding Humor Experiences from Brain Activity of People Viewing Comedy Movies. *PLoS One*. 2013;8:e81009.

[5] Dr. Howard Mierzwiak (Tom Wilkinson) is a surrealist invention from the mind of Charlie Kaufman and in *Eternal Sunshine of the Spotless Mind* (2004); see also Glannon W. Brain Implants to Erase Memories. *Front Neurosci*. 2017;11:584.

[6] For studies on pace, rhythm, motion, and luminance over several decades of filmmaking, see Cutting JE, Brunick KL, Delong JE, Iricinschi C, Candan A. Quicker, Faster, Darker: Changes in Hollywood film over 75 years. *Iperception*. 2011;2:569–576 and Cutting JE, Candan A. Shot Durations, Shot Classes, and the Increased Pace of Popular Movies. *Projections*. 2015:40–62.

[7] Sikov E. *Dark Victory: The Life of Bette Davis*. 1st ed. New York: Henry Holt and Company; 2007.

[8] Youngkin SD. *The Lost One: A Life of Peter Lorre*. Lexington, KY: University Press of Kentucky; 2005. For the Brando citation see Mann WJ. *The Contender. The Story of Marlon Brando*. New York: HarperCollins Publishers; 2019.

[9] Whale J. *Frankenstein*. Universal Pictures. November 21, 1931.

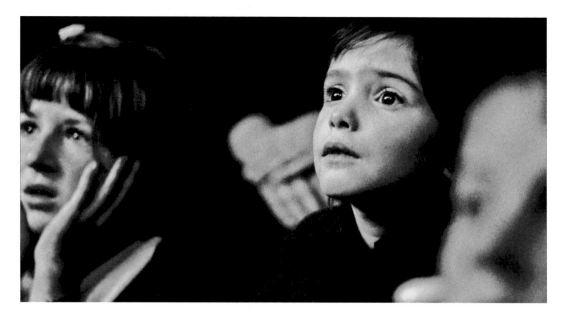

FIGURE 10.1 The gaze of a child in *Spirit of the Beehive* (Everett Collection, Inc.).

precedes nocturnal scares for several girls and an actual trauma for one.[10] The camera pans the full theater and lingers on the children's startled, rapt faces. Some scream. We know that younger children are afraid of symbolic stimuli but will scream and laugh at a loud sound that occurs after a prolonged silence—a "jump scare." Children remain vulnerable to sudden fear because they have no resources to draw upon to protect themselves.[11]

It is different with older, more cognitively aware viewers who are more disturbed by associations. *Fatal Attraction* (1987) offers some great examples, such as the overlap of the child's scream with the whistling kettle containing the boiled rabbit and by Glenn Close's totally unexpected, Lazarus-like sit-up from the bathtub. Exposure to horror films can lead to distress reactions that may require psychological or psychiatric intervention, a condition called cinematic neurosis.[12]

Some movie plots focus on treatments while watching a film. (See also Chapter 2 for *The Mystery of the Kador Cliffs*.) We are shown the aversion therapy of violence pairing with Beethoven in *Clockwork Orange* (Figure 10.2). Alex is strapped into a chair and subjected to forced viewing of violent images while his eyelids are pinned open. The images are linked to Beethoven's Ninth Symphony, which was Alex's musical ambrosia but not anymore. Kubrick's personal disagreement

---

[10] How children react to movies is a bit off the subject. Some studies have shown that real clowns have a beneficial effect on the health outcomes of sick children. But not always. Killer clown movies (*It* [1990]; *Clownhouse* [1989]) may significantly frighten children and become apparent when hospitalized (up to 2%). See Meiri N, Schnapp Z, Ankri A, et al. Fear of Clowns in Hospitalized Children: Prospective Experience. *Eur J Pediatr.* 2017;176:269–272; and Barkmann C, Siem AK, Wessolowski N, Schulte-Markwort M. Clowning as a Supportive Measure in Paediatrics—A Survey of Clowns, Parents, and Nursing Staff. *BMC Pediatr.* 2013;13:166. Be careful Patch Adams!

[11] A complex psychological problem with any rating system that is biased toward nudity and foul language and less on violence and terror. Young SD. *Psychology at the Movies.* 1st ed. New York: Wiley-Blackwell; 2012.

[12] For more on this topic, see Ballon B, Leszcz M. Horror Films: Tales to Master Terror or Shapers of Trauma? *Am J Psychother.* 2007;61:211–230; Straube T, Preissler S, Lipka J, Hewig J, Mentzel HJ, Miltner WH. Neural Representation of Anxiety and Personality during Exposure to Anxiety-Provoking and Neutral Scenes from Scary Movies. *Hum Brain Mapp.* 2010;31:36–47 and Martin GN. (Why) Do You Like Scary Movies? A Review of the Empirical Research on Psychological Responses to Horror Films. *Front Psychol.* 2019;10:2298.

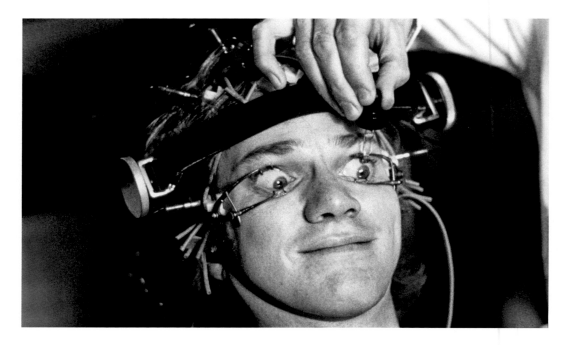

FIGURE 10.2   The forced gaze of a sadistic rapist in *Clockwork Orange* (Photofest).

with Skinner's theories was shown through the satirized Drs. Brodsky and Branom who practice behavioral conditioning.[13]

In *The Parallax View*,[14] rapidly intercut images of American life and family bliss are linked with words such as Family, Country, and Happiness. These visual correlations are then linked with violent images resulting in moral confusion (i.e., happiness with conquest and love with violence and death). Soon we realize that this clever scene essentially exposes the audience to the same hypnotizing indoctrination or brainwashing experienced by the protagonist. Brainwashing, as depicted in this film or *A Clockwork Orange,* does not occur in psychiatry.[15]

Movies have evolved into experiments with the audience as lab animals (or maybe this has always been the situation). Not everyone watches a movie in the same way, and not everyone is interested in perceiving a deeper meaning. If you compare the functional MRIs of analytic thinkers (when defined as persons with a more individualistic world view) with global or holistic thinkers (the ones with more preference for cooperative social orientation), the analytical thinkers, as expected, focus more on little details when watching a film. They may also be more idiosyncratic in how they perceive the movie.[16]

---

[13] Skinner was convinced that despite superior mentality of humans all organisms could be manipulated by positive reinforcement. He claimed that "man was not free in a sense that his behavior is undetermined." See Bjork D. *B. F. Skinner: A Life*. New York: Basic Books; 1993.

[14] Pakula AJ. *The Parallax View*. Paramount Pictures. June 14, 1974.

[15] Brainwashing frightened audiences after *The Manchurian Candidate* (Frankenheimer J. United Artists. October 24, 1962) suggested that the Communists were behind it. The term "Manchurian candidate" has since become synonymous with treason and corruption. The original used drugs to achieve brainwashing. The remake (Demme J. Paramount Pictures. July 30, 2004) actually showed the surgical procedure of a brain implant via a burr hole in a stereotactic frame.

[16] See Lerner Y, Honey CJ, Silbert LJ, Hasson U. Topographic Mapping of a Hierarchy of Temporal Receptive Windows Using a Narrated Story. *J Neurosci.* 2011;31:2906–2915 and Regev M, Honey CJ, Simony E, Hasson U. Selective and Invariant Neural Responses to Spoken and Written Narratives. *J Neurosci.* 2013;33:15978–15988.

Cinema's attraction derives from narratives that depict significant emotional situations that the viewers can recognize and share. Making sense of this narrative content involves associations, memory, self-reflection, and contextualization. Studies have shown that the processing of cinematic narratives occurs in a hierarchical manner. Coherent narrative segments are associated with fMRI signal synchronization in "higher-order" regions (e.g., frontal, temporal, and superior parietal), but unstructured stimuli only activate lower-order sensory regions.[17] A bigger question is what to do with all this MRI information other than understanding how film affects emotions. It is unlikely that movie producers would use it to improve their products and performances.

So how do we, as medical professionals, "experience" the films that encompass neurocinema? "I wish you a disturbing evening!" said Michael Haneke (*Amour*) at a London festival featuring his films. To be sure, neurocinema requires concentration and focused thoughts. I am reminded of the look Nicole Kidman gave us in *Birth*. For a full two minutes, we see her face while she attends a performance of *Die Walküre* at the Metropolitan Opera. It takes a great actress to show subtle, barely notable changes in her face to relay anguish, an outward expression of her inner state. We do not know what she is thinking, but we know it is troubling because something portentous happened before she entered the theater.[18] Kidman gives us an overactive brain retrieving memories and the accompanying emotions. Her brain MRI would have been interesting. It may be how we as neurologists view neurocinema—remembering similar patients and carefully looking at the actors' portrayal, how the family responds to the news, and how decisions are made.

The Neurology of Cinema

Now that we have seen what is offered, can neurologic portrayal in the movies be used in teaching? Is the artistic rendering just entertainment and spectacle, positively esoteric, or can it have an educational purpose?

There has been some interest in what is called *cinemeducation*.[19] "Cinemeducators" advocate the use of film as a teaching tool. This method relies, to a great extent, on the cinematic portrayal of medical and social situations, with teachers finding something important to discuss. Most work done in this field—if there is a field—pertains to virtually everything that can potentially be scrutinized when watching film. Leaving out the major illnesses such as cancer, these interpretations have encompassed a plethora of social- and health-policy issues, couples under emotional duress, strained family behavior, partner violence, aging and frailty, substance abuse, and grieving, as well as the transformative power of loving relationships. These films have been used in college courses on psychology and psychotherapy. Moreover, in counseling sessions, films have been used to provide relief for patients through a technique known as *cinematherapy*. There has been no systematic study of its benefit or how this method of teaching effectively fits within a curriculum. Indeed, finding and creating video clips may be too cumbersome for some educators.

However, as Thomson[20] proclaimed, "see it once, watch it twice," his point being that film watching means absorbing a lot of fleeting images. You may not like the film the first time or even understand it the

---

[17] This process is well explained in Morris G, Cardullo BI, Rosenbaum JF, eds. *Action!: Interviews with Directors from Classical Hollywood to Contemporary Iran*. London: Anthem Press; 2009. Anthem Global Media and Communication Studies, New Perspectives on World Cinema.

[18] One could, of course, argue that she was just conveying the typical misery induced by Wagner's Ring Cycle, even among certain opera devotees (the "Verdi school"). The use of Wagner's overtures in film is well known (*Apocalypse Now*), but the oppressive storm sequence with anticipatory haunting music that opens *Die Walküre* was particularly well chosen here.

[19] See Alexander M, Lenahan P, Pavlov A. *Cinemeducation: A Comprehensive Guide to Using Film in Medical Education*. Abingdon: Radcliffe Publishing Ltd.; 2004 and Alexander M, Lenahan P, Pavlov A. *Cinemeducation: Using Film and Other Visual Media in Graduate and Medical Education*. Boca Raton, FL: CRC Press; 2012.

[20] Thomson D. *How to Watch a Movie*. New York: Knopf Doubleday Publishing Group; 2017.

BOX 10.1   TALKING POINTS

1. Discuss why the portrayal is relevant for physicians and neurologists (who may see this every day).
2. Discuss an inaccuracy and use it as a teaching advantage. Even a film that does not get it right—and perhaps even more so—could prompt a discussion.
3. Discuss several films about one topic. By comparing films, patterns will emerge.
4. Discuss physician behavior and communication and identify common inappropriately portrayed conversations or lack of compassion. Note offensive or sarcastic remarks by healthcare workers.
5. Discuss the major tenets of bioethics in relation to neurologic disease.
6. Discuss neurologic disease and human interaction. How do close relatives respond when facing such a crisis? How can we empathize with them?
7. Discuss relevant neurologic literature (one or two key papers).

---

second time. Movies can become dated or stay fresh after decades. I sometimes watch a film twice in succession and then revisit it later to find more. We viewers may rethink movies more than the film-maker. Be reminded that filmmakers tend to avoid talking about what the film really means. When neurology is portrayed, however, we want to get to the heart of it. Why are we seeing this? Why is it distorted?

Neurologists will have strong subject-matter knowledge about the diseases portrayed. Some films are perceptive, offering a reasonably accurate portrayal of a certain disorder; others are just plain rubbish and absurd. Films with neurologic portrayals really started to emerge in the late 1980s, and there has been a steady increase in each subsequent decade. This likely reflects the gradual visible appearance of neurology as a specialty and the stories about neurologic disability that affect us. Thematic films can help us to appreciate the major challenges confronting those diagnosed with a neurologic disease. Here are some suggestions on how to use these films and the resources most effectively in this book.

Altogether, after separating the wheat from the chaff, the portrayal captures much of what is important to know about neurology. In many films, the portrayal of neurological conditions is excellent, and there is teachable material in many of the films reviewed here (Box 10.1). The films are interesting each in their own way, even if they are (to some degree) inaccurate. Many films highlight and make us aware of the emotional toll neurologic disability has on many family members when caregivers.

Documentaries are ideally suited to discuss the challenges of living with (or dying of) a neurologic disease. Important examples are the documentaries on ALS and Alzheimer's disease. I personally found these documentaries transformative because they show these devastating diseases and their major social consequences in real time.

How can these films best be used for education? One option is to have screenings for medical trainees and professionals.[21] This would allow experts in several subspecialties to evaluate the portrayal and provide context. Films may be watched in small discussion groups; at Mayo Clinic we have an ongoing bioethics film forum. To organize it requires a long-term commitment, and attendance may drop as the novelty wears off. Other options for using neurocinema are shown in Figure 10.3. The interest in this

---

[21] Hassan A, Wijdicks EF. Neurology Book and Film Club: The Mayo Clinic Experience. *Pract Neurol.* 2014;14:68–69.

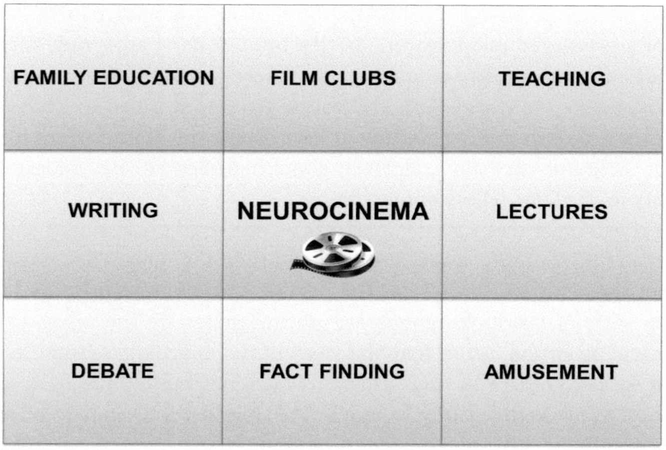

FIGURE 10.3 How Neurocinema can be used and taught.

topic will grow with scholarly lectures, various opinion pieces that look at health and neurology within society as depicted in film, researching why certain choices were made by filmmakers. A forum debate following a screening can be useful when ethical topics come into play. Something has been achieved when a film incites discussion and further reading.

End Credits

There is some great Neurocinema. I would be remiss if I did not close by disclosing my Top 10 list of the finest works (Box 10.2)—because I am asked all the time. Cinephiles, film critics, and filmmakers often indulge in the creation of "Best of" lists. For me, these films are most remarkable and distinguished but there are many more landmark works in this book. The cynicism, pessimism, and moral slide in *The Death of Mr. Lazarescu;* the burden of the elderly left alone to take care of a stroke at home in *Amour;* the heart-breaking, cognitive crumbling, chaos, and unworldliness in *The Father;* the challenges of rehabilitation and extraordinary vulnerability and dependency in *The Diving Bell and the Butterfly;* the celebration of creativity in an individual with severely disabling cerebral palsy in *My Left Foot;* the lack

---

BOX 10.2   TOP 10 NEUROCINEMA

1. *The Death of Mr. Lazarescu* (Puiu C. Tartan, USA, 2005).
2. *Amour* (Haneke M. Les Films du Losange, 2012).
3. *The Father* (Zeller F. Lionsgate, 2020).
4. *The Diving Bell and the Butterfly* (Schnabel J. Pathe/Miramax Films, 2007).
5. *My Left Foot* (Sheridan J. Palace Pictures, 1989).
6. *You Don't Know Jack* (Levinson B. HBO Films, 2010).
7. *The Intouchables* (Nakache O, Toledano E. Gaumont, 2011).
8. *Memento* (Nolan C. Newmarket, 2000).
9. *The Crash Reel* (Walker L. HBO Documentary Films, 2013).
10. *Declaration of War* (Donzelli V. Wild Bunch Distribution, 2011).

of alternative, comprehensive palliative care and the "lone-wolf" final judge in *You Don't Know Jack*; the unlikely caretaker of a privileged quadriparetic in *The Intouchables*; antegrade memory loss and total confusion in *Memento;* the incomplete recovery from severe traumatic brain injury in young athletes and the duress of parents in *The Crash Reel*; and young parents strained to limit during treatment of their child with a brain tumor in the *Declaration of War*. These are all important films that can evoke a new perspective. But these films are not exclusively about neurology or neurologists. They are about us and our responsibility toward our fellow human beings.

Filmmaking, at its best, must seek new perspectives on our lived professional realities, not consumer culture. Neurocinema requires acute, aware viewers, and then the images and experience stay. Can we think carefully about these films? Can we see the poetry? Can we recognize and disregard travesties of the subject matter without overlooking truly significant material? The worth of these films lies not in traditional cinematic invention but in how the story of the neurologic disability provides hope and understanding. Can we take refuge in these stories? How does rapidly progressive neurologic illness affect personal dignity? Why do they suffer so much? We should not hesitate to immerse ourselves and, in the process, understand our own subjectivity and vulnerability.

Appendix: Neurofilmography

This is a full listing and rating of over 180 films with neurology themes that are discussed in this book. Films are arranged by year of wide release. The ratings are again defined below. Most films are both cinematically and neurologically important. Note that films may have poor or questionable accuracy of neurologic portrayal, but of course, this should do nothing to its overall significance in the world of cinema. Some films may be of interest because of their deception or incorrectness, particularly if they create worlds and situations that can be interpreted by the audience as potentially probable.

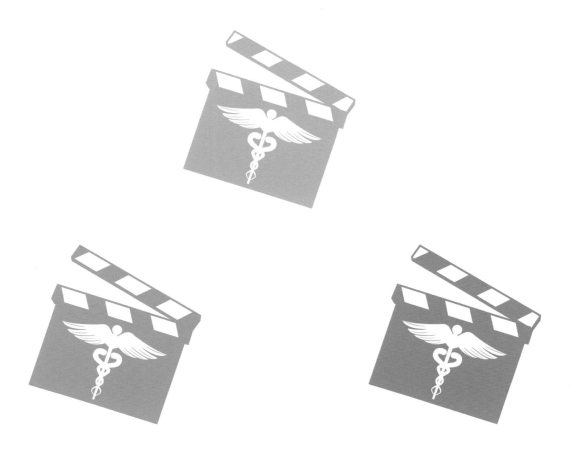

Ratings

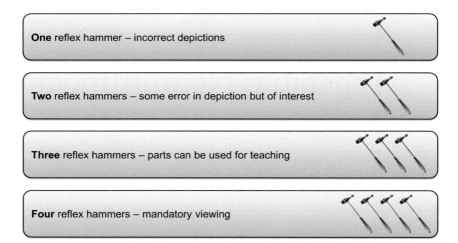

One reflex hammer – incorrect depictions

Two reflex hammers – some error in depiction but of interest

Three reflex hammers – parts can be used for teaching

Four reflex hammers – mandatory viewing

Ratings

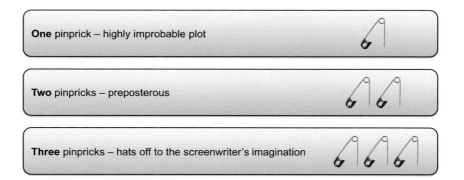

One pinprick – highly improbable plot

Two pinpricks – preposterous

Three pinpricks – hats off to the screenwriter's imagination

Neurocinema (Fiction Films)

Year	Title	Director	Distributor	Rating
1918	*War Neurosis*	Arthur Hurst	Wellcome Trust, London	🎞🎞🎞🎞
1918	*Stella Maris*	Marshall Neilan	Famous Players	🎞🎞
1920	*Pollyanna*	Paul Powell	United Artist	🎞🎞
1920	*High and Dizzy*	Hal Roach	Pathé Exchange	🎞
1932	*Freaks*	Tod Browning	MGM	🎞🎞
1939	*Dark Victory*	Edmund Goulding	Warner Brothers	🎞
1940	*The Courageous Dr. Christian*	Bernard Vorhaus	Stephens-Lang Productions	🎞🎞🎞
1941	*Ich Klage An*	Wolfgang Liebeneiner	Tobis Filmkunst	🎞🎞🎞🎞
1942	*Pride of the Yankees*	Sam Wood	RKO	🎞🎞
1945	*Leave Her to Heaven*	John Stahl	20th Century Fox	🎞🎞🎞
1945	*Rhapsody in Blue*	Irving Rapper	Warner Bros.	🎞
1946	*Let There Be Light*	John Huston	US Army	🎞🎞🎞🎞
1946	*A Matter of Life and Death*	Michael Powell and Emeric Pressburger	Eagle-Lion Films	🎞🎞🎞🎞
1946	*Sister Kenny*	Dudley Nichols	RKO Radio Pictures	🎞🎞🎞🎞
1948	*Shades of Gray*	John Henabery	US Army Professional Medical Films	🎞🎞🎞🎞
1948	*An Act of Murder*	Michael Gorden	Universal Pictures	🎞🎞🎞
1949	*White Heat*	Raoul Walsh	Warner Bros.	🎞🎞
1949	*Home of the Brave*	Mark Robson	United Artist	🎞🎞🎞🎞
1950	*No Way Out*	Joseph Mankiewicz	20th Century	🎞🎞🎞
1950	*Crisis*	Richard Brooks	MGM	🎞
1950	*The Men*	Fred Zinnemann	United Artists	🎞🎞🎞🎞
1958	*The Magician*	Ingmar Bergman	AB Svensk Filmindustri	🎞🎞
1959	*The Five Pennies*	Melville Shavelson	Paramount Pictures	🎞🎞🎞
1961	*Viridiana*	Luis Buñuel	Films Sans Frontières	🎞
1969	*Duet for One*	Andrei Konchalovsky	Golan-Globus Productions Ltd.	🎞
1973	*Turkish Delight*	Paul Verhoeven	VNF	🎞🎞🎞
1975	*The Other Side of the Mountain*	Larry Peerce	Universal Pictures	🎞🎞🎞
1978	*Coming Home*	Hal Ashby	United Artists	🎞🎞🎞
1981	*Whose Life Is It Anyway?*	John Badham	MGM Studios	🎞🎞🎞🎞
1987	*Gaby: A True Story*	Luis Mandoki	TriStar Pictures	🎞🎞
1988	*Rain Man*	Barry Levinson	United Artists	🎞🎞
1989	*Born on the Fourth of July*	Oliver Stone	Universal Pictures	🎞🎞
1989	*Drugstore Cowboy*	Gus Van Sant	Avenue Pictures	🎞🎞🎞
1989	*My Left Foot*	Jim Sheridan	Granada Miramax Films	🎞🎞🎞🎞
1989	*Steel Magnolias*	Herbert Ross	TriStar Pictures	🎞

(Continued)

Neurocinema (Fiction Films) (Continued)

Year	Title	Director	Distributor	Rating
1990	*Awakenings*	Penny Marshall	Columbia Pictures	✓✓✓✓
1990	*Hard to Kill*	Bruce Malmuth	Warner Bros.	✓
1990	*Reversal of Fortune*	Barbet Schroeder	Warner Bros.	✓✓✓✓
1991	*Frankie and Johnny*	Garry Marshall	Paramount Pictures	✓
1991	*My Own Private Idaho*	Gus Van Sant	Fine Line Features	✓✓✓✓
1991	*Regarding Henry*	Mike Nichols	Paramount Pictures	✓
1992	*City of Joy*	Roland Joffé	TriStar Pictures	✓✓
1992	*Lorenzo's Oil*	George Miller	Universal Pictures	✓✓
1992	*The Waterdance*	Neal Jimenez	Samuel Goldwyn Company	✓✓
1994	*Legends of the Fall*	Edward Zwick	TriStar Pictures	✓
1994	*The Madness of King George*	Nicholas Hytner	Samuel Goldwyn Company	✓✓
1995	*While You Were Sleeping*	John Turteltaub	Buena Vista Pictures	✓
1995	*Safe*	Todd Haynes	Sony Pictures Classics	✓✓✓✓
1995	*Go Now*	Michael Winterbottom	Gramercy Pictures	✓✓✓✓
1996	*Breaking the Waves*	Lars von Trier	October Films	✓✓✓✓
1996	*Extreme Measures*	Michael Apted	Columbia Pictures	✓✓
1996	*Persona*	Ingmar Bergman	AB Svensk Filmindustri	✓✓
1997	*Critical Care*	Sidney Lumet	Mediaworks	✓✓✓✓
1997	*Firelight*	William Nicholson	Miramax	✓✓✓✓
1997	*First Do No Harm*	Jim Abrahams	Walt Disney Video	✓✓
1997	*Hugo Pool*	Robert Downey, Sr.	Northern Arts Entertainment	✓
1997	*Niagara, Niagara*	Bob Gosse	The Shooting Gallery	✓
1997	*The Tic Code*	Gary Winick	Lions Gate Entertainment	✓✓✓
1998	*Gods and Monsters*	Bill Condon	Lions Gate Films	✓✓
1998	*Hilary and Jackie*	Anand Tucker	Channel 4 Films	✓✓
1998	*Pi*	Darren Aronofsky	Artisan Entertainment	✓✓✓✓
1998	*The Dreamlife of Angels*	Erick Zonca	Sony Pictures	✓✓✓✓
1998	*The Theory of Flight*	Paul Greengrass	Fine Line Features	✓
1999	*Deuce Bigalow: Male Gigolo*	Mike Mitchell	Buena Vista Pictures	✓
1999	*Flawless*	Joel Schumacher	MGM	✓
1999	*Tuesdays with Morrie*	Mick Jackson	Harpo Productions	✓
2000	*Memento*	Christopher Nolan	Summit Entertainment	✓✓✓✓
2001	*A Song for Martin*	Bille August	Film i Vast	✓✓✓✓

(Continued)

Neurocinema (Fiction Films) (Continued)

Year	Title	Director	Distributor	Rating
2001	*Iris*	Richard Eyre	Miramax Films	✓✓✓✓
2001	*The Royal Tenenbaums*	Wes Anderson	TouchStone	✓✓
2002	*Hollywood Ending*	Woody Allen	Dreamworks	✓✓
2002	*Door to Door*	Steven Schachter	AOL Time Warner Company	✓✓
2002	*Oasis*	Lee Chang-Dong	CJ Entertainment	✓✓
2002	*28 Days Later*	Danny Boyle	Fox Searchlight	✓
2002	*Talk to Her*	Pedro Almodóvar	Sony Pictures Classics	✓✓
2003	*Finding Nemo*	Andrew Stanton, Lee Unkrich	Buena Vista Pictures	✓✓✓
2003	*Goodbye Lenin!*	Wolfgang Becker	Sony Pictures Classics	✓
2003	*Blind Horizon*	Michael Haussman	Columbia Pictures	✓
2003	*Matchstick Men*	Ridley Scott	Warner Bros.	✓✓
2004	*In Enemy Hands*	Tony Giglio	Lions Gate Entertainment	✓
2004	*Million Dollar Baby*	Clint Eastwood	Warner Bros.	✓
2004	*The Machinist*	Brad Anderson	Paramount Vintage	✓
2004	*Garden State*	Zach Braff	Camelot Pictures	✓
2004	*The Motorcycle Diaries*	Walter Salles	Focus Features	✓✓✓
2004	*The Notebook*	Nick Cassavetes	New Line Cinema	✓
2004	*Napoleon Dynamite*	Jared Hess	Fox Searchlight Pictures	✓✓
2004	*The Sea Inside*	Alejandro Amenábar	Fine Line Features	✓✓✓✓
2004	*Trauma*	Marc Evans	Warner Bros.	✓
2004	*Million Dollar Baby*	Clint Eastwood	Warner Bros.	✓
2005	*The Aura*	Fabián Bielinsky	Buena Vista International IFC Films	✓✓✓
2005	*The Death of Mr. Lazarescu*	Cristi Puiu	Tartan USA	✓✓✓✓
2006	*Away from Her*	Sarah Polley	Lions Gate Films	✓✓✓✓
2006	*Dreamland*	Jason Matzner	Echo Lake Productions	✓
2006	*Memories of Tomorrow*	Yukihiko Tsutsumi	ROAR	✓✓
2006	*That Beautiful Somewhere*	Robert Budreau	Loon Films	✓
2007	*The Diving Bell and the Butterfly*	Julian Schnabel	Pathé Renn Productions, Miramax Films	✓✓✓✓
2007	*The Lookout*	Scott Frank	Miramax Films	✓✓✓
2007	*The Savages*	Tamara Jenkins	Fox Searchlight Pictures	✓✓✓✓
2009	*Adam*	Max Mayer	Fox Searchlight Pictures	✓✓✓✓
2009	*The Cake Eaters*	Mary Stuart Masterson	7–57 Releasing	✓
2010	*Extraordinary Measures*	Tom Vaughan	CBS Films	✓✓
2010	*Small World*	Bruno Chiche	Rezo Films	✓
2010	*Love & Other Drugs*	Edward Zwick	20th Century Fox	✓

(Continued)

Neurocinema (Fiction Films) (Continued)

Year	Title	Director	Distributor	Rating
2010	*You Don't Know Jack*	Barry Levinson	HBO Films	✓✓✓✓
2011	*Declaration of War*	Valérie Donzelli	IFC Films	✓✓✓✓
2011	*Fly Away*	Janet Grillo	New Video Group	✓✓✓✓
2011	*The Descendants*	Alexander Payne	Fox Searchlight Pictures	✓✓✓✓
2011	*The Intouchables*	Olivier Nakache	Gaumont Film Company	✓✓✓✓
2011	*Extremely Loud & Incredibly Close*	Stephan Daldry	Warner Bros.	✓✓✓✓
2011	*The Music Never Stopped*	Jim Kohlberg	Essential Pictures	✓✓✓✓
2011	*Contagion*	Steven Soderbergh	Warner Bros.	✓✓✓✓
2012	*Augustine*	Alice Winocour	ARP Sélection	✓✓✓✓
2012	*A Late Quartet*	Yaron Zilberman	Entertainment One	✓✓✓✓
2012	*A Simple Life*	Ann Hui	Distribution Workshop	✓✓✓
2012	*Amour*	Michael Haneke	Artificial Eye, Sony Pictures Classics	✓✓✓✓
2012	*Barbara*	Christian Petzold	Schramm Film Koerner & Weber	✓✓
2012	*Dormant Beauty*	Marco Bellocchio	Emerging Pictures and Cinema Made in Italy	✓
2012	*Fred Won't Move Out*	Richard Ledes	Rainwater Films, Ltd.	✓✓✓✓
2012	*The Sessions*	Ben Lewin	Fox Searchlight Pictures	✓✓
2012	*The Vow*	Michael Sucsy	Screen Gems	✓
2013	*Nebraska*	Alexander Payne	Paramount	✓✓
2013	*The Past*	Asghar Farhadi	Memento Films	✓
2013	*Side Effects*	Steven Soderbergh	Open Roads Films	✓✓✓
2014	*The Theory of Everything*	James Marsh	Focus Features	✓✓✓
2014	*Still Alice*	Richard Glatzer	Sony Pictures Classics	✓✓✓✓
2014	*Run & Jump*	Steph Green	Sundance Select	✓
2014	*You're Not You*	George Wolfe	Entertainment One	✓✓
2014	*Electricity*	Bryn Higgens	Soda Pictures	✓✓✓✓
2015	*Concussion*	Peter Landesman	Sony Pictures	✓✓✓✓
2015	*Floride*	Philippe LeGuay	Gaumont	✓✓✓
2017	*Every 21 Seconds*	Kuba Luczkiewicz	Two9 Productions	✓✓✓
2017	*Brain on Fire*	Gerard Barrett	Netflix	✓✓✓✓
2018	*Yomeddine*	AB Shawky	Desert Highway Pictures	✓✓✓✓
2019	*Extremely Loud & Incredibly Close*	Stephen Daldry	Warner Bros.	✓✓✓✓
2019	*The Meyerowitz Stories*	Noah Baumbach	Netflix	✓✓✓
2020	*Ode to Joy*	Jason Winer	Netflix	✓✓✓
2020	*Falling*	Viggo Mortensen	Netflix	✓
2020	*The Father*	Florian Zeller	Lionsgate	✓✓✓✓
2020	*Relic*	Natalie Erika James	IFC	✓
2021	*Everything Went Fine*	Francois Ozon	IFC	✓✓✓
2021	*Dr Death*	Patrick McManus	Peacock	✓✓✓✓
2021	*Supernova*	Harry McQueen	DiaphanaStudio Canal	✓✓
2021	*Memoria*	Apichatpong Weerasethakul	Cineplex	✓✓✓

Neurocinema (Documentary Films)

Year	Title	Director	Distributor	Rating
1991	*A Brief History of Time*	Errol Morris	Triton Pictures	✓✓✓
1996	*Breathing Lessons*	Yessica Yu	Fairlight Productions	✓✓✓✓
1998	*A Paralyzing Fear*	Nina Gilden Seavey	PBS Home Video	✓✓✓✓
2005	*Martha in Lattimore*	Mary Dalton	Wake Forest University	✓✓✓
2006	*Picturing Aphasia*	Mores McWreath	CreateSpace	✓✓✓✓
2006	*So Much So Fast*	Steven Ascher and Jeanne Jordan	West City Films	✓✓✓✓
2007	*Coma*	Liz Garbus	Moxie Firecracker Films	✓✓
2007	*Living with Lew*	Adam Bardach	Cinetic Media	✓✓
2010	*Aphasia*	Carl McIntyre	Little Word Films	✓✓
2010	*The Forgetting: A Portrait of Alzheimer's*	Elizabeth Arledge	PBS	✓✓
2012	*Do You Really Want to Know?*	John Zaritsky	Optic Nerve Films	✓✓✓✓
2012	*Extreme Love*	Dan Child	BBC2	✓✓
2012	*You're Looking at Me Like I Live Here and I Don't*	Scott Kirschenbaum	You're Looking at Me, LLC	✓✓✓✓
2013	*After Words*	Vincent Staggas	Flag Day Productions	✓✓✓✓
2013	*I Am Breathing*	Emma Davie and Morag McKinnon	Scottish Documentary Institute	✓✓✓✓
2013	*The Crash Reel*	Lucy Walker	HBO Films	✓✓✓✓
2013	*The Genius of Marian*	Banker White	Capital Film Fund	✓✓✓✓
2013	*When I Walk*	Jason DaSilva	Long Shot Factory	✓✓✓✓
2014	*Alive Inside*	Michael Rossato-Bennett	Bond 360	✓✓✓✓
2014	*Glen Campbell … I'll Be Me*	James Keach	PCH Films	✓✓✓✓
2019	*Oliver Sacks: My Own Life*	Ric Burns	Zeitgeist Films	✓✓✓✓
2020	*Out of My Head*	Susanna Styron	Eleventh Hour Films	✓✓✓
2020	*Robin's Wish*	Tyler Norwood	Vertical Entertainment	✓
2020	*Dick Johnson Is Dead*	Kristen Johnson	Netflix	✓✓✓✓
2021	*Muhammad Ali*	Ken Burns	PBS	✓✓✓

Neurocinema (Neurofollies)

Year	Title	Director	Distributor	Rating
1920	*The Penalty*	Wallace Worsley	Goldwyn Pictures	🧠
1953	*Donovan's Brain*	Felix Feist	United Artist	🧠🧠🧠
1959	*The Brain That Wouldn't Die*	Joseph Green	International Pictures	🧠🧠🧠
1968	*Charly*	Ralph Nelson	Cinerama Releasing Corporation	🧠🧠🧠
1973	*Crimson*	Juan Fortuny	Eurociné	🧠🧠🧠
1974	*The Terminal Man*	Mike Hodges	Warner Bros.	🧠🧠
1983	*Brainwaves*	Ulli Lommel	Motion Pictures Marketing	🧠🧠🧠
1983	*The Dead Zone*	David Cronenberg	Paramount	🧠🧠🧠
1990	*Groundhog Day*	Harold Ramis	Pictures	🧠🧠🧠
1994	*Clean Slate*	MIke Jackson	Columbia Pictures	🧠🧠🧠
1996	*Phenomenon*	Jon Turteltaub	MGM	🧠🧠🧠
1999	*The World Is Not Enough*	Michael Aptad	Touchstone Pictures	🧠🧠🧠
1999	*Post Concussion*	Daniel Yoon	Blue Water Films	🧠
2000	*The Cell*	Tarsam Singh	MGM	🧠🧠🧠
2004	*50 First Dates*	Peter Segal	Sony Pictures Releasing	🧠🧠
2010	*Limitless*	Neil Burger	Relativity Media Rating	🧠
2014	*Lucy*	Luc Besson	Universal Pictures	🧠
2019	*Isn't It Romantic*	Todd Strauss-Schulson	Warner Bros.	🧠

Index

Note: *Italicized* pages refer to figures and **bold** pages refer to tables.